Ophthalmology

A
DIAGNOSTIC
TEXT

Editor: Carol-Lynn Brown
Associate Editor: Victoria M. Vaughn
Copy Editor: Linda Forlifer
Design: Norman W. Och
Illustration Planning: Ray Lowman
Production: Raymond E. Reter

Accurate indications, adverse reactions, and dosage schedules for drugs are provided
in this book, but it is possible that they may change. The reader is urged to review
the package information data of the manufacturers of the medications mentioned.

Printed in the United States of America
Library of Congress Cataloging in Publication Data
Coles, William H.
    Ophthalmology: a diagnostic text / William H. Coles.
      p. cm.
    Includes index.
    ISBN 0-683-02056-0
    1. Eye—Diseases and defects—Diagnosis.   2. Ophthalmology.
I. Title.
    [DNLM: 1. Eye Diseases—diagnosis. 2. Ophthalmology. WW 141
C693o]
RE46.C645 1989
617.7′15—dc19
DNLM/DLC
for Library of Congress
                                      88-20900
                                         CIP
                              89 90 91 92
                      1 2 3 4 5 6 7 8 9 10

PREFACE

This textbook is a primer for ophthalmology. It is a primer in two senses. In the old educational sense, primers were the bases for expanded learning. In another sense, primer relates to the pump for a well. To prime the pump, one adds water before pump action starts to produce a full flow of water.

Producing a primer for the nonspecialist is probably more difficult in ophthalmology than any other specialty. Ophthalmology includes a number of disciplines almost totally foreign to other physicians or students. Foremost among these are optics and its bases in physics, the complexity of ocular movements, and the terminology of unique biochemical and physiologic concepts that are generally unparalleled in other parts of the body.

In spite of these difficulties, ophthalmology has very strong associations with other aspects of medicine. The study of vascular disease and the association of eye changes with systemic diseases are examples. In addition, ophthalmology includes direct visualization of pathology; the study of ophthalmologic disease can provide an additional dimension to the diagnosis and management of systemic disease.

I have divided this textbook into two parts: Part 1, Concepts, and Part 2, Essential Topics and Definitions. The concepts section covers the basic knowledge of every ophthalmologist. Understanding these concepts is necessary for the student or physician rotating through an ophthalmology service for a brief period. Reading the concepts section prepares the student.

Concepts are presented in a style that is brief and easily understood. No attempt has been made to suggest completeness of coverage of the subject. The desire is to provide for the reader a background that will be useful in listening to a lecture, understanding a more knowledgeable person from whom the student may learn, or reading a more complex coverage of the subject. The danger in such a presentation is that the material may seem too simplified for those who are knowledgeable. This is a risk that I have accepted to maintain a primer concept.

The essential topics and definitions section is a reference section. A number of topics needed to be developed but only confused the development of certain basic concepts. Others are not encountered frequently enough during a brief exposure to ophthalmology or an early learning of ophthalmology to warrant coverage in a major section. An attempt was made to make this section uniformly brief, but many topics were developed for better understanding. These include illustrations and as much description as is necessary for comprehension. Inclusion in the essential topics section was based on the relative importance of a concept. Once a subject was included, enough information was given to satisfy a primer concept for that topic.

This is a diagnostic text. Disease processes are covered with emphasis on signs, symptoms, and diagnosis. Treatment is mentioned only where it may expand knowledge of the disease. By strictly addressing diagnosis, I intend that the excitement of clinical ophthalmology as a specialty in which one develops and practices clinical skills will be passed to the reader.

I have written this textbook to benefit medical students, interns, ophthalmology residents beginning their training, nonophthalmology physicians who may want to expand their knowledge of ophthalmology, and foreign medical graduates whose first language is not English and who may want to review their knowledge of ophthalmology in the English language.

ACKNOWLEDGMENTS

A single-author textbook implies working alone; that is, of course, untrue. There are many people whom I acknowledge for special contributions.

Illustrators. Illustrations were completed by three very talented professionals: Molly Dunker, Baltimore, Maryland; Nancy Matthews, Atlanta, Georgia, who also did the color drawings; and Sharon Teal, St. Louis, Missouri.

Manuscript Preparation. Elaine Taylor's efficiency and thoroughness provided a completed manuscript. Cindy Campagne started the process.

Illustrations. Mary Atkinson helped to organize illustrations. Many illustrations were generously lent by the following clinicians: Drs. George Waring, Paul Sternberg, Ted Wojno, Louis Wilson, George Alker, Louis Lobes, Peter Forgach, and Louis Antonucci.

Portions of the manuscript were reviewed by Drs. Patricia A. Jaros and Travis A. Meredith. Dr. Robert Spector also reviewed selected illustrations. Drs. Bruce Shield and John Keltner allowed use of illustrations and material. Dr. Dawn Jedrzejewski gave a student's view of abbreviations.

Also thanks to Vicki Vaughn, Carol-Lynn Brown, Kim Kist, John Gardner, and Linda Forlifer.

Cover. The cover painting is *Vega-Nor* by Victor Vasarely (1969, oil on canvas, 78¾ × 78¾″) and is used with the permission of the Albright-Knox Art Gallery, 1285 Elmwood Avenue, Buffalo, New York (gift of Seymour H. Knox, 1969).

CONTENTS

PART 1

PART 2

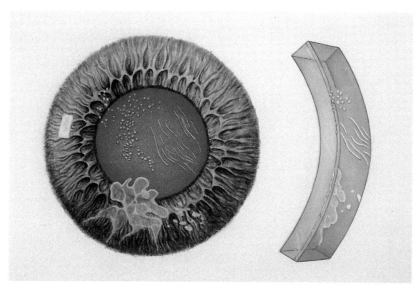

Figure C.1. Basement membrane dystrophy. The basement membrane of the corneal epithelium shows multiple changes: finger-print lines, microcystic dots, and broad geographic opacities. In almost all cases, facility with the slitlamp is necessary to make the diagnosis. Basement membrane changes are frequently associated with recurrent epithelial erosions.

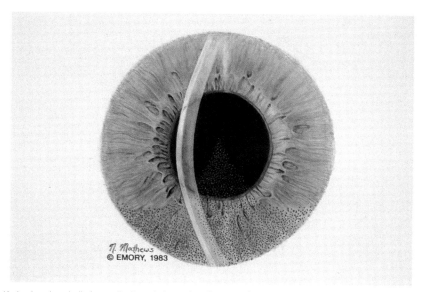

Figure C.2. Krukenberg's spindle is a collection of pigment on the posterior portion of the cornea. Although the pigment may be dispersed, because of the aqueous pattern flows it most often deposits in a roughly triangular shape with a base at the inferior cornea. Although seen in many conditions in which pigment is found in the anterior chamber, Krukenberg's spindle is often associated with pigmentary glaucoma (see page 57).

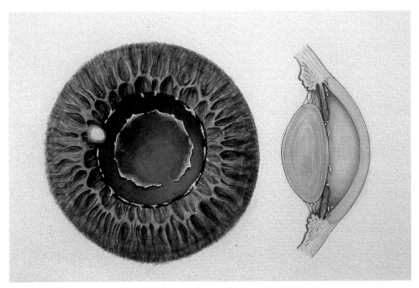

Figure C.3. Exfoliation syndrome is a common syndrome in which the characteristic slitlamp picture is dandruff flakes on the pupillary margin. With dilation, there are irregular, translucent zones on the lens. The condition is associated with glaucoma.

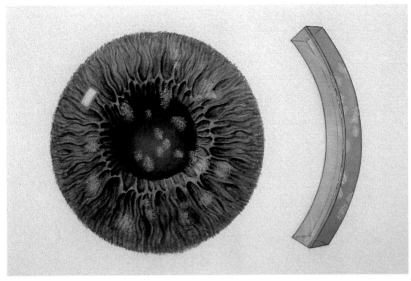

Figure C.4. Epidemic keratoconjunctivitis is caused by an adenovirus. After acute conjunctivitis (see page 34), subepithelial opacities can occur, as illustrated. These are just below the epithelium. Although they are not permanent, they can persist for a number of months and visual acuity may decrease.

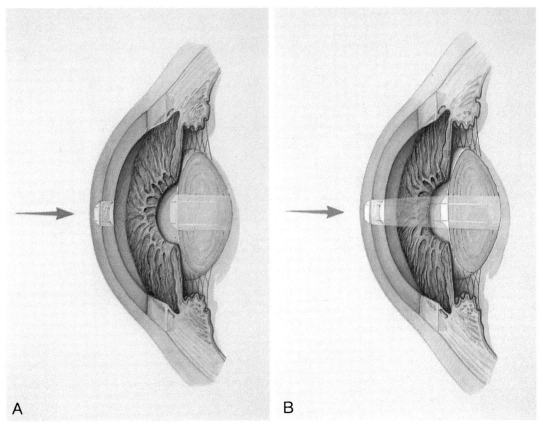

Figure C.5. Anterior chamber flare (aqueous flare). Flare in the anterior chamber is due to protein in the aqueous. When a pencil of light is directed into the anterior chamber, a cloudy or hazy beam appears. This is flare. Its visualization is analogous to the projection from a movie projector into the slightly smoke-filled air of a theatre. Protein is released from the vessels because of inflammation within the eye. Slight increases of flare are difficult to observe, and distinguishing flare requires experience. **A,** Clear aqueous; **B,** Anterior chamber flare.

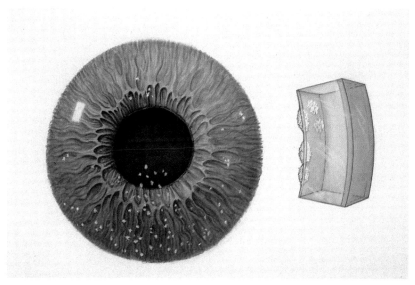

Figure C.6. Keratic precipitates are found on the back of the cornea and are associated with inflammation. They are most often seen inferiorly due to gravity. They are degenerating inflammatory cells.

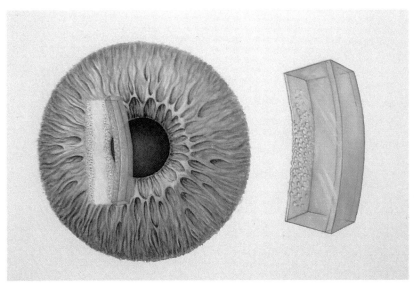

Figure C.7.   Fuchs' dystrophy is a common condition. It is associated with central corneal guttata, corneal increase in thickness due to edema, and subcorneal epithelial bullae. The slitlamp is usually necessary to establish the diagnosis.

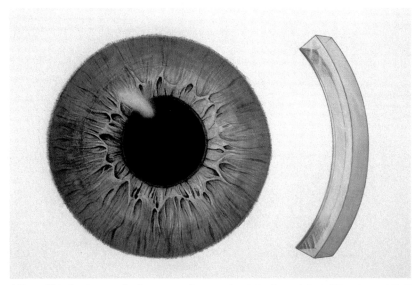

Figure C.8.   A Kayser-Fleischer ring, usually of a copper or bronze color, circles the periphery of the cornea and is found at the level of Descemet's membrane. It is associated with hepatolenticular degeneration (Wilson's disease).

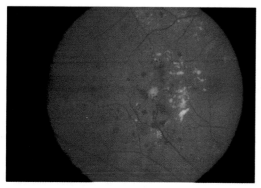

Figure C.9. Background diabetic retinopathy. Small red dots representing microaneurysms as well as yellow-white exudates are seen in the perimacular region. These findings are easily detected with the direct ophthalmoscope.

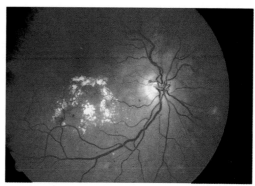

Figure C.10. Background diabetic retinopathy with microaneurysms and perimacular exudates is frequently referred to as circinate retinopathy. Approximately 20% of diabetics will have diabetic retinopathy. (Credit: Paul Sternberg, M.D.)

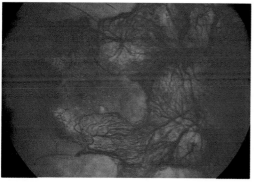

Figure C.11. Proliferative diabetic retinopathy is a stage of diabetic retinopathy in which new vessel response to ischemia occurs. It is the most destructive type of diabetic retinopathy. Approximately 5% of diabetics will have proliferative changes. (Credit: Paul Sternberg, M.D.)

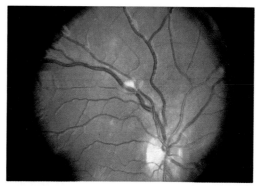

Figure C.12. Atherosclerotic plaque. Emboli from an atherosclerotic plaque in the carotid system can lodge in the arteriole system of the eye. These plaques are also called Hollenhorst plaques.

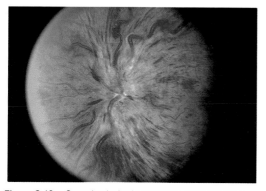

Figure C.13. Central retinal vein occlusion with hemorrhages, venous tortuosity and enlargement, and intraretinal hemorrhages. (Credit: Paul Sternberg, M.D.)

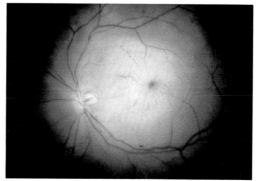

Figure C.14. Central retinal artery occlusion presents with a dramatic, sudden decrease in vision. Within a few hours, the retina opacifies to a whitish coloration. The darker dot in the middle of the edema is the foveola—called a cherry red spot. (Credit: Paul Sternberg, M.D.)

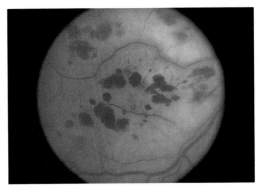

Figure C.15. An example of the ischemic changes seen with Purtscher's retinopathy. Purtscher's retinopathy is associated with chest trauma or trauma to the long bones and is thought to be secondary to embolic fat release and embolization of the ocular structures.

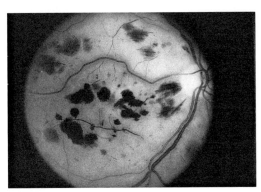

Figure C.16. A fluorescein angiogram (p. 87) of the Purtscher's retinopathy illustrated in Figure C.15. The arteries and veins and areas of red hemorrhage appear black against the lighter flush of fluorescence from the choroidal circulation.

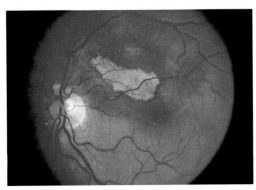

Figure C.17. Traumatic choroidal rupture. Injury to the eye, especially blunt injury, can produce ruptures in the choroid. Here the rupture appears as a white area surrounded by the red discoloration from bleeding. These ruptures can cause visual loss if they are close to the macula and may also be a source of new vessel growth.

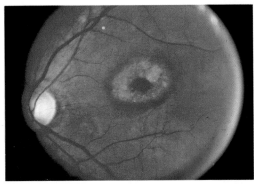

Figure C.18. Chloroquine retinopathy has a lesion that is characteristic and has been called "bull's eye." (Credit: Paul Sternberg, M.D.)

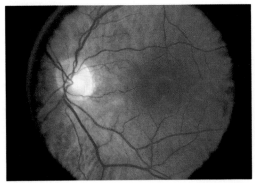

Figure C.19. Macular holes are seen primarily in older patients and may or may not be associated with other pathologic conditions. Macular holes cause significant decrease in central vision. The macular hole here can be seen to the right of the disc; it appears in the macular region and looks dark in the center with a cratered appearance. (Credit: Paul Sternberg, M.D.)

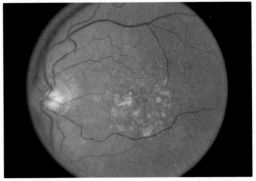

Figure C.20. Macular drusen, a frequent finding, is often associated with aging macular degeneration. These drusen appear as yellow single and confluent spots in the macula. (Credit: Paul Sternberg, M.D.)

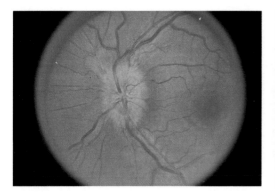

Figure C.21. Papilledema is swelling of the optic nerve. This photograph illustrates blurring of the optic disc margins, hyperemia (increased redness) of the disc, loss of the central physiologic cup, and early tortuosity of the retinal veins.

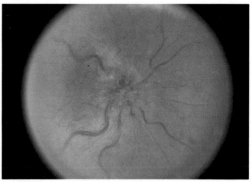

Figure C.22. Advanced papilledema. The disc margins are completely obliterated, and the tortuosity of the vessels is marked. An abnormal artery with an increased light reflex (copper wire) is also visible superiorly.

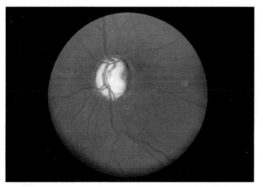

Figure C.23. Optic atrophy. The optic nerve is pale white, and a loss of nerve tissue causes displacement of the vessels nasally. Optic nerve atrophy can be caused by intracranial and orbital diseases as well as intraocular diseases such as glaucoma.

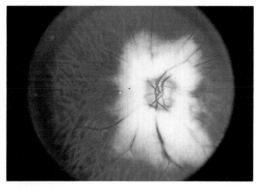

Figure C.24. Myelinated nerve fibers. These changes, although not common, occur around the disc and as patches in the periphery. Normally, eye nerve fibers are not myelinated. When myelinated, they appear white. Myelination is extensive and completely encircles the disc, which is unusual.

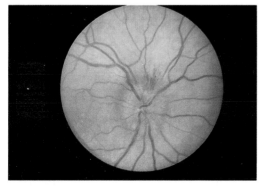

Figure C.25. Optic neuritis is an inflammatory condition of the optic disc. Characteristically, when compared to papilledema, optic neuritis causes decrease in vision, whereas papilledema is not associated with a visual loss until later. Optic neuritis is localized inflammation of the optic nerve; papilledema is swelling around the optic nerve secondary to increased intracranial pressure and the hindrance of normal axoplasmic flow.

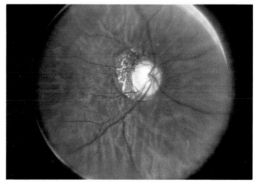

Figure C.26. Characteristic changes can occur in the posterior pole with myopia. Disc changes are referred to as myopic crescents. Notice also the prominence of the choroidal vasculature, which is visible because of changes in pigmentation of the retinal pigment epithelium.

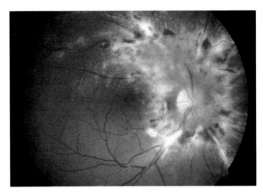

Figure C.27. Cytomegalovirus retinitis is now most frequently found in patients compromised by the acquired immune deficiency syndrome (AIDS). (Credit: Louis Lobes, M.D.)

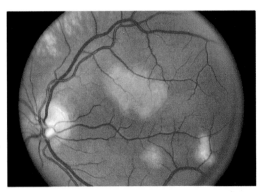

Figure C.28. Acute posterior multifocal placoid pigment epitheliopathy (AMPPE) appears acutely as plaque-like areas of inflammation in the posterior pole. (Credit: Paul Sternberg, M.D.)

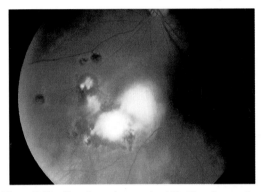

Figure C.29. Toxoplasmosis corneal retinitis. There is a small satellite lesion next to the major lesion. (Credit: Paul Sternberg, M.D.)

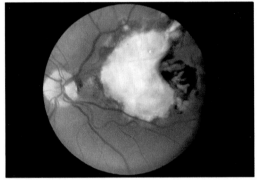

Figure C.30. This large, inactive toxoplasmosis scar shows a white, atrophic, scarred retina with a surrounding halo of pigment that makes the diagnosis highly likely. Such scars can be from congenital or acquired toxoplasmosis (see page 80). (Credit: Paul Sternberg, M.D.)

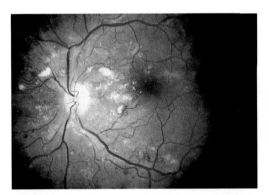

Figure C.31. Hypertensive retinopathy is often superimposed on the more chronic changes of arteriolar sclerosis. Hemorrhages and cotton-wool spots are present. (Credit: Paul Sternberg, M.D.)

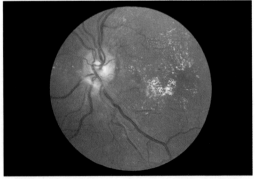

Figure C.32. Hypertensive retinopathy illustrated by changes in the arterioles. In the inferior arteriole, there is an increase in light reflex, a suggestion of focal constriction, and a change in the artery/vein ratio from 2/3 (normal) to 1/2. Also note the lipid residues in the retina due to edema.

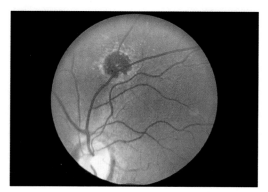

Figure C.33. Retinal pigment epithelial hyperplasia is a collection of pigment that is benign. Note the distinct borders and the undistorted passage of the vessel over the pigment area.

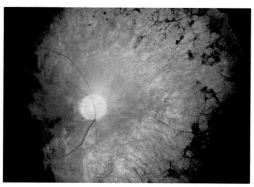

Figure C.34. Retinitis pigmentosa refers to a spectrum of diseases with variable fundus pigmentary changes, disruption of night vision, and visual field constrictions. In this figure, peripheral pigment changes can be seen. Disc pallor and arteriolar attenuation are additional findings. (Credit: Paul Sternberg, M.D.)

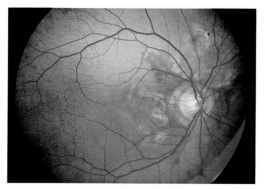

Figure C.35. Angioid streaks are breaks in Bruch's membrane and appear to radiate out from the disc. They are associated with pseudoxanthoma elasticum, Paget's disease, and sickle cell disease. (Credit: Paul Sternberg, M.D.)

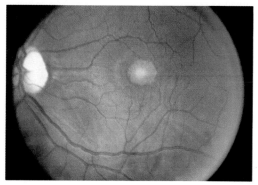

Figure C.36. Best's macular degeneration is a hereditary macular degeneration that can be diagnosed by characteristic macular changes. This figure shows the earlier stage of presentation, which has been likened to a fried egg. (Credit: Paul Sternberg, M.D.)

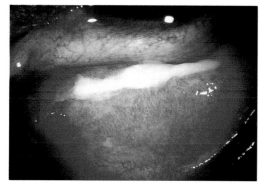

Figure C.37. Epidemic keratoconjunctivitis—pseudomembrane. Epidemic keratoconjunctivitis (adenovirus) presents as an acute conjunctivitis with preauricular adenopathy. Pseudomembrane, also not common, can be present. A pseudomembrane can be removed without causing underlying bleeding, which differentiates it from a true membrane. (Credit: George Waring, M.D.)

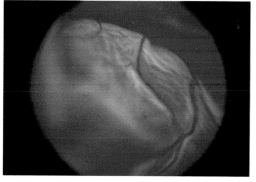

Figure C.38. Retinal detachment. When retinal detachment occurs, the retina separates from underlying structures. Usually, in the space that is created, there is a collection of fluid. Here the retina is detached and appears as a grayish membrane with folds. Note the vessels coursing over the area of the retinal detachment.

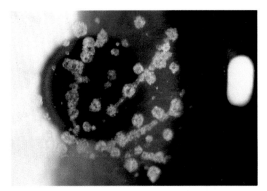

Figure C.39. Granular dystrophy is an autosomal dominant dystrophy of the stroma of the cornea. It is characterized by discrete white lesions in the stroma. It rarely progresses to a point where vision is severely affected. (Credit: George Waring, M.D.)

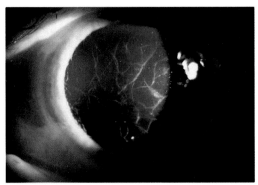

Figure C.40. Lattice dystrophy is an autosomal dominant corneal stromal dystrophy with lattice-like opacifications of the cornea. This dystrophy is often associated with epithelial erosions and may cause pain and tearing. (Credit: George Waring, M.D.)

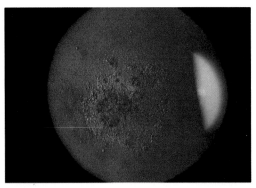

Figure C.41. Posterior subcapsular cataract. By illuminating the eye behind the lens and focusing the camera on the posterior lens, one can see the irregularities of a posterior subcapsular cataract. Normally, the red reflex glows evenly without shadows or disruption. This cataract is due to prolonged steroid use.

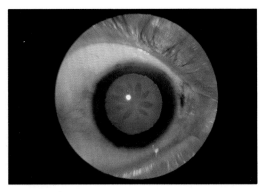

Figure C.42. A cataract with opacification of the cortex and a stellate pattern is referred to as a stellate cataract.

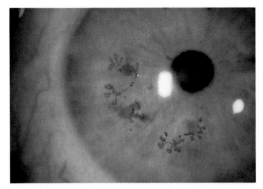

Figure C.43. Herpes simplex can be diagnosed by the characteristic dendrite. Dendrites are branching filamentous patterns in the corneal epithelium. These dendrites on the superficial corneal epithelium are stained red by rose bengal stain, a stain that is taken up by devitalized cells. Note the bulb-like appearance at the end of the dendrites. Although many conditions may cause dendrite-like figures, herpes simplex is associated with dendritic patterns most frequently.

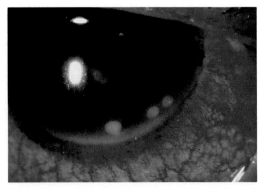

Figure C.44. Staphylococcal marginal ulcers are seen in the anterior stroma. Characteristically, there is a clear zone between the ulcer and the limbus. These may vascularize. (Credit: George Waring, M.D.)

PART
1

1

Cornea

Corneal Anatomy	Corneal Dystrophies	Interstitial Keratitis/Congenital
Corneal Physiology	Fuchs' Endothelial Dystrophy	Syphilis
Describing Corneal Disease	Epithelial Basement	Band Keratopathy
Testing Corneal Sensation	Membrane Dystrophy	Iron Lines
Keratitis (Corneal Ulcers)	Stromal Dystrophies	Salzmann's Nodular
Bacterial Corneal Ulcers	Keratoconus	Degeneration
Fungal Keratitis (Ulcer)	Recurrent Epithelial Erosion	Corneal Blood Staining
Herpes Simplex Keratitis	Mooren's Ulcer	Dellen

To diagnose corneal disease, you need not only a thorough knowledge of disease processes and an understanding of anatomical composition and physiology but also a knowledge of unique concepts and specialized skills for diagnosis. To establish a diagnosis, you need to

- Use the slitlamp (see page 360); should be able
  —to use retroillumination, slit illumination, and broad beam illumination and
  —to differentiate corneal layers with the slit beam.
- Also use frequently (although less important than the slitlamp)
  —keratoscope—measures corneal curvature
  —Placido's disk (see page 341)
  —keratometer—measures power of refraction of the cornea
- Understand astigmatism (see page 235) and how it affects visual acuity (see page 379).

Once these concepts and technical skills are mastered, the cornea provides a dynamic opportunity for the rewarding practice of clinical ophthalmology.

CORNEAL ANATOMY

The Layers

The cornea is classically divided into five layers. These five can be seen on histologic section and can also be seen with slitlamp evaluation. These layers are the epithelium, Bowman's layer, the stroma, Descemet's membrane, and the endothelium.

Epithelium

The epithelial layer is five or six cells thick. Cylindrical cells, which replicate, are at the base; wing cells are between the basal layer and the superficial cells; and flat cells are on the surface. Ultrastructural study shows microplicae and microvillae on the surface. Corneal nerves emerge from the stroma through Bowman's membrane to pass between the epithelial cells. The epithelial basal cells attach to the underlying Bowman's membrane by a basement membrane and complex connections.

Bowman's Layer

Bowman's layer is a condensation of the anterior stromal collagen and lamellae between the epithelium and stroma. In the periphery of the cornea, the termination of Bowman's layer marks the margin of the corneal scleral limbus (see frontispiece).

Stroma

Stroma represents 90% of the corneal thickness and consists of bundles of collagen fibers of uniform thickness that are meshed in a mucopolysaccharide ground substance. The collagen bundles form 200 lamellae arranged parallel to the corneal surface. These lamellae alternate layers crossing at right angles, producing a lattice structure.

Descemet's Membrane

Descemet's membrane is a basement membrane at the base of the endothelial cells. The membrane consists of fine collagenous filaments in the upper or anterior layer with an amorphous posterior layer. The membrane thickens with age, being three to four times thicker in the adult (10 to 12 μm) than in the infant at birth (3 to 4 μm). Descemet's membrane is produced by the endothelial cells.

Endothelium

The endothelial layer is a single cell thick and has approximately 500,000 individual, polygonal cells. These cells are uniformally spread across the posterior portion of the cornea. An intact endothelial layer is essential for maintaining a relatively dehydrated state of the corneal stroma which, along with the collagen arrangements in the stroma, assures the clarity of cornea.

Gross Anatomy

The corneal surface area is 1.3 cm². From the inside of the eye, it is a circle. On the outside, however, the horizontal diameter is larger than the vertical diameter (horizontal, 11.6 mm; vertical, 10.6 mm). The cornea is 0.52 mm thick at the center but becomes thicker toward the periphery (0.70 mm).

The normal horizontal diameter of the cornea is 12 mm. A horizontal diameter greater than 12.5 mm is known as *megalocornea*, and a horizontal diameter of less than 11 mm is termed *microcornea*.

CORNEAL PHYSIOLOGY

Tear Film

The precorneal tear film, because of its importance in maintaining an optically smooth surface to the cornea as well as acting as a wetting agent to prevent dryness of the corneal epithelium, is considered an essential part of corneal physiology. The tear film has three layers: (*a*) an outer *oil* layer, which is produced by the meibomian glands in the lid margins; (*b*) the *aqueous* layer, which makes up the bulk of the tear film and is produced by the lacrimal gland and accessory lacrimal glands; and (*c*) the *mucous* layer, which acts to hold the tear film on the cornea and tends to repel water. The mucous coating is produced by the goblet cells. (For further details about the tear film, see page 000.)

Function of the Cornea—Optical Clarity

To maintain a clear cornea, the structures of the cornea provide a constant balance between opposing forces. One force is the carefully oriented collagen lamellae of the stroma, which are optically clear only if they are maintained in a dehydrated state. Collagen naturally takes on water, a state not compatible with clarity. A state of dehydration is maintained by both the epithelium and the endothelium. Both act as barriers to fluid flow from aqueous and tears, but the endothelium has an additional pump function to move water actively from the stroma. Endothelial pump function depends upon glucose metabolism in the normal state and provides the major dehydrating force for the cornea to maintain optical clarity.

Loss of dehydration of the corneal stroma clouds the cornea and decreases vision. Common conditions in which this occurs are Fuchs' endothelial dystrophy; injuries to the corneal endothelium, as may occur during surgical procedures; and certain inflammatory processes.

DESCRIBING CORNEAL DISEASE

Stromal edema—characterized by cloudy stroma, thick cornea, and folds in Descemet's membrane

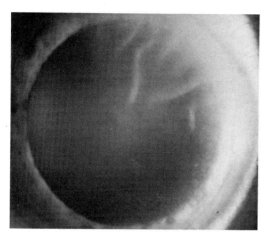

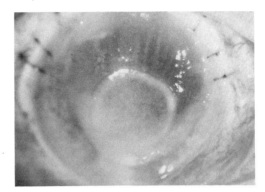

Figure 1.3. Central corneal ulcer secondary to infection with a streptococcal organism. (Credit: George Waring, M.D.)

Figure 1.1. Corneal edema with folds in Descemet's membrane. With corneal thickening due to edema, folds in Descemet's membrane occur. Here the folds are seen in the *upper right quadrant* of the cornea as grayish, irregular lines. (Credit: George Waring, M.D.)

Folds in Descemet's membrane—associated with corneal stromal edema (Fig. 1.1)

Epithelial bullae—subepithelial collection of fluid that causes "blisters"

Keratitis—inflammation of the cornea (Fig. 1.2)

Stromal ulcer—excavation of the cornea, usually associated with inflammation (keratitis) (Fig. 1.3)

Stromal neovascularization—blood vessels in the stroma

Corneal perforation (see Fig. 16.40)

Endothelial guttata—drop-like excrescences on Descemet's membrane, best seen by retroillumination with the slit-lamp; associated with endothelial cell disease

Dendrite (epithelium)—linear branching defect most often seen with herpes simplex virus infection (see color Fig. C.43)

Neovascularization—new vessel response due to irritation or inflammation (see Fig. 1.7)

TESTING CORNEAL SENSATION

Use

Detecting decreased or absent corneal sensation is primarily useful in the diagnosis of *herpetic keratitis* or *fifth cranial nerve* involvement in cases of acoustic neurinoma.

Technique

The end cotton of a cotton-tipped applicator is fluffed slightly and drawn out so that one or two strands of cotton fiber form a point (Fig. 1.4). It is helpful, at first, to touch the scleral portion of the eye with the fiber of cotton to allow the patient to relax, knowing that there will not be severe pain. One usually tests

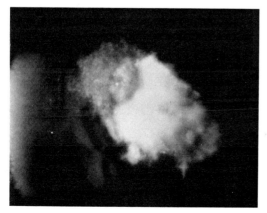

Figure 1.2. Fungal keratitis. These ulcers tend to be slow-growing. In some infections, satellite lesions may be seen, as suggested by the inferior part of this lesion. (Credit: George Waring, M.D.)

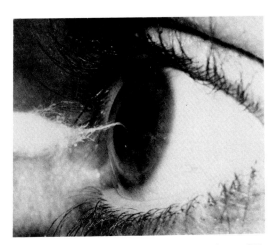

Figure 1.4. Corneal sensitivity testing shows fifth nerve sensation and seventh nerve motor function. Using a wisp of cotton from a cotton-tipped applicator, the investigator touches the central cornea. In a patient with a normal cornea, the touch initiates an immediate blink. With an abnormal cornea, the blink reflex is diminished. With a little practice, a clinician can judge the degree of corneal sensation with considerable accuracy. Usually only one eye is abnormal, and the normal eye serves as a standard.

the normal eye before the suspected abnormal eye. In the actual test, the apex of the cornea, where corneal sensation is the greatest, is touched with the cotton wisp. The normal eye blinks, and the patient sometimes jerks backward after the cotton touches the cornea. An abnormal response is no blink or a reduced blink. With experience, the response can be roughly graded (no, reduced, and normal sensation).

Other Causes of Decreased Corneal Sensation

- Herpes zoster
- Corneal ulcer
- Prolonged contact lens wearing
- Medication such as timolol and topical anesthetics such as proparacaine or tetracaine
- Previous cataract extraction in that eye

Overall corneal sensitivity decreases with age, and there is a noticeable decrease in diabetics.

KERATITIS (CORNEAL ULCERS)

Inflammation of the cornea has three major causes:

- Bacterial infections and immune reactions related to those infections
- Fungal infections
- Herpes simplex keratitis

There are, of course, many other causes.

Bacterial Corneal Ulcers

Infiltrations and inflammation accompanying bacterial invasion produce changes that may not always allow diagnosis on clinical findings. The clinical characteristics of various bacterial causes of inflammation are often distinctive enough, however, to allow therapy to be initiated before the laboratory results of tests for specific bacteria are known.

Staphylococcus aureus *and* Staphylococcus epidermidis

S. aureus and *S. epidermidis* are the most common causes of keratitis in most parts of the United States. The ulcers are usually superficial and often follow topical corticosteroid therapy or disease compromising the cornea. Hypopyon (see page 173) is variable. *S. epidermidis* is associated with minimal anterior chamber reaction, and *S. aureus* is associated with mild inflammation ulcers. The ulcers tend to remain localized with distinct borders and nonedematous corneal stroma. They tend to bore deeply and may cause intrastromal abscess.

Pseudomonas *Corneal Ulcer*

A *Pseudomonas* ulcer starts as a gray to yellow infiltrate at the site of a break in the corneal epithelium and is usually accompanied by severe pain. The infiltrate and exudate may develop a bluish to greenish hue. (The blue-green color is caused by pigment produced by the organism and is pathognomonic of *Pseudomonas aeruginosa*). These ulcers spread rapidly, and there is a large hypopyon. *Pseudomonas* ulcers tend to be central and may be more common in compromised hosts.

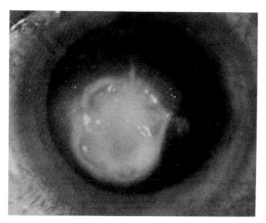

Figure 1.5. *Pseudomonas* corneal ulcer. *Pseudomonas* destroys corneal collagen and is rapidly progressive. Because of its virulence, it requires rapid recognition and early treatment. (Credit: George Waring, M.D.)

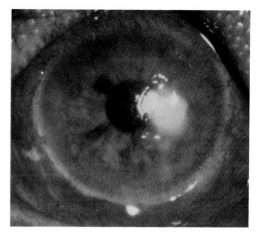

Figure 1.7. Peripheral corneal vascularization. Vessels grow in superficially as a response to the corneal ulcer secondary to *Streptococcus.* (Credit: George Waring, M.D.)

Contaminated solutions, such as liquid fluorescein, traditionally have been indicated as common sources. A mucopurulent discharge frequently adheres to the cornea (Fig. 1.5).

Pneumococcal Corneal Ulcer (Acute Serpiginous Ulcer)

This type of ulcer occurs in corneas that have been abraded and have lost epithelium. The ulcer is gray with a well-circumscribed edge. Its spread is erratic, with an active edge on the advancing border. There is moderate hypopyon. The ulcer begins superficially and progresses deep into the stroma. If the ulcer is

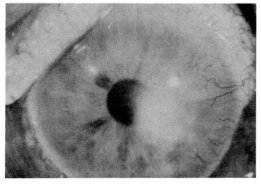

Figure 1.6. Central corneal ulcer due to *Pneumococcus.* (Credit: George Waring, M.D.)

untreated, perforation of the cornea is common (Fig. 1.6).

Moraxella liquefaciens Corneal Ulcer (Diplobacillus of Petit)

This is an oval ulcer that is slow to progress. It involves the inferior cornea and progresses to the deep stroma over a period of days. There is no hypopyon. Most of these ulcers are seen in debilitated patients such as chronic alcoholics, diabetics, and those with immunosuppression due to disease.

β-Hemolytic Streptococcus

The β-hemolytic streptococcus causes severe infections without typical features (Fig. 1.7).

Fungal Keratitis (Ulcer)

Fungal ulcers grow very slowly. Their most marked characteristic is hypopyon, and the globe generally is inflamed. Ulcerations tend to be superficial, and satellite lesions are characteristic. Satellite lesions occur away from the main area of ulceration and are usually smaller. There may be a severe anterior chamber reaction, and the cornea may be abscessed. An endothelial plaque with irregular edges can be seen under the superficial corneal ulcer.

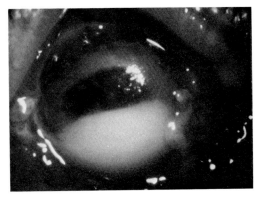

Figure 1.8.   Fungal keratitis. Example of an ulcer with hypopyon due to the fungus *Aspergillus*. (Credit: George Waring, M.D.)

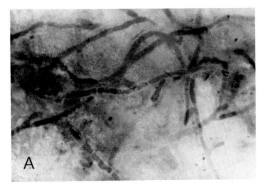

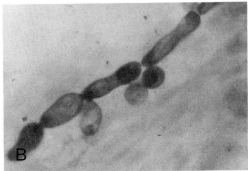

Figure 1.10.   A, Fungal elements illustrated on a stained smear from a corneal ulcer. **B,** Material taken from a corneal ulcer and stained, showing typical *Candida* organisms. (Credit: George Waring, M.D.)

Fungal ulcers are also associated with trauma and agricultural settings. There is a common association with topical corticosteroid drug usage in the eyes. Fungi penetrate into the anterior chamber and can be isolated from the anterior chamber. Common causes of fungal ulcers are *Candida, Fusarium, Aspergillus, Cephalosporium,* and *Penicillium* (Figs. 1.8 to 1.10).

Herpes Simplex Keratitis

An entire section is devoted to changes in the cornea due to herpes simplex (see page 32). In the differentiation of disciform keratitis, a form of common herpes simplex virus infection, from other corneal infections, these clinical features are helpful:

- Common association with immunosuppression;
- Presentation as a midcorneal round lesion with edema (Fig. 1.11);

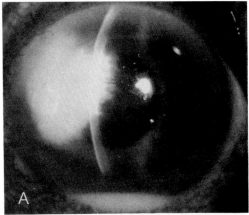

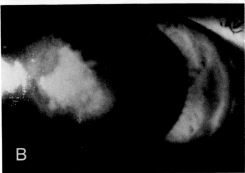

Figure 1.9.   A, Fungal corneal ulcer with a fluffy margin and hypopyon. **B,** Fungal ulcers may show satellite lesions. (Credit: George Waring, M.D.)

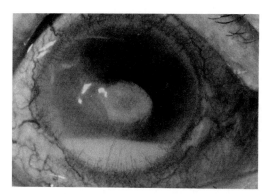

Figure 1.11. Herpes simplex corneal ulcer with hypopyon. This is herpes simplex keratitis in the acute stage. Hypopyon is present, but is a rare finding with herpes simplex keratitis. (Credit: George Waring, M.D.,)

- Possible presence of keratitic precipitates (see page 173); common association with iridocyclitis;
- Rare occurrence of hypopyon (see page 173);
- Decreased corneal sensation.

CORNEAL DYSTROPHIES

The corneal dystrophies are classified as anterior, stromal, or posterior. The following list of the corneal dystrophies highlights the conditions of strong clinical importance with italics.

I. Anterior dystrophies
  A. *Anterior basement membrane dystrophies*
    1. Cogan's microcystic epithelial dystrophy
    2. Fingerprint dystrophy
    3. Map or dot dystrophy
    4. Recurrent epithelial erosion
  B. Meesman's epithelial dystrophy
II. Stromal dystrophies
  A. Granular dystrophy
  B. Lattice dystrophy
  C. Macular dystrophy
  D. Fleck dystrophy
  E. Schnyder's crystalline dystrophy
  F. Congenital hereditary stromal dystrophy

III. Posterior dystrophies
  A. *Fuchs' epithelial-endothelial dystrophy*
  B. Posterior polymorphous dystrophy
  C. Congenital hereditary endothelial dystrophy

Many of the dystrophies have little or no clinical consequence. However, two dystrophies require thorough understanding: the anterior basement membrane dystrophies and Fuchs' endothelial dystrophy. Both are common.

Fuchs' Endothelial Dystrophy

Fuchs' epithelial-endothelial dystrophy (Fig. 1.12) is common and is diagnosed more frequently in women during the fifth to sixth decades of life. It is known to be transmitted in a dominant mode.

Clinical Findings

Fuchs' dystrophy is a progressive condition characterized by increasing corneal thickness due to edema. As the corneal stromal edema increases, epithelial edema results, with collections of fluid under the epithelium causing blisters or bullae (bullous keratopathy).

With progression, complications occur as the edema becomes chronic. Vascularization of the cornea may occur. Vision is decreased. Rupture of bullae may be painful. The con-

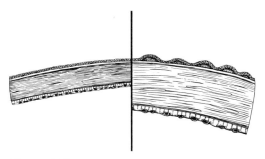

Figure 1.12. Fuchs' dystrophy. The changes of Fuchs' dystrophy *(right)* are compared to a normal cornea *(left)*. In Fuchs' dystrophy, the cornea is thickened by edema, the endothelium is abnormal, guttata are seen on the posterior surface of Descemet's membrane, and epithelial bullae with subepithelial edema are present.

dition is associated with a high incidence of cataract changes as well as an increased incidence of chronic open-angle glaucoma.

Microscopy

The endothelial layer has fewer cells than normal as well as irregularities in the characteristic polygonal shape of the individual endothelial cell. The altered endothelial cells may produce corneal guttata, which are excrescences of collagenous material secreted on the back of Descemet's membrane. Gutta, meaning drop-like, is a clinical description of the appearance of these excrescences by slitlamp examination. They appear as little drops of water on a smooth glass surface (Descemet's membrane), with a fair degree of variation. The presence of guttata centrally in the cornea is an indication of compromised endothelium. Peripheral guttata (Hassall-Henle warts) are physiologic. Important clinical signs of Fuchs' corneal dystrophy are:

- Guttata;
- Stromal thickening;
- Stromal edema;
- Subepithelial edema;
- Epithelial bullae (see color Fig. C.7).

Epithelial Basement Membrane Dystrophy

Other names for epithelial basement membrane dystrophy are map-dot-fingerprint dystrophy, Cogan's microcystic dystrophy, and fingerprint dystrophy.

Clinical Characteristics

Slitlamp Characteristics. Epithelial basement membrane dystrophies have three major signs: dots, superficial corneal lines (fingerprint), and maps (geographic areas) (see color Fig. C.1). These have been described independently, but only recently have they been included under a single title.

Dots. Many types of dots occur in this dystrophy. There are large, putty-gray cysts (described by Cogan) and also fine, clear blebs. The putty-gray cysts are discrete and may be round or comma-shaped. They may also be clustered in the central cornea.

The clear or empty cysts are unusual. These cysts discharge their content through the epithelial surface. Only at the time of discharge do they stain with fluorescein; usually, there is no staining.

Superficial Corneal Lines Superficial corneal lines are the least frequent of the three major signs of epithelial basement membrane dystrophy. Fingerprint lines, which are roughly parallel refractile lines, are seen in elongated and swirl patterns. Tear film breakup (see page 31) over these fingerprint lines may be decreased.

Maps. Map patterns appear as diffuse patches of gray. These gray sheets may have sharp edges or may blend with the normal cornea. Thick microcysts may be seen within the grayish map changes, but are not seen in the clear zones. These patches contain clear lacunae.

Blebs. Blebs are fine, closely clustered, round dots that are clear centrally.

Association with Recurrent Epithelial Erosions

Of patients who present with recurrent epithelial erosions (see page 13), about one-half will exhibit epithelial basement membrane dystrophy. In general, epithelial basement membrane dystrophy occurs in about 2% of the population.

No systemic or ocular diseases are associated with recurrent epithelial erosions. The condition is probably inherited as an autosomal dominant trait. Although epithelial basement membrane dystrophies can be seen in children, they are seen most commonly after the age of 30.

Slitlamp Diagnosis

Special skills with the slitlamp are needed to make the diagnosis. Of the three major types of changes—maps, dots, and fingerprint lines—fingerprint lines and dots are best seen by retroillumination. Retroillumination is best accomplished by shining the slitlamp's small direct beam into the pupil to form a red reflex while the cornea is kept in focus. Broad, tangential illumination is needed to see the map areas best. (See the slitlamp section, page 360.)

Pathology

There are three elements of epithelial basement membrane dystrophy: (*a*) a thickened basement membrane with extension into the epithelium, (*b*) abnormal epithelial cells and intraepithelial microcysts, and (*c*) a collection of fibrillar material between the epithelial basement membrane and Bowman's layer.

Maps are actually thick epithelial basement membrane. Putty-gray dots are intraepithelial pseudocysts that contain nuclear and cytoplasmic debris. Blebs are an accumulation of fibrillogranular material between the basement membrane of the epithelium and Bowman's layer. Blebs are not actually microcysts or micropseudocysts, but are indentations in the overlying basal epithelial cell. Fingerprint lines are formed by sheets of subepithelial and intraepithelial material composed of both fibrils and a granular material.

In epithelial basement membrane dystrophy, Bowman's layer, the stroma, Descemet's membrane, and the endothelium are normal.

Cause

The cause of epithelial basement membrane dystrophy is probably abnormal basement membrane synthesis. The common association with erosions is probably due to poor epithelial adhesion to the abnormal basement membrane.

Stromal Dystrophies

Granular Dystrophy

Inheritance. Autosomal dominant

Clinical Appearance. Lesions of granular dystrophy are usually in the central portion of the cornea and in the anterior stroma. They are fine and whitish and are usually distinct. The stroma between the lesions is clear. Epithelial erosion is not common (Fig. 1.13).

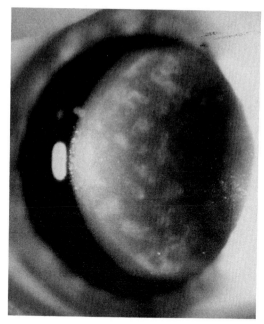

Figure 1.13. Granular dystrophy is a stromal dystrophy that is bilateral and autosomal dominant. It presents as discrete lesions with clear zones in the corneal stroma. It is most often confused with the early stages of macular dystrophy. As macular dystrophy progresses, however, more generalized clouding occurs, and between the lesions of macular dystrophy there is grayish opacification (see color Fig. C.39).

Onset. Granular dystrophy is first seen during the first 10 years of life.

Progression. Progression is fairly slow throughout life. Granular dystrophy frequently does not require medical therapy or surgery (penetrating keratoplasty).

Histologic Findings. The cornea has a uniform deposition of *hyaline* material. Table 1.1 shows the staining characteristics of stromal dystrophies.

Macular Dystrophy

Inheritance. Autosomal recessive

Clinical Appearance. Dense gray-white

Table 1.1.
Histologic Staining Characteristics of Stromal Dystrophies

Dystrophy	Masson's Trichrome	Periodic Acid-Schiff	Congo Red	Birefringence
Granular	Red	0	0	0
Macular	0	Pink	0	0
Lattice	Red	Pink-red	Red	Yes

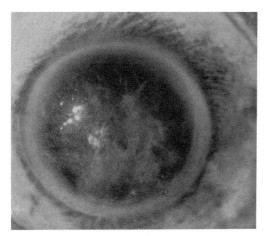

Figure 1.14. Lattice dystrophy is an inherited stromal dystrophy. Typical latticework can be seen, especially in the periphery of this central opacification of the cornea. As the condition progresses, epithelial erosions of the cornea may occur. Amyloid is the cause. (See also color Fig. C.40.)

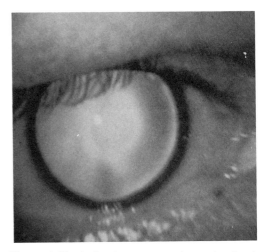

Figure 1.15. In keratoconus, an abnormal reflex is seen when the red reflex from the posterior pole is used as retroillumination. Note the bright central cone area, with the cone faintly outlined in the center and surrounded by a halo of bright light.

central opacities start at Bowman's layer but, later in the disease, spread to the periphery and involve deep stroma. The corneal stroma between the lesions is often cloudy. The lesions tend to be indistinct. There may be recurrent corneal epithelial erosions.

Onset. Macular dystrophy begins between ages five and nine.

Progression. The disease may progress with significant effects on vision. Corneal transplantation is frequently necessary.

Cause. There is a deposition of *mucopolysaccharides* in the stroma around keratocytes.

Lattice Dystrophy

Inheritance. Autosomal dominant

Clinical Appearance. This dystrophy appears as branching linear opacities in Bowman's layer early and later spreads to the periphery and the deep stroma (Fig. 1.14). These opacities do not reach the level of Descemet's membrane. The filaments form an irregular latticework and show dichotomous branching. Between the filaments, there may be other opacities, such as fine dots, flakes, and snowflake opacities. Recurrent erosions and decreased visual acuity are common.

Cause. Histopathologically, the deposits are *amyloid.*

Onset. Lattice dystrophy begins at 2 to 20 years of age.

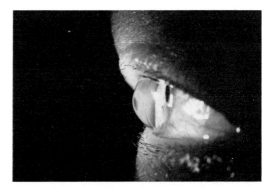

Figure 1.16. Side view of keratoconus. The clear cornea comes to a cone shape pointing to the left. This cone would appear from the front as shown in Figure 1.15.

Progression. As the disease progresses, visual acuity is often severely affected, and penetrating keratoplasty may be necessary during the fifth decade.

KERATOCONUS

Keratoconus is a degenerative bilateral disease of the central cornea in which corneal thinning results in a cone-shaped deformity (Figs. 1.15 and 1.16).

Characteristics

Keratoconus may have a familial pattern, but is most often erratic with no definite inheritance pattern. It is associated with a number of other conditions. Most important are Down's syndrome, atopic dermatitis, aniridia, and vernal conjunctivitis. Keratoconus has additionally been associated with Marfan's syndrome, neurofibromatosis, Addison's disease, Ehlers-Danlos syndrome, retinitis pigmentosa, blue sclera, cataract, ectopia lentis, optic atrophy, and Apert's syndrome.

Establishing the Diagnosis

The following clinical features can help establish the diagnosis of keratoconus.

Onset. Symptoms usually start during the patient's 20's.

Myopic Astigmatism. Progressive refractive error, usually an irregular myopic astigmatism, is an early sign.

Conical Cornea. As corneal thinning occurs, the cornea takes on a cone shape (Fig. 1.16) instead of its normal spherical shape. This abnormal shape will distort the lower lid margin when the patient looks down. This is called Munson's sign.

Iron Deposition. An iron ring is deposited in the corneal stroma around the base of the cone in many patients. This is called Fleischer's ring.

Thinning of the Central Cornea. The central cornea will be less than the normal thickness of 0.52 mm.

Linear Scars. At the apex of the cone, superficial and irregular linear scars can be seen. Superficial scarring is at the level of Bowman's membrane.

Prominent Corneal Nerves. Stromal corneal nerves are more visible in most patients with keratoconus.

Stromal Lines. Very fine, fibrillary lines are seen posteriorly at the internal edge of Fleischer's ring (when present).

Abnormal Reflex. Because of the conical distortion of the superficial surface, reflections are distorted. Corneascope (keratoscope) and Placido's disk, as well as keratometry, all use or record the corneal reflex, and all will show distortion in keratoconus.

Acute Corneal Edema. Acute corneal edema in keratoconus causes a sudden and severe visual loss with slow clearing over a period of months. Ruptures in Descemet's membrane from the distortion of the cornea allow fluid to invade the cornea immediately, with resulting corneal edema and swelling of the stromal fibers. This is called *acute hydrops.*

Course

The condition most commonly progresses slowly over a number of decades. However, it may arrest in its progression at any time and remain stable. Usually, vision can be corrected during the early stages with spectacles and, during more advanced stages, vision can be improved with the use of contact lenses to provide a smooth corneal surface. If the distortion becomes extreme or scarring occurs, the result with penetrating keratoplasty is excellent (success rate as high as 95%).

RECURRENT EPITHELIAL EROSION

Clinical Appearance

Patients with recurrent epithelial erosions report consistent and distinct clinical symptoms. They awake in the morning with a searing, exquisite pain accompanied by redness of the eye (perilimbal injection), excessive tearing, marked light sensitivity, and lid spasms. Characteristically, the erosion will clear within a few days to a week. Acute pain is usually gone within 24 to 48 hours after patching and treatment with pupil-dilating medicines.

Recurrent epithelial erosions are called recurrent because they tend to come back over time. Erosions may occur every few months. The condition is almost always self-limited and, after a few months to years, completely resolves without further recurrence.

Epithelial Appearance with Erosion

After the acute pain of recurrent epithelial erosion, examination shows an area of the cornea that stains with fluorescein and rose bengal. If still present, the epithelium is loose and wrinkled. There may be a flap of epithelium hanging below the visual axis. The anterior stroma has a grayish brown granular edema. As the erosion heals over 12 to 24 hours, the disrupted epithelium will appear gray and thickened and may have white cystic spaces that stain with fluorescein or rose bengal.

Posthealing

After healing of the epithelium in some cases of recurrent erosion, small pinpoint microvacuoles can be seen just below the epithelium. These are visualized by retroillumination techniques with a slitlamp (see page 360).

Although many erosions have no known cause or association, two associations should be remembered and looked for:

- Association with epithelial basement membrane dystrophy and
- Association with ocular trauma, always minor.

Epithelial basement membrane dystrophy is found in one-half of the patients with recurrent epithelial erosions. Careful examination of both the involved cornea and the normal cornea for dots, fingerprint lines, and maps is important (see page 10).

Patients with recurrent epithelial erosions may have a history of trauma. The characteristic injury is by a fingernail (for example, a mother accidentally swiped by a baby's fingernail), by a piece of paper (such as a file clerk injured by the edge of a sheet of typing paper), or by a twig or leaf (such as a gardener injured by a broadleaf plant or a hunter swiped by a twig).

MOOREN'S ULCER

Definition

Mooren's ulcer is a corneal ulcer near the limbus that is not caused by infection.

Clinical Appearance

Pain is most often associated with the condition, although it is variable. It is unilateral in 60 to 80% of cases, usually older individuals. The more severe, bilateral type occurs in younger patients.

This marginal ulcer is a progressive excavation in the peripheral cornea near the limbus. The stroma shows melting, which leaves a typical overhanging edge of cornea. The central area of the cornea is frequently spared ulceration, although it may have mild edema. The area of ulceration may vascularize.

Onset

Mooren's ulcer tends to occur in older individuals, but is not associated with any aging process.

Cause

This is thought to be an autoimmune phenomenon. It is unresponsive to steroid medication, but immune suppression has been useful.

Progression

The ulcer may remain localized or progress to 360° around the cornea. The course of the disease continues over a number of weeks to a few months. Perforation, although not the rule, is not uncommon. Perforation is a serious complication that may cause loss of useful vision; grafting may be necessary.

Excision of the limbal conjunctiva has provided some therapeutic results. Response to recessing or removing conjunctiva has supported a local autoimmune theory of cause. Recently, immune suppression drugs have been used in therapy, but we do not have a full understanding of the action of their effectiveness.

INTERSTITIAL KERATITIS/CONGENITAL SYPHILIS

Characteristics

- Bilateral, although it may start unilaterally
- More common in female patients
- Onset between 5 and 20 years of age
- Self-limited because it is a topical allergic reaction to early infestation with *Treponema pallidum.*

Symptoms

In the acute phase, which may last weeks or months, the patient has extreme photophobia and decreased vision. There is often a severe intraocular inflammation (uveitis), and there is danger of the formation of intraocular scars (posterior synechiae). (Most patients have their pupils dilated to prevent posterior synechiae near the visual axis.) The central cornea is edematous and vascularized, which often gives a pinkish coloration ("salmon patch").

After a few weeks, the inflammation resolves. Scarring of the cornea with ghost vessels remains for a lifetime.

Diagnosis

The clinical ocular signs are accompanied by other possible signs of congenital syphilis: deafness, notched teeth, and saddle nose. A serological test (FTA-ABS) will be positive.

BAND KERATOPATHY

Appearance

Band keratopathy begins as a fine, dusty opacity in the superficial cornea at the level of Bowman's membrane. There is a clear zone at the limbus between the corneal deposition and the sclera. The early peripheral deposits tend to coalesce with time, causing a broad band horizontally across the cornea that involves the visual axis. Characteristically, there are translucent areas that are round, oval, or irregular, similar to the holes in a slice of Swiss cheese.

Histology

Band keratopathy is calcific degeneration of the superficial cornea. It primarily involves Bowman's layer.

On occasion, a band keratopathy secondary to the deposition of urates in the cornea may appear. This urate keratopathy is brown, in contrast to the characteristic grayish appearance of calcific degeneration.

Associations with Numerous Conditions

Band keratopathy is a nonspecific finding and is associated with:

- Chronic ocular disease, such as uveitis, interstitial keratitis, phthisis bulbi, and chronic superficial keratitis
- Hypercalcemic conditions, such as hyperparathyroidism, vitamin D toxicity, sarcoidosis, and conditions with elevated serum phosphorus but normal serum calcium (for example, renal failure)
- Inherited band keratopathy
- Exposure to mercurial vapors or mercury preservatives, which occur in some ophthalmic medications. (Mercury causes collagen corneal changes, which result in the deposition of calcium.)

Removal

Removal is unnecessary unless there is chronic epithelial nonhealing due to the deposits or unless visual acuity is threatened.

Deposits are removed by the application of disodium ethylenediaminetetraacetic acid (EDTA) and gentle scraping of the cornea to remove the calcium. The EDTA binds the calcium, and the scraping removes it. EDTA application and scraping will not affect scarring, which may be a late change in band keratopathy degeneration.

IRON LINES

Deposition of iron in the corneal epithelium occurs often. Iron depositions are given special names when they are associated with certain conditions or with characteristic distributions. An iron line (Fig. 1.17) can be:

- Horizontal, at a point where the middle and lower thirds of the cornea join, approximately corresponding to the line of lid closure. These are frequently found in elderly people (Hudson-Stähli line).
- Circular, in a ring that surrounds the base of the cone in keratoconus patients (Fleischer's ring).
- Vertical, at the edge of pterygium (Stocker's line).
- Around the edge of a filtering bleb after glaucoma filtering surgery (Ferry's line).
- Central and horizontally oriented after radial keratotomy.

SALZMANN'S NODULAR DEGENERATION

Clinical Appearance

Salzmann's nodular degeneration appears as multiple, gray-white, elevated, round lesions in the central or paracentral cornea. These lesions may also occur at the end of the vessels in a corneal pannus.

Characteristics

Salzmann's nodules usually occur in older people and are more frequent in women. They may be unilateral or bilateral.

Histology

There is a localized replacement of Bowman's membrane by a hyaline and fibrillar material.

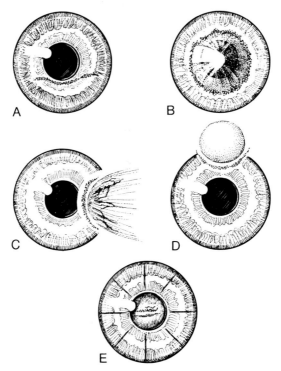

Figure 1.17. Corneal iron lines are deposits of iron in the superficial layers of the cornea. Their position and their association with certain processes allow a loose classification. **A,** a Hudson-Stähli line is commonly seen in elderly individuals. **B,** Fleischer's ring is seen with keratoconus. **C,** Stocker's line is seen with pterygium. **D,** Ferry's line is seen with glaucoma filtration blebs. **E,** Iron lines have also been seen after radial keratotomy.

Cause

Salzmann's nodular degeneration is a noninflammatory condition that frequently follows inflammatory conditions of the cornea by months or years. Inflammatory conditions that may precede Salzmann's degeneration include trachoma, interstitial keratitis, and phlyctenulosis.

CORNEAL BLOOD STAINING

Blood staining of the corneal stroma is almost always associated with trauma, usually blunt trauma to the globe with blood in the anterior chamber (hyphema), and with high intraocular pressure, although it is also seen with low intraocular pressure and least commonly with normal intraocular pressure. Initially, there is evidence of mild to moderate corneal edema. The cornea takes on a bloody, bronze coloration that is characteristic of corneal blood staining.

Cause

The cause of the blood staining is breakdown products deposited in the corneal stroma. How these breakdown products are transported into the cornea is not clear; however, it is thought that a compromised endothelium is necessary before corneal blood staining can occur.

Course

Once the blood staining is present, it remains for months. Clearing always progresses from the periphery toward the center. Severe blood staining has been known to take more than a year to clear entirely. In some cases of severe trauma, fibrosis due to prolonged staining and edema in the cornea may cause permanent scarring.

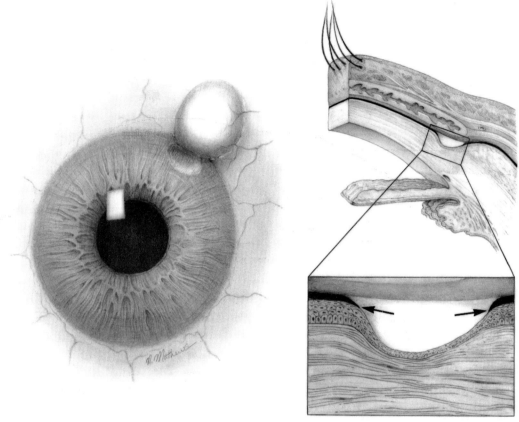

Figure 1.18.   A dellen is an excavation in the cornea that occurs usually next to an elevated lesion, especially one at the limbus. The illustration shows an elevated conjunctival mass with dellen formation on the cornea. The dellen is caused by lack of tear distribution by the lid over the area next to the raised lesion. Lack of tear distribution results in alterations of the stroma from improper wetting. The epithelium is usually intact.

Dellen

A dellen is an excavation in the cornea, usually at the limbus. The dellen is always adjacent to a raised area in the conjunctiva cornea such as a pinguecula or pterygium. This elevation prevents the lids from distributing the tear film at the edge of the elevation and at the area of the excavation. The stroma becomes dehydrated from lack of tear film and thins, resulting in excavation. The epithelium may show erosions, but generally the epithelium is intact (Fig. 1.18).

2

External Disease

NORMAL CONJUNCTIVA (FIGS. 2.1 TO 2.3)

- Episcleral vessels
- Bulbar conjunctiva
- Limbal arcade of blood vessels
- Conjunctival vessels
- Lower fornix
- Lower tarsus
- Upper tarsus
- Palpebral arcade

ESSENTIAL DIAGNOSTIC TERMS FOR EXTERNAL DISEASE

Hyperemia

Hyperemia (Fig. 2.4) is due to an increase in the number, the caliber, and the tortuosity of vessels (see injection, Fig. 2.5) in the conjunctiva. The result is a reddish appearance of the conjunctiva. Hyperemia is frequently associated with edema of the conjunctiva. On occasions, small subconjunctival hemorrhages can be seen with the hyperemia. Hyperemia can be seen with both acute and chronic inflammatory processes in the conjunctiva.

Congestion

Congestion is caused by poor conjunctival venous drainage. It produces a dusky red discoloration. This discoloration is due to prolonged circulation time within the conjunctival vessels. Congestion of the conjunctiva is most frequently associated with allergic states, when the pale, swollen, dusky red conjunctiva takes on a jelly-like appearance (Fig. 2.6).

Exudates

Exudates are byproducts produced with conjunctival inflammations and may vary in their characteristics. Exudates may be purulent, watery, catarrhal, ropy, mucoid, or bloody. Exudates collect on the lid margins and in the corners of the eye and are seen on the conjunctiva when the lid is pulled away from the eye.

Follicles

A follicle is a collection of lymphocytes in the conjunctiva. Follicles appear pink or gray and are elevations beneath the conjunctival epithelium. There is frequently a small net-

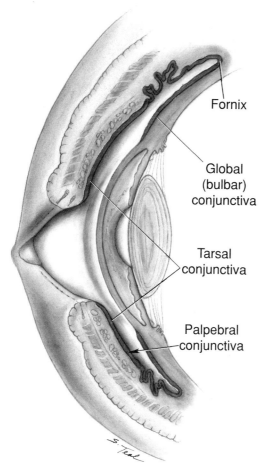

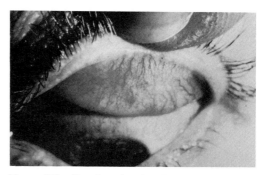

Figure 2.3. Tarsal conjunctiva. The technique of lid eversion is used to examine the character of the conjunctiva on the tarsal surface as well as to examine for foreign bodies. The lid is everted by pulling the upper lid downward and then placing countertraction (usually with a cotton-tipped applicator) on the skin. The lid is then folded back over the applicator as gentle pressure is exerted downward.

Figure 2.1. Conjunctival anatomy. Conjunctiva in the lid is known as the palpebral conjunctiva (that in front of the tarsus is called the tarsal conjunctiva), conjunctiva on the globe is called global (bulbar) conjunctiva, and conjunctiva deep in the recesses between the lid and the globe is called "fornix" conjunctiva.

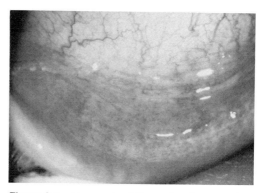

Figure 2.4. Hyperemia of the conjunctiva associated with acute infection. (Credit: George Waring, M.D.)

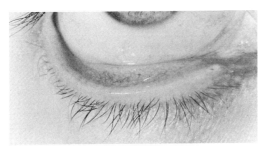

Figure 2.2. Normal lid margin. The lacrimal punctum where the tears drain is noted at the right margin of the lid. The base of the lashes shows no evidence of inflammation or swelling. The vessels of the conjunctiva on both the globe and the lid are normal. Note also the normal thickness of the lid margin.

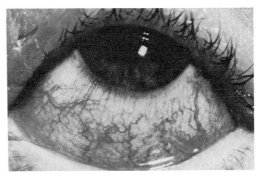

Figure 2.5. Injection is a clinical sign due to changes in vessel size, shape, and tortuosity. Injection of the conjunctiva may be differentiated from deeper injection of the episclera by diluted solution of a vasoconstrictor, which will blanch conjunctival vessels but not deeper vessels. Injection is an indication of conjunctival inflammation. (Credit: George Waring, M.D.)

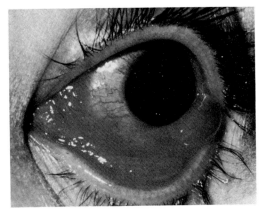

Figure 2.6. Congestion of the conjunctiva causes a dusky appearance of the conjunctiva due to a lack of venous drainage. It is frequently associated with injection. (Credit: George Waring, M.D.)

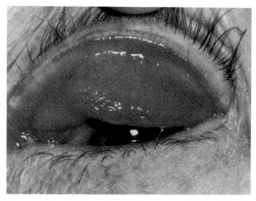

Figure 2.7. Conjunctival edema associated with acute infection of the conjunctiva. Also present are papillae, follicles, and hyperemia at the lid margin. (Credit: George Waring, M.D.)

work of blood vessels on the surface. Follicles are seen most frequently and characteristically in the recesses of the conjunctiva (fornices). They may involve the tarsal conjunctiva and can be seen infrequently on the bulbar conjunctiva, especially near the limbus. They are often seen with edema (Fig. 2.7). Follicles are most often associated with viral infections and drug hypersensitivity (Figs. 2.8 to 2.13).

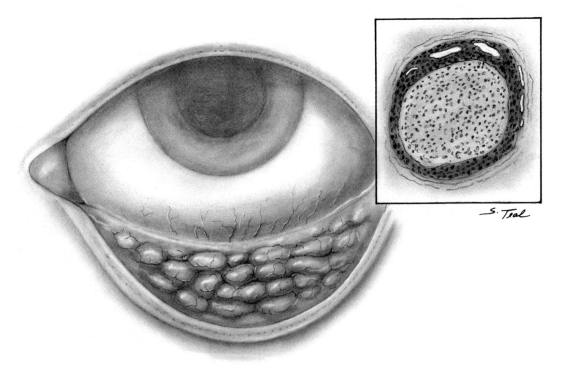

Figure 2.8. Follicles are collections of lymphocytes in the conjunctiva, typically surrounded by vessels. This differentiates them from papillae, which tend to have a central vascular core. Follicles may be seen with allergy, toxic reactions, and viral conjunctivitis.

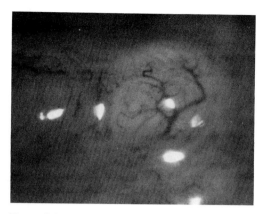

Figure 2.9. A large follicle under high magnification shows vessels outside the lymphocytic collection. (Credit: George Waring, M.D.)

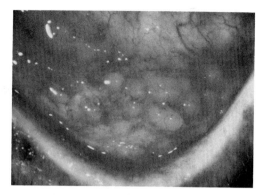

Figure 2.11. Follicular conjunctivitis on the lower palpebral conjunctiva. Follicles are collections of lymphocytes and are associated with certain causes of conjunctivitis. (Credit: George Waring, M.D.)

Papillae

Papillae are reactions of the conjunctiva on the upper and lower lids. They occur during both acute and chronic inflammatory states. When small, they produce a velvety appearance on the surface of the conjunctiva.

Under magnification, papillae are seen to

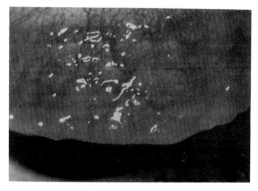

Figure 2.12. Follicles on the upper palpebral conjunctiva. The presence of follicles helps establish the diagnosis of specific disease processes. (Credit: George Waring, M.D.)

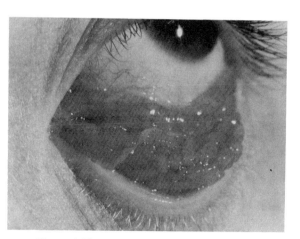

Figure 2.10. Follicular conjunctivitis. Follicles are a collection of lymphocytes within the conjunctiva. Those illustrated are exceptionally large. Follicles are often associated with allergy, viral conjunctivitis, and toxicity to topical medications. A characteristic diagnostic point is the vessels on the outside of each follicle. This is in contrast to papillae, which have vessels as a central core (see Figs. 2.14 and 2.15).

Figure 2.13. The caruncle, at the inner canthus, can show localized changes similar to those in other areas of the conjunctiva. Illustrated are follicles on the caruncle of unknown but suspected bacterial etiology. (Credit: George Waring, M.D.)

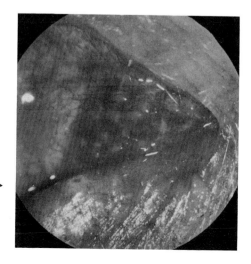

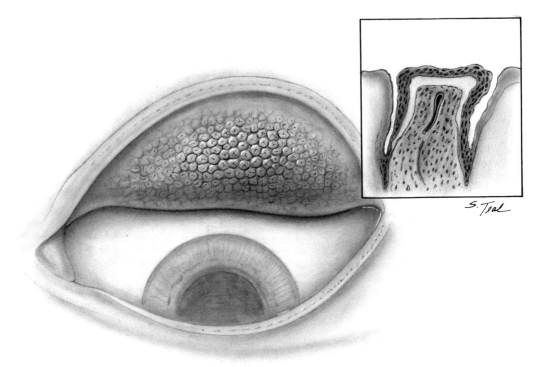

Figure 2.14. Papillae are changes in the conjunctiva showing a central vessel core surrounded by chronic inflammatory cells such as eosinophils. Illustrated are papillae on the tarsal conjunctiva, a common place for large papillae. Epithelial cells line the papillae. Papillae can be seen with contact lens wear, chronic irritation as from a suture, or conditions such as vernal conjunctivitis.

be elevations on the conjunctiva with a central vascular core. Around the core is a clear area of conjunctival swelling.

Giant papillae are seen easily without magnification (Figs. 2.14 and 2.15). These are associated with contact lens wear, irritation from sutures after operation, and vernal conjunctivitis (page 35).

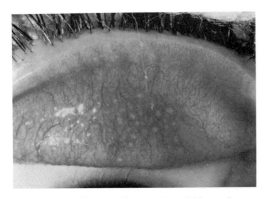

Figure 2.15. Giant papillary conjunctivitis on the superior tarsal conjunctiva. Papillae (page 21) are differentiated from follicles (page 18) by the presence of a central vascular core. (Credit: George Waring, M.D.)

Membranes and Pseudomembranes

Membranes and pseudomembranes are coagulam formed by the inflammatory reaction to an infection. *Pseudomembranes* (Figs. 2.16 and 2.17) are fine coagula that cover the conjunctival surface and can be stripped off without damaging the underlying conjunctiva. *Membranes* (Fig. 2.18) are coagula that are attached to the underlying conjunctiva; when removed, a membrane takes portions of the conjunctiva with it, leaving a rough, bloody base.

Pseudomembranes are seen in epidemic keratoconjunctivitis, primary herpes simplex virus conjunctivitis, streptococcal conjunctivitis, alkali burns, and erythema multiforme. *Membranes* are most often associated with diphtheria, but are also seen in streptococcal conjunctivitis, alkali burns, and erythema multiforme.

Giemsa Stain of Conjunctival Tissue

A Giemsa stain on a smear or scraping (Fig. 2.19) of the conjunctiva (Fig. 2.20) will show

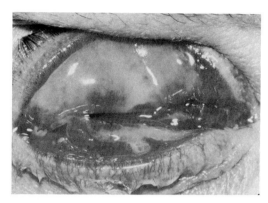

Figure 2.16. Pseudomembranes are seen in conjunctivitis produced by a number of different organisms. Pseudomembranes may be stripped without causing underlying bleeding, a feature that differentiates them from true membranes. (Credit: George Waring, M.D.)

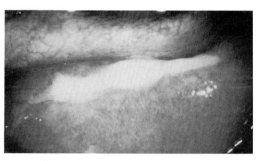

Figure 2.17. Epidemic keratoconjunctivitis (adenovirus) presents as an acute conjunctivitis with preauricular adenopathy. Pseudomembrane (shown here), although not common, can be present. A pseudomembrane can be removed without causing underlying bleeding, which differentiates it from true membranes. (See also color Fig. C.37.) (Credit: George Waring, M.D.)

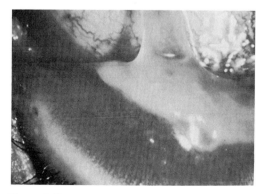

Figure 2.18. Membranous conjunctivitis. A conjunctival membrane is an exudative collection of cells that is firmly attached to the underlying conjunctiva. Membranes, when peeled, will bleed. Pseudomembranes, in contrast, can be removed without producing bleeding from the underlying tissue. (Credit: George Waring, M.D.)

inflammatory cells, the state of the epithelial cells, and the presence of inclusion bodies (see Fig. 2.22, **I** to **L**).

Cellular Response

Polymorphonuclear Response (Fig. 2.21). This cellular response predominates in the following conditions:

- Bacterial infections;
- Infections from fungi and actinomyces canaliculus;
- Infections with chlamydia (trachoma, lymphogranuloma venereum, or inclusion conjunctivitis);

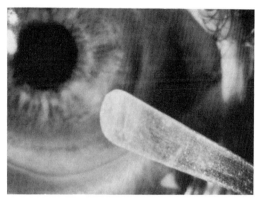

Figure 2.19. Scraping the cornea for laboratory diagnosis. A platinum spatula is used to scrape infected corneal tissue. This is used for culture directly on an agar plate, or tissue may be smeared on a glass slide for staining and examination under the microscope. (Credit: George Waring, M.D.)

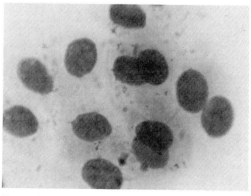

Figure 2.20. Normal conjunctival cells are important to identify on smears on the conjunctiva when diagnosing inflammatory conjunctival disease. The nucleus is usually full and oval or round, and there is significant pale cytoplasm.

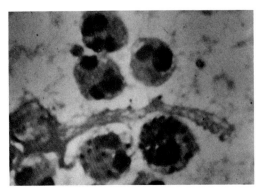

Figure 2.21. Smear showing gonococcus. Example of a smear stained for diagnosis. Present are bacteria of *Neisseria gonorrhoeae.* Inflammatory cells (polymorphonuclear leukocytes) are present. (Credit: George Waring, M.D.)

- Other less common conditions:
  —Stevens-Johnson syndrome;
  —Reiter's syndrome;
  —Ocular pemphigoid in early stages;
  —Medicamentosus;
  —Conjunctivitis with membranes or pseudomembranes.

Mononuclear Response. Mononuclear cells predominate in the following conditions:

- Viral conditions:
  —Epidemic keratoconjunctivitis;
  —Other adenoviruses;
- Herpes simplex conjunctivitis;
- Other less common conditions:
  —Newcastle disease;
  —Conjunctival inflammation with molluscum contagiosum;
  —Conjunctivitis associated with verruca vulgaris;
  —Chronic chemical irritation.

Eosinophilic Response. Eosinophils predominate in the following conditions:

- Vernal conjunctivitis;
- Chronic allergic conjunctivitis, both atopic and contact;
- Parasitic infestation;
- Ocular pemphigoid in its late stages.

Cell Changes

Changes are seen in the epithelial cells of the conjunctiva. *Keratinization* is seen in dry

eye, scarring from chronic conditions such as trachoma, ocular pemphigoid, and exposure of the conjunctiva as seen with ectropion. *Multinucleated epithelial cells* are seen in viral infections and are suggestive of herpes simplex. Increase in the *goblet cells* is seen with keratoconjunctivitis sicca, with most chronic conjunctivitis, and also with phlyctenular conjunctivitis. Intracytoplasmic basophilic *inclusion bodies* are seen in trachoma, lymphogranuloma, and inclusion conjunctivitis (all chlamydial infections). Specific changes can be seen with Giemsa smear cytological examination (Fig. 2.22):

A. Normal conjunctival cell;
B. Polymorphonuclear cell;
C. Eosinophil;
D. Lymphocyte;
E. Plasma cell;
F. Keratinized conjunctival cell;
G. Multinucleated giant cell;
H. Leber cell;
I. Prowazek inclusion bodies;
J. Guarnieri inclusion bodies;
K. Lipschütz inclusion bodies;
L. Henderson-Patterson inclusion bodies.

Clues to Diagnosis on Giemsa Stain

- Vaccinia—Guarnieri bodies
- Trachoma—Leber cells (these are giant macrophages with debris)
- Trachoma—Basphilic inclusion bodies (Prowazek)
- Molluscum Contagiosum—Cytoplasmic eosinophilic inclusion body (Henderson-Patterson)
- Dry Eye—Keratinized cells with increase in goblet cells
- Herpes simplex—Multinucleated giant cells, Lipschütz inclusion bodies
- Chlamydia—Basophilic cytoplasmic inclusion bodies
- Allergy—Eosinophil
- Bacterial infections—Polymorphonuclear cell responses
- Viral infections—Lymphocytic or monocytic responses

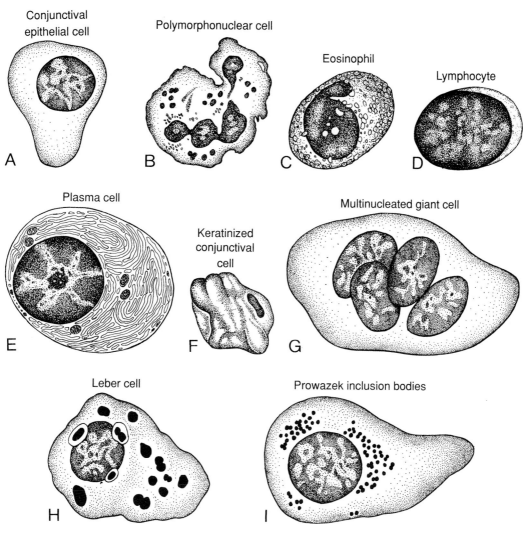

Figure 2.22. Cell types and intracellular changes on conjunctival smears that are associated with specific diagnoses. To emphasize characteristics, we show a stylized appearance on smears, which is variable. **A,** Normal conjunctival cell. **B,** Polymorphonuclear cell. **C,** Eosinophil. **D,** Lymphocyte. **E,** Plasma cell. **F,** Keratinized conjunctival cell. **G,** Multinucleated giant cell. **H,** Leber cell. **I,** Prowazek inclusion bodies. **J,** Guarnieri inclusion bodies. **K,** Lipschütz inclusion bodies. **L,** Henderson-Patterson inclusion bodies.

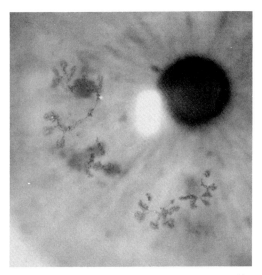

Figure 2.23. Dendrite of cornea. Dendrites are epithelial corneal defects. They are linear with characteristic branching. They stain with rose bengal and to a lesser extent with fluorescein. This dendrite is due to herpes simplex, its most common cause. (See color Fig. C.43.) (Credit: George Waring, M.D.)

Dendrites

Corneal epithelial lesions with a branching pattern similar to a tree are termed dendriform or dendrites. In adults, dendrites are almost always associated with herpes simplex virus (Fig. 2.23; see also color Fig. C.43). Other causes of dendrites that can be confused with herpetic dendrites are healing epithelial defects, zoster ophthalmia, and tyrosinemia.

Filaments

Corneal filaments are sheets of desquamated epithelial cells attached to abnormal surfaces of the drying cornea. Filaments are associated with keratoconjunctivitis sicca (dry eye).

Mucous Threads

Mucous threads are seen in patients with dry eye (keratoconjunctivitis sicca). These threads can be seen across the cornea or primarily in the inferior fornix.

Punctate Epithelial Erosions

Punctate epithelial erosions are fine lesions of the cornea that are slightly excavated. They

stain with both rose bengal and fluorescein and are a nonspecific response to many conditions, including light damage, minor chemical injuries, staphylococcal blepharoconjunctivitis, dry eye, toxicity to drugs, and neuroparalytic keratitis.

Punctate Epithelial Keratopathy

These are round lesions in the epithelial layer of the cornea that vary in size; some are large enough to be seen with the naked eye. In punctate epithelial keratopathy, accumulations of epithelial cells are surrounded by an inflammatory cell infiltrate. The lesions stain poorly with fluorescein but well with rose bengal. These lesions occur in multiple conditions including staphylococcal blepharokeratoconjunctivitis, viral ocular infections, chlamydial disease, dry eye, exposure keratitis, and molluscum contagiosum.

INFECTIOUS AGENTS

Bacteria

Staphylococcus Species

Staphylococcus is commonly cultured from the eye. Both *Staphylococcus aureus* and *Staphylococcus epidermidis* are pathogenic to the eye and can produce toxins, indirectly causing signs and symptoms. Staphylococcal organisms can be cultured in 75% of conjunctival specimens from asymptomatic individuals.

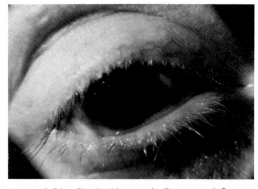

Figure 2.24. Blepharitis marginalis means inflammation of the lid margins. This is illustrated by desquamated cells that appear as debris at the lash bases. The lids are thickened and red, with hyperemia. Blepharitis is most often related to staphylococcal organisms.

Characteristics. Staphylococcal organisms are Gram-positive cocci that are seen singly or in pairs but may also be in clumps or strings.

Clinical Importance. Staphylococcal organisms may cause:

- Lid margin infection (blepharitis) (Fig. 2.24);
- Marginal corneal infiltrates (Fig. 2.25);
- Conjunctivitis;
- Keratitis with ulcer;
- Phlyctenules (see page 36);
- Localized infection of the lid margin (hordeolum; also called sty);
- Infection within the meibomian glands [resulting in chalaza (see page 209)];
- Inflammation of the lacrimal system (dacryocystitis);
- Postoperative infection inside the eye (endophthalmitis);
- Toxic marginal infiltrates (also called toxic or staphylococcal ulcers)—usually associated with blepharitis or other evidence of staphylococcal disease.

Pseudomonas aeruginosa

Characteristics. Pseudomonas is a Gram-negative rod.

Clinical Importance. Pseudomonas produces a number of clinical entities. It is especially dreaded in ophthalmology because of its rapid progression and devastating effects on the eye if not diagnosed and treated early. It causes in the eye:

- Ulcers of the cornea with keratitis, when the organism lyses corneal and scleral collagen and spreads rapidly;
- Endophthalmitis, a not uncommon complication of cataract surgery, is postoperative inflammation.

Haemophilus

Characteristics. This is a Gram-negative rod and may also be seen as cocci.

Clinical Importance. In children, haemophilus is a not uncommon cause of conjunctivitis with purulent mucous production.

Streptococcus pneumoniae (Pneumococcus)

Characteristics. Pneumococcus is a Gram-positive diplococcus.

Clinical Importance. This organism produces a conjunctivitis that is sometimes associated with conjunctival hemorrhages. The differential diagnosis for conjunctivitis associated with hemorrhage includes acute hemorrhagic conjunctivitis (see page 000) and some types of viral conjunctivitis, including adenovirus infections [epidemic keratoconjunctivitis and pharyngeal conjunctival fever (PCF)]. Pneumococcus can also produce a keratitis with ulceration of the cornea, ocular infection in the newborn (ophthalmia neonatorum), and postoperative infection (endophthalmitis).

Neisseria (N. gonorrhoeae, N. meningitidis, N. catarrhalis)

Characteristics. Any of the *Neisseria* organisms are Gram-negative diplococci that have a characteristic kidney bean shape.

Clinical Importance. Clinical ocular problems include:

- Purulent hyperacute conjunctivitis that occurs both in adults and in newborns;
- Keratitis that produces ulceration of the cornea and that may perforate;
- Postoperative infection (endophthalmitis).

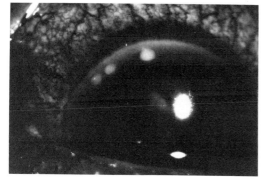

Figure 2.25. Staphylococcal marginal ulcers are seen in the anterior stroma. They characteristically have a clear zone between the ulcer and the limbus. These may vascularize. A conjunctival limbic reaction of injection is common. (Credit: George Waring, M.D.) (See also color Fig. C.44.)

Moraxella

Characteristics. *Moraxella* are Gram-negative, dumbbell-shaped or flat-ended diplobacilli.

Clinical Importance. Ocular changes include an angular blepharitis (inflammation and infection of the lids at the corners) and a conjunctivitis that is usually mucopurulent. Corneal inflammation (keratitis) may occur with ulceration.

Actinomyces

Characteristics. Actinomyces is a Gram-positive branching filament. It does not have terminal clubs. Sometimes the filaments occur as fragmented pieces.

Clinical Importance. This organism is important in inflammation of the lacrimal system, especially the canaliculi (canaliculitis). *Actinomyces* also produces conjunctival infections (conjunctivitis) and corneal infections (keratitis with ulceration).

Treponema pallidum

Characteristics. This is a spirochete.

Clinical Importance. Spirochetes can produce inflammation within the eye. This is a common differential diagnosis for prolonged, especially unresponsive, uveitis. Interstitial keratitis (see page 14) is also produced by treponema.

Fungi

There are a number of fungi that are important in ophthalmology. Fungi can produce corneal infections (keratitis) and intraocular infections both postoperatively and without previous operation (endogenous). Organisms vary greatly with various climates and geographic locations.

Both filamentous fungi and yeast are involved. Of the filamentous fungi, aspergillus, fusarium, and cephalosporium are commonly implicated. Of the yeast, candida is the most important.

Viruses

Viruses play an important role in infectious insults to the eye. Herpes simplex virus (see page 32), adenoviruses (see page 34), molluscum contagiosum (see page 210), and varicella zoster viruses are all important in external ocular disease.

Chlamydia

Chlamydial agents cause conjunctivitis and ocular infection. They should be suspected in long-standing cases of chronic conjunctivitis, especially in unilateral chronic conjunctivitis.

Conjunctival changes are follicular (see page 000). Corneal inflammation and ulceration with vascularization can occur. Lid margins and lid changes can occur.

For further information regarding chlamydial infections, look under specific disease processes such as:

Trachoma (page 269);
Adult inclusion conjunctivitis (page 35);
Opthalmia neonatorum (page 325).

EXTERNAL DISEASES AND DEGENERATIONS

Dry Eye (Keratoconjunctivitis sicca)

Physiology

In the normal state, the eye is kept moist by tears distributed over the ocular surface by the lids during a normal blink. An abnormal wetting process is referred to as dry eye. Abnormal wetting may be due to (*a*) disturbances of tear composition or volume or (*b*) disruption of tear distribution over the eye because of decrease or lack of a blink.

Tear Film. The tear film is a complex layer of fluid that is drawn over the surface of the cornea by the lids. Any disruption in this tear film can result in corneal drying. Severe disruption can cause scarring and loss of vision.

Layers. The tear film is conveniently divided into three layers.

1. Oil. The outer layer is the *oil layer.* This is produced by the meibomian glands, modified sebaceous glands in the lid margins.

2. Aqueous. The second largest and the middle layer is the *aqueous layer.* Aqueous is produced primarily by the lacrimal gland. Additional aqueous production comes from the conjunctival glands of Wolfring and Krause.

3. Mucin. The third or inner layer is the *mucin layer.* Mucin is produced by the goblet cells, which are concentrated primarily in the inferior conjunctival regions but are found throughout the conjunctiva.

Distribution. Tear film is distributed over the cornea, where it remains intact for 20 to 30 seconds. As the tear film begins to lose integrity, a phenomenon known as *breakup,* the sensitive cornea is stimulated and, by a reflex pathway (fifth nerve and seventh nerve) a blink occurs. The blink carries the tear film at the edge of the lids in a specific, and visible, line called the meniscus. The meniscus (of tears) is dragged across the cornea during the blink and reestablishes the wetness of the corneal surface.

Abnormalities of the Tear Film. Dry eye can occur from abnormalities of specific tear film layers. Loss of the lipid layer causes rapid evaporation of the aqueous layer. Decrease in the volume of the aqueous layer causes insufficient wetting. Lack of mucin results in loss of adhesion of the aqueous part of the tear film to the corneal surface, and drying occurs.

Irregular Surfaces. Localized drying of the cornea can occur because of irregularities in the corneal or conjunctival surfaces. These irregularities do not allow even distribution of the tear film, and corneal drying occurs at a specific point (for example, next to a raised lesion, where tears are insufficient).

Blink Abnormalities. Abnormalities of blink also occur due to lack of stimulation from decreased corneal sensation, lack of eyelid closure (as in seventh nerve dysfunction), or eyelid disease, where the lids may not touch the globe and distribute tears, causing a localized or generalized drying.

Causes of Dry Eye

Dry Eye from Decreased Aqueous Production.

Congenital
  Riley-Day syndrome (familial dysautonomia)
  Anhidrotic ectodermal dysplasia
  Cri-du-chat syndrome
  Absence of lacrimal nucleus
  Congenital familial sensory neuropathy with anhidrosis
  Adie syndrome
  Multiple endocrine neoplasia
Acquired
  Trauma to the lacrimal gland (surgery, injury, irradiation)
  Inflammation
    Sjögren's syndrome
    Primary amyloidosis
    Mumps
    Trachoma
  Infiltrations
    Sarcoidosis
    Lymphoma, leukemia
    Amyloidosis
Drugs
  Antihistamines
  Thiabendazole
  Antimuscarinics
  General anesthetics
Neuroparalytic hyposecretion
  Brain stem lesions
  Cerebellopontine angle and petrous bone lesions
  Middle fossa floor lesions
  Lesions of the sphenopalatine ganglion

Dry Eye Due to Decreased Mucin Production (Goblet Cells).

- Goblet cell dysfunction—vitamin A deficiency
- Goblet cell destruction
  —Alkali burn
  —Cicatricial pemphigoid
  —Stevens-Johnson syndrome
  —Trachoma
- Drug-induced
  —Practolol
  —Echothiophate iodide

Lipid Abnormalities.

- Deficiency—only in anhidrotic ectodermal dysplasia, where meibomian glands are congenitally absent
- Alteration—blepharitis (bacterial lipases break down lipids to free fatty acids)

Lid Abnormalities Causing Dry Eye.

- Entropion (rolling inward of the lid)
- Ectropion (rolling outward of the lid)
- Symblepharon
- Lid notch
- Lagophthalmos

Surface Abnormalities Causing Dry Eye, Localized.

- Keratinized lid margin
- Dellen
- Contact lens wear
- Topical anesthesia

Symptoms and Signs of Dry Eye

General. The symptoms of the early stages of dry eye are common and are often found in women in later life. The distinctive symptoms are recognizable by the patient, who describes them in general terms such as tiredness, irritation, heaviness, or fullness of the eyes. Additional signs, such as redness and swelling, can help diagnosis if they accompany symptoms.

At times, excess tearing may occur. Although this seems paradoxical to dry eye, the inability of the tear film to cover the cornea adequately may cause reflex tearing in excess.

Signs on Physical Examination of Dry Eye.
1. Filaments. The slitlamp with magnification is needed to see filaments. Filaments are thin lines of epithelial cells and are seen on the superficial cornea.
2. A Decreased Meniscus. The meniscus is best examined on the lower eyelid. The meniscus is the area of tear collection on the inner eyelid next to the globe. The meniscus is normally approximately 0.2 to 0.3 mm in height. When the height of the meniscus is less than 0.1 mm, it is considered abnormal.
3. Mucous Strands. Rolled mucous strands frequently occur to the inferior fornix of the conjunctiva. These strands sometimes are blinked up onto the cornea and may cause visual dysfunction.
4. Meniscus Floaters. Debris in the meniscus is a common finding in dry eye patients. The normal meniscus is clear.
5. Papillary Conjunctivitis. A nonspecific conjunctivitis may occur with dry eye pa-

tients. Because it occurs with many other conditions, it is not diagnostic without other signs and symptoms.

Establishing the Diagnosis of Dry Eye

1. Rose Bengal Staining. Rose bengal is a red dye that stains devitalized cells both on the cornea and on the conjunctiva. Corneal rose bengal staining appears as punctate red dots usually in the inferior one-third of the cornea. Staining is more extensive with severe dry eye.

Rose bengal staining of the conjunctiva is usually limited to the areas of conjunctiva exposed when the eyes are open. These are triangular areas with the base at the limbus and the point in either the temporal or nasal direction. This triangular staining is characteristic of dry eye.

2. Fluorescein Staining. Fluorescein staining is not usually helpful in the diagnosis of conjunctival drying. Fluorescein staining can be positive when the cornea is eroded by drying and is usually found in the lower half of the cornea.

3. Shirmer Test. Shirmer test (Figs. 2.26 and 2.27) is accomplished by placing filter paper strips between the lower lid and the globe. Portions of the filter paper strip then project outward from the eye. The degree of

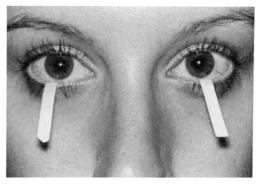

Figure 2.26. Shirmer test strips are placed along the lower lid. Tears wet the strips so that normal or abnormal tear function can be determined. The wetting is seen along the strip, more in the right eye and less in the left eye. After 5 minutes, the left eye would be considered abnormal and the right eye normal. Usually the strips are placed slightly more laterally to avoid corneal stimulus.

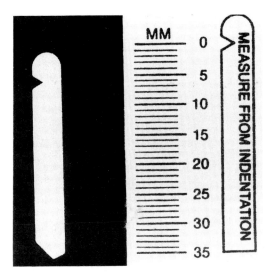

Figure 2.27. The filter paper Shirmer test strip on the left is used for tear film evaluation. To measure wetting, the millimeter rule provided with the strips can be used. As indicated, measurement starts from the indentation, which represents the point at which the inner portion of the lid touches the strip.

wetting of the strip during a 5-minute period is measured.

The test can be done with or without anesthesia. If topical anesthesia is used, there is about a 40% reduction in the Shirmer test values. There is controversy in the literature about the way the test should be monitored. Repeated experience with a single technique is usually most helpful for the individual practitioner.

4. Tear Film Breakup Time. To determine the tear film breakup time (see page 4), one uses enough fluorescein to stain the tear film. After a blink, the fluorescein-stained tear film can easily be seen with a cobalt blue filter on the slitlamp as the lid spreads the film over the cornea. Normally, the tear film will remain intact and be seen as a uniform layer of greenish blue. As the tear film breaks up, it assumes one of two patterns—lines or dots. Lines or dots of breakup show as black or blue-black against the background of blue-green. During the test, the patient blinks and is told to hold the eye open. The time from blink until breakup is then recorded. Anything over 10 seconds is considered normal.

Differential Diagnosis of Dry Eye

1. Decreased or absent aqueous
   A. Congenital absence of the lacrimal gland, either an isolated finding or, more frequently, secondary to anhidrotic ectodermal dysplasia (X-linked recessive)
   B. Trauma to the lacrimal gland from injury, surgery, or infection
   C. Neurogenic changes—congenital changes such as familial dysautonomia (Riley-Day syndrome)
   D. Cri-du-chat syndrome
   E. Trauma, infection, neoplasm, use of anticholinergic drugs, or vascular insufficiency
   F. Lacrimal gland infiltration as seen in the sicca syndrome, Sjögren's syndrome, and tumors
2. Changes in the mucous layer of the tear film
   A. Conjunctival scarring (causes poor tear film integrity due to loss of mucus production)
      1) Chemical burns
      2) Radiation
   B. Disease processes
      1) Stevens-Johnson syndrome
      2) Ocular pemphigoid
      3) Meibomian gland destruction from any source
      4) Vitamin A deficiency
3. Abnormal blink mechanism
   A. Facial palsies
   B. Corneal hyposensitivity
   C. Partial blinks, frequently seen in elderly patients
   D. Abnormal external anatomy, such as ectropion
   E. Tumors causing lid distortion
   F. Corneal irregularities causing improper tear distribution
   G. Conjunctival irregularities also causing poor tear distribution

Complications of Dry Eye

Complications of dry eye include sterile ulcers (also known as stromal melt or sterile melt), blepharitis, conjunctivitis, and keratinization of cornea and conjunctiva. Band keratopathy, although unusual, does occur.

Sterile Corneal Ulcers. Corneal ulcers (or corneal melt) are characteristic. They are often associated with dry eye in patients with rheumatoid arthritis. The ulcers are frequently inferior and oval, with the long diameter of the ulcer being parallel to the limbus. The ulcers are at or below the visual axis and often progress to perforation. They are seen much more frequently in women than in men.

Other. Blepharitis and conjunctivitis, which are commonly associated with dry eye, are thought to be due to loss of the enzymatic bacterial protection of the tear film. Lysozyme, an enzyme with antibacterial properties, is the enzyme most widely known to be decreased in dry eye syndrome. Without physiologic enzymatic protection, opportunistic infections take over.

Herpes Simplex

Herpes Simplex Virus and Humans. Herpes simplex virus is a ubiquitous parasite. It is so prevalent that, by age 60, 97% of the population have antibodies to this virus. Antibodies to the virus cross the placental barrier and are generally protective to the newborn for the first 6 months of life. After that time, children may be infected. By age 5, 70% of children have titers against herpes simplex virus. Most infections are unrecognized by the patient or the parents. Of the symptomatic primary infections that occur in children, a systemic illness or a focal lip lesion are most common.

Primary ocular infections as the first herpetic infection are uncommon but do occur. When they occur, both inflammation of the cornea (keratitis) and conjunctival inflammation (conjunctivitis) may be seen. The primary ocular infection is frequently accompanied by vesicles on the skin that may be obvious or that may need to be searched for carefully. Preauricular adenopathy may also occur.

Congenital and Neonatal Ocular Herpes

Ocular herpes can occur at birth or just after birth. Conjunctivitis, keratitis, cataracts, and necrotizing chorioretinitis may occur in the eye and are almost always accompanied by a vesicular eruption of the skin. This is a serious infection in neonates and may be fatal. The majority of the ocular conditions due to herpes occur after a person has had a primary infection, usually nonocular, and has developed antibody titers to the virus.

Recurrent Herpetic Infections (When Patient Has Humoral and Cellular Immunity)

1. Epithelial Herpetic Disease. Epithelial herpetic disease is characterized by the dendrite (see Fig. 2.23). A dendrite is caused by invasion of the epithelium by live virus. Additional epithelial disease with large defects in the superficial cornea is described as geographic. Geographic areas may cover large portions of the cornea. In epithelial disease with the live virus present, polymorphonuclear cells are present. There are no lymphocytes.

2. Trophic Changes. Trophic corneal defects are chronic, nonhealing, sterile ulcers in the stroma and epithelium. They have characteristic gray, thickened borders. The ulcer base is irregular, and the epithelium fails to heal over the damaged ulcer base.

3. Stromal Disease. Necrotizing viral keratitis occurs where active virus is present. Interstitial keratitis, immune rings (Wessely's rings) (see page 381), and limbic vasculitis occur with immune complex hypersensitivity that may result in deep vascularization.

Disciform keratitis is a delayed hypersensitivity to the herpes simplex virus. It may cause focal bullous edema or may be generalized. Focal bullous epithelial changes can accompany the edema. Keratitic precipitates may occur on the endothelium with little or no anterior chamber reaction. The edema of the cornea may also be accompanied by folds in Descemet's membrane.

4. Endothelialitis. At times the endothelium can be specifically affected with inflammation.

5. Iridocyclitis and Trabeculitis. Nongranulomatous inflammation may or may not occur with corneal disease. More frequently, the inflammation occurs without prior keratitis. With trabeculitis, glaucoma often occurs. The exact mechanism of trabeculitis in herpes simplex virus infection is unknown.

Diagnosis

Diagnosis by Conjunctival Smear. Giemsa stain is the most common stain used when conjunctival scrapings are taken for evaluation. The following characteristics are helpful when establishing herpes simplex virus infection:

- Multinucleated giant epithelial cells;
- Viral intranuclear inclusion bodies (Lipschütz);
- Mononuclear cell infiltration.

Viral Cultures. Viral cultures can be used to establish the presence of the virus. As the virus is commonly present and sheds periodically in different individuals, this may not always be helpful in confirming the diagnosis of herpes simplex as a cause of a specific infection.

Sera Titers. A rising serum titer can help establish a primary infection. It is very rarely used clinically by the ophthalmologist because most ocular infections are not primary. If sera titers are to be used, two titers are taken 4 to 6 weeks apart. Titers should be requested for both type 1 and type 2 viruses.

Ocular Herpes Simplex Virus Types

Ocular herpes simplex is primarily type 1 (oral). On occasion, type 2 (genital) is involved.

Concept of Latency

The virus is known to be harbored in the neural system in humans. The trigeminal nerve ganglion is probably the major source for ocular herpes recurrent infections. The virus remains latent most of the time but can be stimulated by a number of trigger mechanisms. Trigger mechanisms are important when taking a patient history to aid in the diagnosis of herpes.

Trigger mechanisms that activate latent virus in the ganglion are:

- Exposure to sunlight;
- Fever;
- Menstruation;
- Emotional stress;
- Surgery;

- Infection;
- Local trauma to the cornea;
- Heat.

There are a number of antiviral drugs that affect herpes simplex:

- Trifluridine;
- Idoxuridine;
- Vidarabine;
- Acyclovir.

Recurrence

After a second ocular herpes infection, there is a 25 to 30% chance that there will be another recurrence. After two recurrences, there is a 50% chance of having a third or more. When informing patients about recurrences, the most important, clinically useful risk factor is the presence of a former ocular herpetic infection.

Sjögren's Syndrome (Sicca Syndrome)

Cause

This is an autoimmune, multisystem disease process.

Characteristics

The classic triad described by Sjögren was keratoconjunctivitis sicca, xerostomia, and connective tissue disturbance, usually arthritis. There are two categories: *primary,* which is the sicca syndrome alone or combined with xerostomia, and *secondary,* which is the sicca syndrome and a connective tissue disorder with or without xerostomia.

Pathology

With Sjögren's syndrome, there is a mononuclear infiltration into the lacrimal and salivary glands. This infiltration causes decreased tear and saliva production and eventual dry eye and dry mouth.

Clinical Characteristics

There is a high female to male predominance of 9:1. Approximately 25% of the patients with Sjögren's syndrome will have rheumatoid arthritis. The onset is commonly between 40 and 60 years of age.

Connective Tissue Disorders Associated with Sjögren's Syndrome

- Rheumatoid arthritis
- Systemic lupus erythematosus
- Hashimoto's thyroiditis
- Polymyositis
- Polyarteritis nodosa
- Waldenström's macroglobulinemia
- Progressive systemic sclerosis

Importance

Dry eye is a common condition. Sjögren's syndrome should be considered in any patient with dry eye.

Adenovirus

Different types of adenovirus produce conjunctival and corneal changes that vary significantly. In general, there are two clinically definitive infections caused by adenovirus: (*a*) epidemic keratoconjunctivitis and (*b*) pharyngoconjunctival fever (PCF) (Table 2.1). Epidemic keratoconjunctivitis is not preceded by systemic symptoms but has a much higher incidence of corneal involvement than PCF. In PCF, previous upper respiratory infection is common and the incidence of corneal involvement is very low. The conjunctival signs and symptoms are similar in both types of adenovirus infection.

Epidemic Keratoconjunctivitis (EKC)

Clinical Characteristics. EKC is characterized by watery discharge. The eye tends to be moderately painful and sensitive to light. The conjunctiva is swollen and red.

Enlarged, nontender or slightly tender lymph nodes, which can be felt in the preauricular area, are common. There is inflammation on the superficial epithelium of the cornea in approximately 80% of patients (superficial keratitis). There are usually no systemic symptoms (compare the presence of systemic signs in PCF).

Cause. The cause is adenovirus, most often types 8 and 19.

Late Corneal Involvement. With EKC, subepithelial corneal opacities may occur just under the epithelium, appearing coarse and white-gray. They are actually intraepithelial infiltrates. They tend to be round and somewhat snowflake-like (see color Fig. C.4). These corneal changes start about 2 weeks after the more acute epithelial involvement early in the infection. They may persist for months or even years. These may affect visual acuity but are self-limited and are frequently treated only symptomatically. The size of the lesions is reduced by corticosteroid therapy. Once corticosteroid therapy is stopped, however, the lesions return to pretreatment size or larger. Steroids do not shorten the time that the intraepithelial opacities are present.

Pharyngoconjunctival Fever (PCF)

Cause. The cause is adenovirus types 3, 7, and others.

Clinical Characteristics. This conjunctivitis usually follows an upper respiratory infection and fever. The conjunctivitis shows (*a*) redness from increased vessel diameter and (*b*) general edema of the conjunctiva. The eye may be painful and very light-sensitive.

Table 2.1.
Comparison of EKC and PCF

	EKC	PCF
Adenovirus type	8 and 19	3 and 7
Keratitis	80%	30%
Fever and sore throat	rare	common
Spread by office contamination	yes	yes
Intraepithelial corneal involvement	common	unusual
Preauricular nodes	yes	yes
Contagious	yes	yes
Length of conjunctivitis	10–14 days	10–14 days
Discharge	watery	watery
Hemorrhages	yes	yes
Light-sensitive symptoms	yes	yes

The discharge is watery. There may be some subconjunctival hemorrhages and occasionally membrane formation. *Lymph node enlargement* (slightly tender) in the preauricular area is present.

Corneal Involvement. Corneal involvement is unusual in PCF (compare the corneal involvement in EKC).

Adult Inclusion Conjunctivitis

Cause

Adult inclusion conjunctivitis is caused by chlamydial organisms and is frequently associated with venereally transmitted chlamydial urethritis or cervicitis.

Epidemiology

The chlamydial organisms can be transmitted by direct or indirect ocular contact with genital secretions. They can also be transmitted through improperly chlorinated water in swimming pools contaminated with the organism.

Incubation Time

Ocular findings occur 1 to 2 weeks after exposure.

Clinical Manifestations

Conjunctival Changes. There is an acute follicular conjunctivitis. The follicular reaction is more prominent in the lower conjunctival recess (fornix) and in the conjunctiva of the lower lid (see Fig. 2.1).

Corneal Changes. Spotty breakdown of the corneal epithelium (epithelial keratitis) is common. Small marginal and central infiltrates occur in the superficial stroma. Follicles are seen at the limbus. Preauricular adenopathy is present.

Laboratory Diagnosis

In contrast to inclusion conjunctivitis of a newborn (see Chapter 14, Special Considerations in Children), stained scrapings of the conjunctival epithelium rarely show inclusion bodies in epithelial cells. When the condition is acute, however, inclusion bodies may be seen occasionally in adults and assist in the diagnosis.

Allergic Conjunctivitis

Other Name

Immunological conjunctivitis

Hay Fever Conjunctivitis

Clinical Symptoms. Itching of the eye is an important feature of allergic conjunctivitis. Itching is not seen in bacterial or viral conjunctivitis.

Signs. There is tearing and redness of both eyes. The conjunctiva tends to be chemotic. Discharges tend to be firm and ropy. No papillae or follicles are seen on the conjunctival surfaces. There is no preauricular lymph node enlargement.

Diagnosis. Epithelial scraping reveals eosinophils.

History. There is usually a history of recurrent, nonocular allergy to pollens, grasses, or other seasonal antigens.

Vernal Keratoconjunctivitis

Vernal keratoconjunctivitis is an immediate, or humoral, hypersensitivity reaction.

Characteristics. This type of conjunctivitis is bilateral. It begins during the prepubertal years and is much more frequent in boys than in girls.

Course. Vernal keratoconjunctivitis lasts 5 to 10 years and then regresses. It is more common in warm climates and more severe during spring and summer.

Other Manifestations of Allergy. Hay fever, asthma, or allergies to specific pollens are common. Itching is extremely common and should be questioned specifically in any patient with inflammation. There is usually a family history of allergy, asthma, or eczema.

Signs. There is a fine papillary reaction on the lower lid (tarsal) conjunctiva. The upper lid conjunctiva shows giant papillae. These are large enough to be easily visible without slitlamp manification, and they are sometimes called *cobblestone papillae*. An individual papilla is polygonal, has tuffs of capillaries inside, and has a flat top. There is a fine, stringy discharge, and a pseudomembrane (see Fig. 2.16) may occur (called Maxwell-Lyons sign).

In vernal keratoconjunctivitis, a fine subepithelial infiltration (micropannus) can be seen. Conjunctival scarring does not occur.

Superficial corneal ulcers that tend to be superior and oval may occur, probably from the direct rubbing effect of the palpebral giant papillae. Also, a diffuse keratitis may be present.

Limbic Vernal Keratoconjunctivitis

This is common in the black race and presents as nodular swellings at the limbus. Pseudogerontoxon (arcus), Trantas's dots (white dots at limbus), and eosinophils on conjunctival smears can be seen.

Association with Keratoconus

Both vernal keratoconjunctivitis and limbic keratoconjunctivitis may be associated with *keratoconus* (see page 12).

Atopic Keratoconjunctivitis

Characteristics.

- Atopic keratoconjunctivitis is seen in patients with *atopic dermatitis* (eczema) (Fig. 2.28). There is usually a history of allergic conditions such as asthma or hay fever.
- *Fine papillae* are found on the conjunctival surfaces. Giant papillae are very unusual and, when they do occur, they are on the lower tarsus rather than the upper tarsus, as seen in vernal keratoconjunctivitis.
- The lid margins are flushed red (erythematous).
- Conjunctival tissue is swollen with edema.
- There is an association with *keratoconus.* Concomitant with keratoconus, when present, there may be increased flexure of wrists and knees and creases in the axillary skin folds.
- Conjunctival scrapings show eosinophils.
- Corneal signs include keratitis followed by vascularization. Scarring of the conjunctiva and cornea is seen. In advanced cases, the cornea may become entirely opacified. Atopic cataract may be associated (a posterior subcapsule cataract and an anterior subcapsule cataract in the shape of a shield).

Course. The disease becomes inactive in later life.

Common Secondary Complications and Associations. These may be keratoconus, retinal detachment, herpes complex keratitis, bacterial blepharitis, and conjunctivitis.

Giant Papillary Conjunctivitis (GPC) (Pseudovernal Conjunctivitis)

Signs. These are giant papillar changes that occur on the palpebral conjunctiva, usually on the superior tarsus.

Cause. Patients wearing certain types of contact lenses can develop this giant papillary reaction from tissue contact with lens substances.

Phlyctenulosis (Phlyctenular Keratoconjunctivitis)

Description. This is a delayed or cellular hypersensitivity reaction.

Cause. Phlyctenulosis is a hypersensitive response to microbial proteins. Most common is staphylococcus, although tuberculous bacillus and a number of other oranisms have been responsible.

Clinical Appearance. Phlyctenulosis starts as a 1- to 3-mm-diameter lesion that is elevated, hard, and red. The lesion is in the conjunctiva, usually near the limbus. It may have a triangular shape with an apex toward the cornea. The surrounding area is hyperemic. As it progresses, the center tends to ulcerate and become grayish white. On rare occasions, the phlyctenules may develop on other areas of the global conjunctiva and on the palpebral conjunctiva.

The conjunctival phlyctenule leaves no scar. In contrast, corneal phlyctenules do

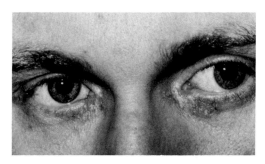

Figure 2.28. Atopic dermatitis of the lids is illustrated on the inner canthus of both eyes. (Credit: Ted Wojno, M.D.)

leave scars; at first, they appear as gray infiltrates and they end as triangular scars with the base at the limbus.

Associations. Phlyctenulosis can be seen with *lid margin infections* (blepharitis), in patients compromised by *dietary deficiencies,* and in acute *bacterial conjunctivitis.* Corneal involvement may be followed by Salzmann's nodular degeneration (see page 15).

Histology. The phlyctenule is a collection of small, round cells. An infiltration of polymorphonuclear cells follows. This is a reaction characterized by the delayed cellular tuberculin type hypersensitivity reaction.

Normal Course. Untreated, the course of a phlyctenule lasts 10 to 12 days.

Sensitivity to Steroids. The response of these lesions to steroids is so dramatic as to be helpful in making the diagnosis. Symptoms disappear and the lesion is gone within 24 hours after the application of topical steroids.

Dacryocystitis

Dacryocystitis is a common cause of unilateral conjunctivitis. Dacryocystitis is an inflammation of the lacrimal system (see page 000), usually bacterial or fungal. In chronic eye inflammation involving one eye, it is wise to press on the lacrimal sac to determine whether yellow mucus (which is associated with dacryocystitis) comes out of the punctum and also to irrigate the lacrimal system, assuring normal function and absence of infection.

3

Glaucoma

DEFINITION

Glaucoma is loss of vision due to increased pressure inside the eye.[a] The concept of increased pressure associated with visual loss (or potential loss) has significant clinical importance because some eyes can tolerate relatively high pressure without visual loss, whereas others succumb to visual loss at relatively low intraocular pressures.

Significance

Glaucoma is the second leading cause of blindness in the United States; 2% of the population over the age of 35 have glaucoma. In the very elderly, the prevalence is as high as 10%. Glaucoma is also a significant worldwide public health problem. Because the condition is painless and almost always without symptoms until the late stages, it requires education and screening of the populace. The diagnosis of glaucoma is as challenging as it is important: first, to find those unaffected patients who are at high risk and, second, to halt progression in those with existing damage.

Multiple Causes

Glaucoma, although often thought of as a single entity, has more than 40 different causes.

Distribution and Importance of Intraocular Pressure

The average pressure in an eye without glaucoma is 16 mm Hg, with a normal range of 13.5 to 18.5 mm Hg. The average intraocular pressure increases with age and is slightly higher in women than men. Hereditary factors are also important. For example, high pressures are often measured in relatives of patients with open angle glaucoma.

---

[a]The term *ocular hypertension* has been used when intraocular pressures are above the usual established standards but are not associated with evidence of tissue destruction (visual field loss or optic nerve changes).

Glaucoma can be difficult to diagnose. A single normal pressure does not necessarily rule out glaucoma because pressure fluctuates over 24 hours. Glaucoma diagnosis requires not only multiple pressure readings, but also optic nerve observation and visual field examinations.

Known risk factors help identify patients in potential danger. Factors that make certain individuals more susceptible to visual loss from increase of intraocular pressure are large physiologic cups in the optic nerve; asymmetrical optic nerve cupping; compromised vascular flow to the eyes; and a strong family history of glaucoma. Myopia, cardiovascular disease, and diabetes are additional risk factors for damage from elevated pressures.

Every eye has an intraocular pressure level that will produce visual loss. Although the level for each individual eye is different, there is enough similarity among eyes that guidelines can be used, even as we remember that there will be exceptions. The accepted guidelines are that pressure of less than 20 mm Hg poses a slight risk of causing glaucomatous changes, pressures between 20 and 30 mm Hg present a moderate risk, and pressures above 30 mm Hg present a high risk.

In general, pressures above 21 mm Hg should be followed for a lifetime at routine intervals of approximately 1 year. After age 40, the interval should be shortened to every 6 months or even less if additional individual risk factors are present.

THE PHYSIOLOGY OF AQUEOUS FLOW AND GLAUCOMA

Aqueous, the fluid that fills the anterior portion of the eye, is produced by the ciliary body (see Frontispiece) by two mechanisms:

- *Ultrafiltration.* This process is affected by the systemic blood pressure, intraocular pressure, and osmotic (oncotic) pressure within the plasma.
- *Secretion.* This is a metabolic process within the ciliary epithelium and is independent of pressure, either intraocular or systemic blood, but is affected by hypoxia, hyperthermia, and other factors that decrease metabolism.

Flow of Aqueous

The aqueous formed by the ciliary body flows from the posterior chamber (from behind the iris) through the pupil into the anterior chamber. The fluid leaves the anterior chamber at the chamber angle, which is formed by the iris and the junction of the cornea and sclera. Evaluation of this chamber angle provides a general differential diagnosis for most types of glaucoma (Fig. 3.6).

Aqueous leaves the anterior chamber through the chamber angle by filtration through a sieve-like, layered structure called the *trabecular meshwork.* The aqueous then flows into Schlemm's canal which, like the trabecular meshwork, circles the eye. From Schlemm's canal, aqueous drains through the collection channels of the sclera into the scleral vessels, where aqueous mixes with blood.

Intraocular pressure is maintained by a balance between a production of aqueous by the ciliary body and the outflow of aqueous from the chamber angle through the trabecular meshwork. Change in this balance causes changes in the intraocular pressure. Blockage of outflow is the most common cause for increases in intraocular pressure in most forms of glaucoma.

Variation of Pressure over 24 Hours (Diurnal Curve)

Intraocular pressure fluctuates throughout the day. The peak time varies from individual to individual. These swings of intraocular pressure are wider in glaucomatous eyes. Usually, the diurnal curve peaks during the early morning hours.

MEASUREMENT OF INTRAOCULAR PRESSURE

Ideally, to measure intraocular pressure a device should be within the eye. Manometry, in which a pressure-measuring device is inserted into the anterior chamber, is used experimentally and to calibrate the accuracy of other types of measuring devices. A variety of pressure measuring devices are available. These are called tonometers.

Shiötz Tonometer

The Shiötz tonometer measures pressure by the amount of indentation of a plunger on the surface of the eye. The Shiötz tonometer (Figs. 3.1 to 3.3) has a footplate that fits over the cornea. In the center of the footplate is a hole for a plunger. The degree that the plunger indents the eye is proportional to the amount of pressure within the eye. The movement of the plunger is indicated on a directly connected scale. The scale reading is noted and translated into millimeters of mercury of intraocular pressure. If the plunger does not indent the eye because of high pressure, additional weights are used. Appropriate scale readings are then correlated with the higher weights on the plunger.

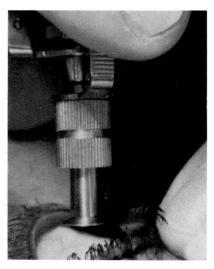

Figure 3.2.   A Schiötz tonometer, showing the position of the footplate of the tonometer on the eye.

This method of intraocular pressure measurement has been accepted for decades. In the usual range of measurement, it is accurate. However, it is inaccurate at the extremes of pressure measurement and if the sclera is distended. In high myopia, a condition where the sclera is often thin, falsely low pressure readings may be observed.

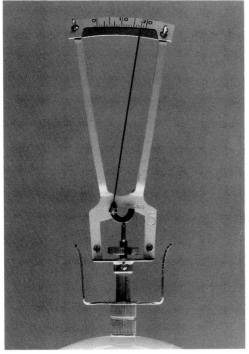

Figure 3.1.   The Schiötz tonometer is used to measure intraocular pressure. The base is placed directly on the anesthetized eye. The apparatus is held by the two curved prongs extending from the base. The plunger in the center, only a portion of which can be seen above the base plate, projects upward to touch the curve connected to the needle and adjusts according to the tension within the eye. The scale above does not show a direct pressure reading. The scale numbers are translated with a chart to determine the pressure in millimeters of mercury. (See the technique of holding the tonometer, Fig. 3.3.)

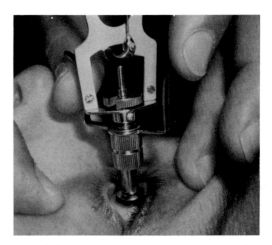

Figure 3.3.   Eyelid retraction with fingers while holding the Schiötz tonometer. To hold the Schiötz tonometer with the thumb and the forefinger and accurately place the tonometer on the eye, one must have the other fingers free. With the middle finger for retraction of either the upper or the lower lid, depending upon where the examiner is standing, and the opposite hand for retraction of the other lid, the Schiötz tonometer can be used with relative ease.

Applanation Tension

In applanation tonometry (see Chapter 16), a small plastic device is placed against the cornea. The end of the applanation tonometer is flat and round. A calibrated amount of pressure allows this small, round plastic area to flatten the cornea. When flattened, there is an endpoint viewed with the slitlamp, which appears as two semicircles. (Fluorescein dye in the tears is used to help visualize the endpoint using a slitlamp with the cobalt blue light.) These semicircles are lined up accord-ing to a pressure gauge that measures the pressure directly (Fig. 3.4).

Pneumotonography

Tensions are also measured by the amount of air required to distort the corneal surface. These devices are noncontact tonometers and require, in most cases, no anesthesia. Pneumotonography requires skill by the examiner, and there may be error until a significant skill level is acquired.

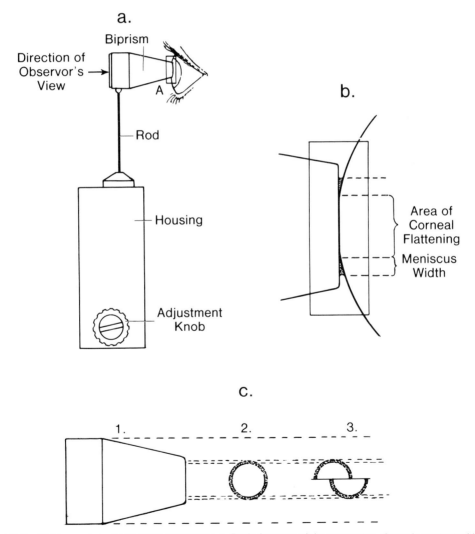

Figure 3.4. Goldmann-type applanation tonometry. **a**, Basic features of the tonometer, shown in contact with patient's cornea. **b**, Enlargement shows the tear film meniscus created by contact of the biprism and cornea. **c**, View through the biprism (*1*) reveals circular meniscus (*2*), which is converted into semicircles (*3*) by prisms. (From Shields MB: Textbook of glaucoma. 2nd ed. Baltimore: Williams & Wilkins, 1987:55.)

Other Types

A variety of other tonometers are available but are not used widely.

VISUAL FIELD TESTING

Definition

The visual field is the total area of central and peripheral vision. An area of non-seeing within the visual field is called a scotoma. (The *blind spot* is a natural scotoma created by the optic nerve of the eye, where no visual cells are present.)

Visual Field Defects in Glaucoma

Testing Technique

By checking the ability of the eye to perceive objects in the visual field, knowledge of both the extent of peripheral vision and the presence or absence of scotoma is obtained. This knowledge contributes to the diagnosis of glaucoma.

A white test object is commonly used in mapping glaucoma field defects. The size of the test object is adjusted to the patient's vision. For example, a 3-mm test object is used with 20/20 to 20/50 vision, a 6-mm test object is used with 20/60 to 20/100 vision, and a 9- to 12-mm object is used for eyes with less than 20/100 vision. The size of the test object, the test conditions, and the size of the pupil should remain constant from examination to examination to permit accurate assessment of visual field changes.

Small (miotic) pupils secondary to pilocarpine or other antiglaucomatous therapy may produce artifacts in visual field testing. Opacification (cataract), especially if central, may accentuate poor vision when light entrance is decreased by a small pupil.

Characteristics of Glaucoma Visual Field Defects

Glaucoma defects will stop at the horizontal meridian. The horizontal meridian, a quasiline on fields not seen when examining the retina, runs from 0° to 180° on the field. This meridian, which delineates glaucomatous field defects, is created by pathways of the nerve fiber bundles that leave the retina and sweep either superiorly or inferiorly toward the optic nerve without crossing the horizontal meridian. Because of this anatomical feature, a glaucomatous defect will not cross the horizontal meridian until late in the disease process. (This is in contrast to neurologic defects in the visual field, which tend to respect a vertical meridian from 90° to 270°.)

Types of Defects

Arcuate Defect. This arc defect, which is usually superior around the area of central vision but is sometimes inferior, may connect with the blind spot. It can be continuous or interrupted. When interrupted, round or oval visual field defects sweep in an arc above or below the central point of fixation. The arc defect is also called Bjerrum's scotoma (see page 357).

Nasal Step. Because nasal retinal fibers course away from the horizontal meridian in two directions, up and down, glaucoma fields may present with a characteristic appearance. In normal fields, the outer edge that we no longer see is continuous, even when crossing the meridian. Glaucoma fields are often not continuous. The discontinuity in a glaucoma field at the meridian is known as a nasal step. In fields for glaucoma defects, the nasal step is carefully sought by repeated stimulus testing of the nasal area at the horizontal meridian.

Visual Field Testing for Glaucomatous Damage—Methods and Instrumentation

Tangent Screen.
Technique. The tangent screen is 2 m² of black felt, usually mounted on a board or hanging free 1 or 2 meters from the patient. A small fixation point is placed in the center of the black field. For orientation, faint lines marked by dark thread radiate out from the center at 5° intervals and circle the screen at 5° intervals up to 30° from fixation. The examiner uses the marks to map the field and transfer information to a similar outline on paper for a permanent record.

As the patient keeps the eye fixated on the center point, a round, white test object is used to map the visual field. Other colors may be used but not usually in glaucoma testing. Each eye is tested separately.

The blind spot (caused by the optic nerve) is mapped first (it is outlined on the screen) both to educate the patient to the nature of the test and to establish patient reliability. The test object will disappear in the blind spot in the normal patient.

All areas of the central field are tested by moving the test object in the most common non-seeing areas (scotomas). The points of see to non-see and non-see to see areas are tested and recorded to determine peripheral constriction, nasal step (lack of continuity of the edge of the field between the upper and lower non-seeing areas in the nasal periphery), and scotoma.

Use. This is an inexpensive and accurate way of mapping the central 30° of field. It takes a fair amount of training for the examiner as well as time and patience for both the examiner and the patient to provide accurate, reproducible fields. Tangent screen testing is not useful with the uncooperative patient.

Perimetry—Goldmann Perimeter.

Technique. For central and peripheral field measurements, the Goldmann perimeter continues to be a standard in most ophthalmologist's offices. The patient's head is placed inside the center of a half round bowl that corresponds to the field of visual perception for each eye (Fig. 3.5A). Each eye is tested separately, and the patient's head is immobilized in a holder. Instead of a solid test object, as in tangent field testing, the Goldmann perimeter uses a projected light as a test object.

Use. The Goldmann perimeter is espe-

cially useful for controlling illumination of both the background and the test object. The white light is used to reflect against a consistently illuminated background. The patient's fixation is at the center of the bowl. Responses are charted, and reduction or changes of visual field are plotted.

Automated Perimetry (the Octopus, Humphrey Analyzer) (Fig. 3.5B).

Technique. Automated computerized vi-

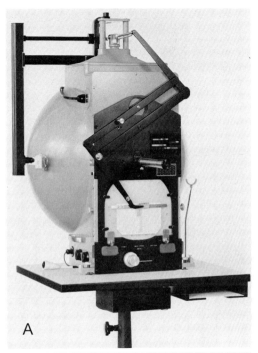

A

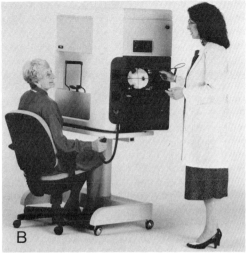

B

Figure 3.5. A, Goldmann visual field perimeter, viewed from the back. The patient would sit in front of this instrument, where there is a hemisphere. Lights are projected on a white background, and the patient responds by pressing a small button (*white triangular handle* on table). A perimeterist observes through the small *telescopic eyepiece*. As the spot of light is flashed, the perimeterist can move the position of the light and record the appropriate findings with a pencil on the *chart*. The *double bar with parallel arms* inferiorly and superiorly is the mechanism for moving the light and marking the appropriate charts. (Credit: Haag-Streit Service, Inc.)

B, Humphrey visual field analyzer. Visual fields are tested by presenting the eye with test objects away from the central visual area. The patient is sitting in a chair and will place her chin in the *chin rest* with her forehead against the *bar* in front of her. Standing is a technician, who will then turn on the analyzer. There is a computer visual field analysis on the *chart* on the side of the machine. The patient is holding a *response button* so that she can subjectively respond when a test object is presented in the peripheral field. (Credit: Allergan Humphrey)

sual field testing units look similar to the Goldmann perimeter, with a bowl in which the patient's head is positioned. Computer-generated programs project a light stimulus on 72 points (Octopus) when the visual fields are tested. When the stimulus is varied in intensity, the threshold of each point can be recorded.

Use. Automated perimeters may detect early field defects on serial examination, and reproducibility is excellent in some patients. They do require patient cooperation, and they are expensive. Patients may fatigue easily while taking the test.

DIAGNOSING TYPES OF GLAUCOMA

Gonioscopy

Principle

Normally, light and the image coming from the chamber angle are not visible. Where the cornea and the air meet, changes in the index of refraction cause total internal reflection of the light and the image from the angle (Fig. 3.6). No light or image passes out. However, the angle can be seen when air is replaced with a substance that has an index of refraction close to that of the cornea. Glass or plastic is most often used. Under these circumstances, total internal reflection does not occur, and the image is viewed (see Fig. 3.8). To understand the basic physical principles, study Snell's law (see page 366).

There are two methods of gonioscopy—indirect and direct. The Goldmann three-mirror prism is used most often for the indirect method of examination (Figs. 3.7 and 3.8). The chamber angle is seen in a mirror 180° from the position where the light is directed. A slitlamp is needed. The image is indirect because it is reflected.

Another type of goniolens, the Koeppe lens, gives direct visualization of the angle. The Koeppe prism forms a dome over the eye, and direct visualization of the chamber angle is possible with a magnifying lens and light source.

Both Koeppe and Goldmann gonioscopy can distort the anatomy of the chamber angle because of pressure on the eye. Experience helps avoid this error. (At times, distortion of the angle can aid in visualization, as with the Zeiss lens). The Goldmann gonioscope requires a facility with a slitlamp (see page 360). The Koeppe

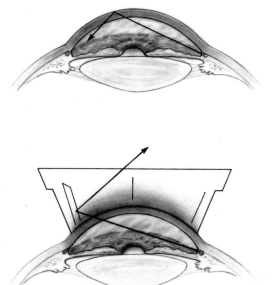

Figure 3.6. Principles of gonioscopy. Normally, because of the difference between the index of refraction in the cornea and the index of refraction of air, all light rays coming from the chamber angle are deflected internally—total internal reflection. In visualizing the chamber angle, the index of air is replaced by a glass or plastic contact lens. This allows visualization of the angle by changing the index of refraction and correcting total internal reflection. The image is reflected in a mirror, in this illustration, to the observer.

lens requires practice with a hand-held slitlamp or holding separate optical and illuminating instruments.

Another type of gonioprism is the Zeiss. This lens allows a 360° angle view. The Zeiss lens is also used to see the obscured angle in narrow

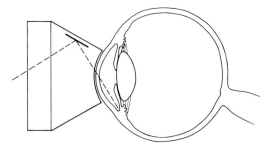

Figure 3.7. Gonioscopy—basic. When a gonioprism (see Fig. 3.8) is placed on the eye, a slitlamp is used to view the chamber angle by a mirror incorporated in the prism. The angle of view is always 180° from the position of the mirror. The angle appears anatomically with the iris below and the cornea above. Illustrated is a standard goniolens, the Goldmann lens.

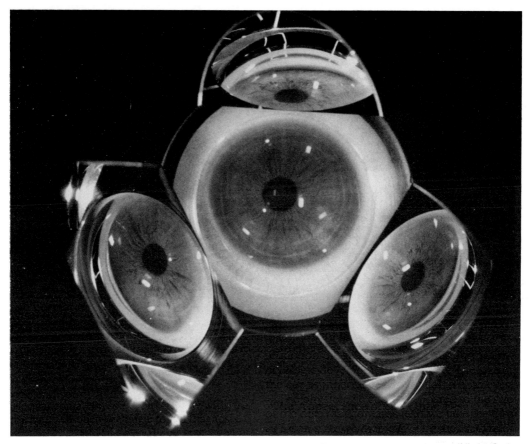

Figure 3.8. The view of the eye with a gonioprism. This is a three-mirror prism. The fundus (posterior pole), if the pupil were dilated, could be directly examined with the slitlamp. In the superior portion of the illustration is a dome-shaped mirror, which is used to examine the chamber angle, seen in the reflection of the mirror. The superior mirror also gives a view of the inferior angle. The rectangular mirrors to the left and right are for examination of the peripheral retina, which requires pupillary dilation.

angle glaucoma. Pressure on the eye with the Zeiss lens will open the angle to aid diagnosis.

The normal chamber angle has the following key anatomical landmarks (Fig. 3.13):

- Cornea;
- Schwalbe's line;
- Trabecular meshwork;
- Scleral spur;
- Ciliary body;
- Iris spur.

Changes in the Chamber Angle

Gonioscopy provides clues that can help with the diagnosis of different types of glaucoma (Figs. 3.13 and 3.16 to 3.22).

The Appearance of the Optic Disc

The Cup/Disc Ratio (Figs. 3.9 to 3.11)

In observing the optic disc, there is often a pale, central depression known as the physiologic cup. The physiologic cup is formed by retraction of the primary vitreous during embryologic development of the eye. The size of the cup is inherited and is equal in both eyes.

The physiologic cup is compared to the size of the disc that contains it. If we take the disc as 1.0 in size, we then can estimate the size of the physiologic cup as 0 (no cup) to 0.9 (large cup with essentially no rim of normal tissue). Measurement is primarily done vertically because the edges of the cup are more distinct superiorly and inferiorly.

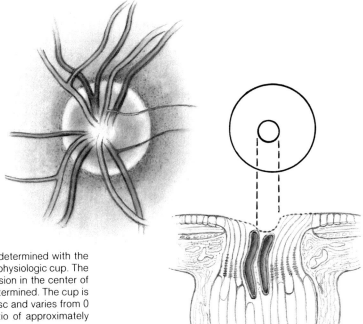

Figure 3.9. The cup/disc ratio is determined with the ophthalmoscope and relates to the physiologic cup. The physiologic cup is a central depression in the center of the disc. The cup is congenitally determined. The cup is graded relative to the size of the disc and varies from 0 to 0.9. Illustrated is a cup/disc ratio of approximately 0.2.

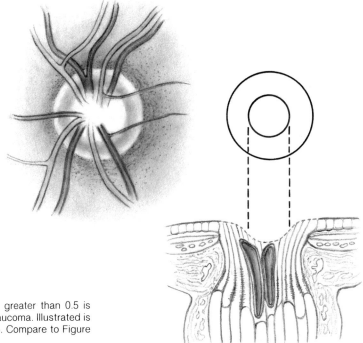

Figure 3.10. A cup/disc ratio of greater than 0.5 is considered highly suggestive of glaucoma. Illustrated is a cup/disc ratio of greater than 0.5. Compare to Figure 3.9.

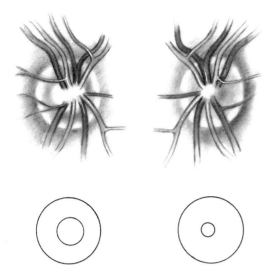

Figure 3.11. Cup/disc ratio asymmetry. Asymmetry between the left eye and the right eye in the cup/disc ratio is considered abnormal. The size of the physiologic cup is congenitally determined and is expected to be the same on both sides. An asymmetry of greater than 0.2 should be investigated for possible glaucoma. Illustrated are two cups, with ratios of approximately 0.4 and 0.1. These would be considered abnormal until proven otherwise. In addition, any cup ratio greater than 0.5 should be investigated.

Changes in cup size in glaucoma are due to loss of nerve tissue.

Instrumentation. The best instruments for optic nerve evaluation and determination of cup/disc ratio are the direct ophthalmoscope or the 90D Volk lens. The indirect ophthalmoscope should not be used for this evaluation because of low magnification and intense light. Also, direct binocular evaluation of the disc by gonioprism lens with the slitlamp is very accurate (a Hruby lens can also be used). Stereophotography of the disc is an excellent way to document and follow cup/disc ratio and has become almost standard in following a glaucoma patient's disc change.

Use of the Cup/Disc Ratio.

Susceptibility. The cup/disc ratio is known to correlate with susceptibility to increased pressures and probability of eventual glaucomatous damage. Any cup/disc ratio greater than 0.5 is highly suggestive of potential or actual glaucomatous damage. Also, the cup/disc ratio in both eyes is the same in normal subjects. Any asymmetry between a pa-

tient's left and right eyes is also indicative of probable glaucomatous damage. Any difference of 0.2 or more should be fully investigated. The cup/disc ratio tends to be larger in blacks than in whites.

Assessment of Damage. Assessment of glaucomatous damage by examining the size and appearance of the cup and by documenting changes in the physiologic cup, especially by means of the accuracy of photography, is extremely useful in determining the success of therapy and the severity of the disease process in an individual eye.

Notches in the cup are important. They frequently appear early in the inferior temporal area of the cup (correlating with a superior nasal scotoma in the arcuate area of the visual field).

The major indications of glaucoma are (a) enlargement of the cup and thinning of the rim and (b) increasing visualization of the anatomical perforated membrane (lamina cribrosa) at the base of the cup.

Nerve Fiber Layer Dropout

Newer techniques of photography, using high contrast black-and-white photography and filters, can outline nerve fiber layer dropout as an early indicator of glaucomatous damage. With some experience and using the red-free (green-colored) filter on the direct ophthalmoscope, the examiner can see changes in the nerve fiber layer that may occur before changes in the optic cup (Fig. 3.12).

Detection of Glaucoma: A Summary

Glaucoma may go undetected and result in severe visual loss for three reasons: (a) primary open angle glaucoma is painless, and there is no warning signal; (b) the vision loss is difficult to detect because it occurs peripherally, away from central vision; and (c) vision loss from primary open angle glaucoma progresses slowly and may occur over a period of years. The patient may not recognize severe visual loss until the late stages, when central vision becomes affected.

Screening processes are important. The most common check for glaucoma is measurement of intraocular pressure. Applanation, Schiötz, or other techniques are most

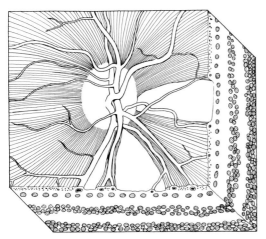

Figure 3.12. Nerve fiber defect. The nerve fibers of the retina are ganglion cell axons that course across the surface of the retina to the optic nerve. Loss of ganglion cell fibers occurs in lesions of the optic nerve, optic chiasm, and optic tract. Segmental dropout of the nerve fibers may be seen. The dropout is more easily visualized with red-free light (green filter on ophthalmoscope).

often used. After the age of 40, routine intraocular pressure readings are suggested every year for all patients. In patients with a strong family history of primary open angle glaucoma, screening should take place earlier and, in selected cases, more frequently. Where there is a high probability of the development of glaucoma, visual fields and careful observation and documentation with photography of the optic disc are recommended.

In screening for glaucoma, a pressure greater than 22 mm Hg is considered suspicious, and further tests, such as visual fields and optic nerve evaluation, should be done. Pressures in the range of 25 to 30 mm Hg should be regarded as highly suggestive. Patients with pressures above 30 mm Hg should receive a thorough workup with consideration for immediate therapy.

How a Patient Is Selected for Treatment after an Initial High Pressure Reading on Screening

After an increased pressure (usually 22 mm Hg or more) is discovered, visual fields are evaluated and optic nerves are observed for cupping sizes and changes. Additional evaluations that can aid in determining glaucoma-

tous damage are: (*a*) tonography in which the amount of aqueous outflow from the eye is measured under controlled conditions over a specific period (see Measurement of Intraocular Pressure, page 39); (*b*) evaluation of the nerve fiber layers with red-free filters or specialized photographic techniques; (*c*) measurement of the intraocular pressures over 24 hours to determine the character of an individual's diurnal curve. This last is done by admitting the patient to the hospital, with pressure checks every 4 hours, or teaching the patient or a member of the family to take and record intraocular pressures at home.

The indications for consideration of diurnal intraocular pressure measurement are:

- In uncontrolled glaucoma, with continued high pressures, where vision loss is continuing despite adequate therapy in a patient who is known to take the drops;
- In the patient who has demonstrated visual loss if the intraocular pressures are below 20 mm Hg; or
- When visual loss progresses despite therapy and apparently well-controlled pressures with maximal available medical therapy.

Dilate or Not Dilate? An Important Point about Dilation of the Pupil

Eyes with open angle glaucoma, the most common type of glaucoma, can be dilated for a complete fundus examination without danger. In narrow angle glaucoma, a relatively unusual condition, acute pressure rise may develop after dilation.

PRIMARY OPEN ANGLE GLAUCOMA

Open angle glaucoma is diagnosed by ruling out other types of glaucoma. In other words, a diagnosis is made by exclusion. Primary open angle glaucoma is *not* secondary to any other eye disease or a previous inflammatory condition or injury. The angle of the iris to the cornea, the iridocorneal angle, must be open and normal as determined by gonioscopy (a nonopen angle is angle closure glaucoma).

Associations

Familial Tendencies

Primary open angle glaucoma runs in families. Any patient with a strong family history should have a detailed baseline examination and careful follow-up. This may mean frequent examinations every 6 months or so after the age of 40 and at least every year in young adulthood. It is also wise to consider periodic visual field determination and optic disc photography.

Diabetes Mellitus

Diabetics have a higher incidence of open angle glaucoma. Screening of glaucoma patients also reveals a higher incidence of positive glucose tolerance tests than in the nonglaucomatous population.

Black Patients

Blacks have optic nerves that are more susceptible to damage from high pressures and have less response to medical treatment of open angle glaucoma than nonblacks.

Treatment of Primary Open Angle Glaucoma

The vast majority of patients with primary open angle glaucoma are treated medically. There are many medical therapies that are additive to help control the intraocular pressure to prevent glaucomatous nerve damage and visual field loss. Some patients do not respond to medical therapy and require either laser treatment or surgery.

Medical Therapy of Primary Open Angle Glaucoma

Pilocarpine. Pilocarpine stimulates the parasympathetic nerves of the eye and causes a small pupil (miosis). It improves the outflow of aqueous from the eye. Pilocarpine has no effect on aqueous production.

Concentrations. Pilocarpine comes in 0.5, 1, 2, and 4% solutions; usually, a 1% solution is used first in therapy. The higher percentages are rarely used because there is slight advantage in increasing the concentration. Higher concentrations produce more side effects.

Side Effects of Pilocarpine.

Induced Myopia. Nearsightedness may be induced, presumably by the parasympathetic action of pilocarpine on the ciliary muscle of the eye. This induced miosis is most prominent in younger patients. It is rarely seen in patients over the age of 50.

Brow Ache. Many patients experience a headache, usually above the eyes. Therapy need not be discontinued because, in most patients, the headache will stop after 2 to 3 days.

Decreased Vision. Because primary open angle glaucoma occurs in older patients who have cataracts, the combination of small pupil (miosis) and cataract causes decreased vision.

Cataracts. Pilocarpine has produced cataracts in young patients.

Synechiae. Prolonged pilocarpine therapy with a long-term miotic pupil may result in posterior synechiae (scarring between the iris and the lens in the pupillary region).

Pupillary Iris Cysts. Prolonged pilocarpine therapy produces cysts on the pupillary margin. These may cause a decrease in vision. This is especially true in children, and the risk can be decreased with Neo-Synephrine drops.

Flare. Pilocarpine affects the blood-aqueous barrier and causes an increase of protein in the anterior chamber (see Fig. C.5).

Conjunctivitis and Blepharitis. Conjunctivitis and blepharitis can be caused by chronic pilocarpine administration.

Beta-Blockers. Timolol, Betagan, and Bataxolol are beta-blockers. Timolol is a nonspecific beta-blocker and has side effects in patients with lung and heart disease. These beta-blockers may precipitate bronchospasm or bradycardia and heart block. Bataxolol and Betagan are specific beta-blockers that have the advantage of not producing some side effects that are often seen with timolol. All beta-blockers decrease aqueous production and are additive to other medical therapies.

Carbonic Anhydrase Inhibitors (Diamox, Neptazane). Carbonic anhydrase inhibitors are given orally. They are not effective topically. These drugs decrease aqueous production. They are not used as a first line treatment for glaucoma. Prolonged usage produces significant side effects in approximately 50% of patients. Loss of libido, depression, gastrointestinal upset, renal stones, and rarely thrombocytopenia occur often enough to make use on a long-term basis practical only in the control of severe glaucoma.

Epinephrine. Epinephrine decreases aqueous outflow. It has a high complication rate with continued use. It causes conjunctivitis and blepharitis. It also results, in some patients, in pigment deposits in the conjunctiva and, on rare occasions, in the cornea. These deposits appear as dark, almost black, spots or patches.

Epinephrine is additive in its effects to pilocarpine. It has the advantage of being used only twice a day. It should not be used in patients who are aphakic (without a lens) because there is a high risk of causing cystoid macular edema (see page 281).

Propine. Propine is a synthetic agent that decrease aqueous outflow. Its dose schedules, effects, and complications are similar to those of epinephrine.

Anticholinesterase Inhibitors. These are strong miotics that decrease intraocular pressure. They may be complicated by cataract and in some patients retinal detachment. They also decrease the cholinesterase levels and, in patients who might require certain types of anesthesia, such as halothane, they are contraindicated. The effects of halothane can be prolonged for hours because of suppression of the cholinesterase level. It is *dangerous* to give *general anesthesia* if patients have been on *topical drops with anticholinesterase action.*

Laser Therapy for Primary Open Angle Glaucoma

Lasers are used to place small spot burns in the trabecular meshwork. This treatment is thought to increase outflow. The argon laser is most commonly used, although the yttrium-aluminum-garnet (YAG) laser is also being evaluated for this therapy. Not all patients respond to laser therapy, and laser therapy may cause only transient decreases in pressure. A pressure rise immediately after therapy requires monitoring and may require therapy.

NARROW ANGLE GLAUCOMA (Figs. 3.13 to 3.15)

Characteristics

Narrow angle glaucoma may be acute or chronic. The acute form presents with high intraocular pressure, pain, halos around lights, and blurred vision. The chronic form may not be as painful and is characterized by intermittent increases in ocular pressure. Acute narrow angle glaucoma usually exhibits redness and hyperemia of the conjunctiva. Photophobia (light sensitivity) and tearing may be present. *Glaukomflecken,* characteristic small anterior subcapsular lens opacities, may develop.

Mechanism

In angle closure glaucoma, the outflow of aqueous is prevented because the iris is against the outflow passage of the trabecular meshwork (Fig. 3.16).

Establishing Diagnosis

The diagnosis of closed angle or narrow angle glaucoma is made by gonioscopy. Gonioscopy of the chamber angle under normal conditions will show all of the structures of the angle (Fig. 3.8). These include Schwalbe's line, the scleral spur, the trabecular meshwork, the ciliary body band, and the iris root. When the angle is closed, these structures are not visible. Rating of the angle is done from 0 to 4. Zero is a closed angle with increased intraocular pressure. The grades from 1 to 4 vary in their prediction of possible angle closure. A grade 4 angle is wide open, and there is no possibility of angle closure. A gross test for narrow angle is shining a light from the side into the eye, causing characteristic shadow in the anterior chamber (Figs. 3.14 and 3.15).

Provocative Testing

Provocative tests are used to help determine the presence of narrow angle glaucoma. By changing the position of the pupil and moving the iris so that the peripheral iris comes closer to the trabeculum, changes in intraocular pressure may be seen, which can determine the diagnosis.

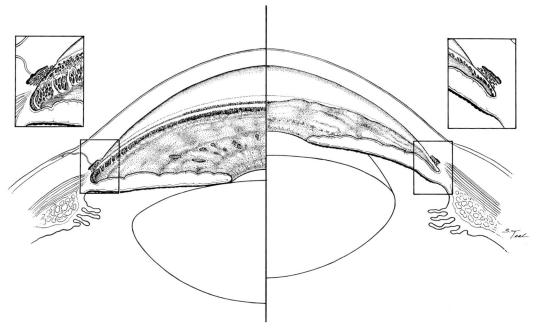

Figure 3.13. Narrow angle glaucoma occurs when the chamber angle is shallow and the angle between the iris and cornea is narrow, causing blockage of the trabecular meshwork, decreased aqueous outflow, and increased intraocular pressure (glaucoma). Illustrated is a normal chamber angle on the *left* with a narrow chamber angle on the *right*. Notice that the iris is forward and the distance between the posterior portion of the cornea and the lens is decreased. For grading of the chamber angle, see Figure 3.16.

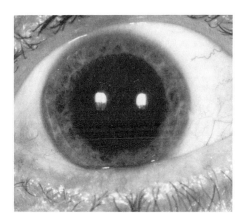

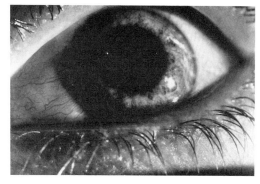

Figure 3.14. This is a normal anterior chamber depth. If we measure the depth from the posterior portion of the cornea to the anterior portion of the lens in terms of corneal thicknesses, the normal anterior chamber is five corneal thicknesses or more in depth. Compare to the shallow anterior chamber (Fig. 3.15).

Figure 3.15. Narrow angle glaucoma, diagnosis by light reflex. In narrow angle glaucoma, the chamber angle between the iris and the cornea is narrowed. In most instances, the entire anterior chamber distance between the iris and the cornea is decreased. When shining a light from the side, as illustrated, there is a distinct shadow on the opposite side due to this bowing forward of the iris. Compare to a normal chamber angle (Fig. 3.14).

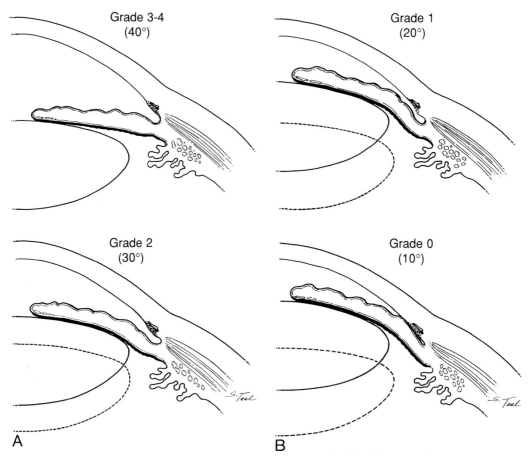

Figure 3.16.   Grading of chamber angles. In narrow angle glaucoma, the chamber angle becomes narrow with eventual blockage of the trabecular meshwork. The angle can be graded from 0 to 4, or it can be graded by degrees according to the angle formed by the cornea and the iris. Both are indicated.

Dark Room

By placing a patient in a dark room for 45 minutes, usually in the prone position, the pupil is dilated and the lens iris diaphragm is therefore brought forward. An increase of 8 mm Hg over the baseline intraocular pressure is considered abnormal.

Pharmacologic Testing

Weak dilating medicines, such as parasympatholytic agents, can be used to dilate the pupil. This pupillary dilation creates increase in pressure in an eye with narrow angle glaucoma in the same way that a dark room dilation test does. Increases of more than 8 mm Hg are considered abnormal.

Important Warning

Patients with narrow angle glaucoma should not have the pupil dilated indiscriminantly. An acute glaucoma attack may result.

Treatment of Angle Closure Glaucoma

Acute episodes of angle closure glaucoma are treated with topical and systemic agents. Oral hypertonic agents, such as glycerine, are used to lower the pressure. After control of the initial pressure increase or if medical therapy does not decrease the pressure, either laser or surgical therapy is required. The goal of this therapy is to produce a hole in the iris so that aqueous can easily get from the posterior chamber to the anterior chamber. This allows equilibrium of the fluids in front of and behind the iris to be reestablished and allows the iris to fall away from the trabecular meshwork, releasing the block. Free drainage of aqueous from the anterior chamber is then restored. The procedure is called iridotomy. This iridotomy hole may be created by a laser (laser iridotomy) or by operation (surgical iridectomy).

PLATEAU IRIS

Plateau iris is a variant of angle closure. The peripheral iris blocks the trabecular meshwork as the iris thickens during pupillary dilation (Fig. 3.17). This is an uncommon mechanism for angle closure glaucoma.

A diagnostician should be aware of this condition because it may cause angle closure without the shallowing of the anterior chamber that is seen with the more conventional type of angle closure. Shallowing of the anterior chamber is caused by pupillary block and a collection of fluid behind the iris that pushes the iris forward. In plateau iris, the pupillary block mechanism is not thought to be present, and it is the special configuration of the iris in the periphery that causes the glaucoma. If a peripheral iridectomy (or a laser iridotomy) relieves the glaucoma, then pupillary block is the mechanism causing angle closure, not plateau iris. Plateau iris can be treated with a mild miotic to keep the pupil small and the peripheral iris configuration normal.

SECONDARY GLAUCOMAS

Secondary glaucomas are caused by other identifiable processes occurring in the eye. There are many secondary glaucomas.

Traumatic Glaucoma

Traumatic glaucoma is caused by a blunt injury to the eye. This blunt injury causes a cleavage at the base of the iris (called angle recession) and destruction of the normal outflow channels of the eye (Fig. 3.18). This glaucoma is usually unilateral. A history of severe

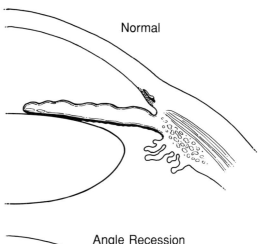

Normal

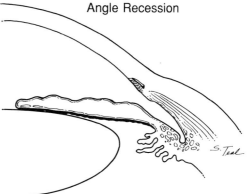

Angle Recession

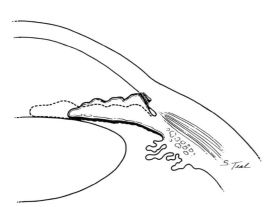

Figure 3.17. In plateau iris syndrome, the peripheral iris has an abnormal plateau configuration. With dilation, aqueous outflow is blocked by iris obstruction of the trabeculum meshwork. Illustrated is a plateau iris with changes on dilation.

Figure 3.18. Angle recession is a tear of the angle due to the pressure effects of blunt trauma. Illustrated is a deep anterior chamber angle on the *bottom* with a normal anterior chamber angle on the *top* for comparison.

or moderately severe injury to the eye usually establishes the diagnosis. The final diagnosis is confirmed by examining the chamber angle by gonioscopy (see page 44) for angle recession.

Neovascular Glaucoma

Definition

Neovascular glaucoma results from new vessel formation in the eye. New vessels grow into the angle and form a fibrovascular membrane that causes the iris to be drawn up over the angle structures, preventing aqueous outflow and resulting in glaucoma. When vessels are in the angle, there is almost always new vessel formation on the iris (Fig. 3.19). New vessels may be diagnosed early at the edge the pupillary margin and in the angle.

Associated Disease Conditions

There are two conditions commonly associated with neovascular glaucoma: (*a*) diabetes and (*b*) central retinal vein occlusion and some branch retinal vein occlusions.

Ghost Cell Glaucoma

Definition

A ghost cell is a red blood cell that has undergone degenerative changes in the vitreous cavity. The normally pliable, biconcave, red cell changes to a more rigid, khaki-colored, spherical cell. When blood enters the vitreous, this change begins within days and is usually completed within a few weeks.

Mechanism

There are two prerequisites for ghost cell glaucoma: (*a*) vitreous hemorrhage and (*b*) breaks in the hyaloid face of the vitreous to permit ghost cells to escape from the vitreous and float into the anterior chamber. The intraocular pressure increases when ghost cells go into the chamber angle and directly block aqueous flow through the trabecular meshwork.

Diagnosis of Ghost Cell Glaucoma

1. Glaucoma Associated with Hemorrhage. There is increased intraocular pres-

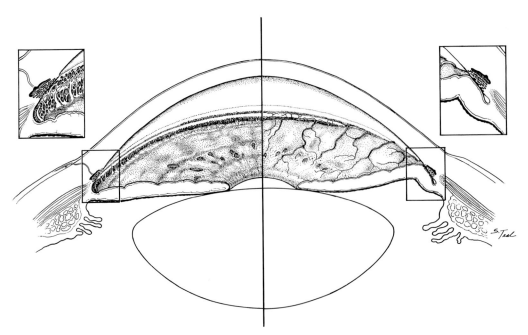

Figure 3.19. Neovascular glaucoma is glaucoma caused by vessels in the chamber angle. It is often associated with diabetes or other conditions that cause retinal ischemia, such as central retinal vein occlusion. Illustrated on the *right* are vessels in the angles, which can be seen only by gonioscopy. *Left*, normal.

sure, usually after trauma, with the vitreous hemorrhage.

2. Cornea and Anterior Chamber. Corneal color may change, with khaki-colored cells collected on the endothelium. These cells float in the aqueous, and many of them layer inferiorly in the anterior chamber (pseudohypopyon).

3. Chamber Angle. Gonioscopy shows an open angle that is covered by the khaki-colored cells, causing a tannish discoloration of the trabecular meshwork. Normal landmarks seen with gonioscopy are obscured.

4. Vitreous. Examination of the vitreous will reveal khaki-colored ghost cells and red blood cells in various stages of transformation.

Congenital Glaucomas

Glaucomas present at birth or immediately postnatal are known as congenital glaucomas. They are discussed in Chapter 14, Special Considerations in Children. They are bilateral and may present with cloudy corneas and tearing.

Drug-induced Glaucoma

Certain drugs cause increases in intraocular pressure:

- Anticholinergics;
- Amphetamines;
- Corticosteroids;
- Hexamethonium;
- Reserpine;
- Tricyclic antidepressants.

Glaucoma Associated with Inflammation (Inflammatory Glaucoma)

1. Iritis

Any inflammation of the anterior segment can cause elevated intraocular pressure. For example, herpes zoster iritis and herpes simplex keratouveitis may frequently be associated with an increase in the intraocular pressure. Later complications from prolonged or severe uveitis, such as scar adhesions in the angle (peripheral anterior synechiae) (Fig. 3.20) or scar adhesions at the pupillary border

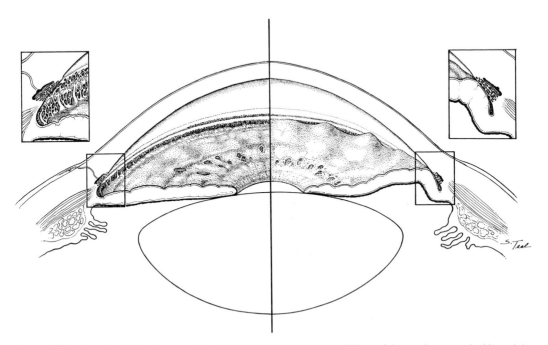

Figure 3.20. Peripheral anterior synechiae are scars that form in the periphery of the eye between the iris and the cornea. If extensive, they may obstruct aqueous outflow and result in glaucoma. These synechiae are due to inflammation. *Left,* normal; *right,* synechiae.

between the iris and the lens (posterior synechiae), may cause increase in pressure. Mechanisms of inflammation include blocking of the trabecular meshwork by debris, swelling of the traumatized endothelial cells in the trabecular meshwork, a change in the viscosity of the aqueous humor, closure of the angle by synechiae, and a pupillary block (the iris comes forward and blocks the trabecular meshwork).

2. Glaucomatocyclitic Crisis (Posner-Schlossman Syndrome)

Glaucomatocyclitic crisis is usually unilateral and may cause pressure rises high enough to cause corneal edema. The signs of intraocular inflammation (cell and flare) are less than would be expected by the degree of pressure rise. (See also page 295.)

3. Fuchs' Heterochromic Cyclitis

Heterochromia (difference in color between the irises), cataracts, and low grade iritis make up a Fuchs' heterochromic cyclitis. The iritis is usually in the eye with the lighter color. Glaucoma occurs in only 5% of these cases. Glaucoma occurs more often in patients with bilateral iritis.

Because iritis is mild, synechiae do not form. Keratitic precipitates (see Fig. C.6) may be present and may have a star-shaped, fibular appearance. Approximately 15% of the cases are bilateral. The condition is seen infrequently in blacks.

Therapy is difficult because of poor response to drugs. The degree of glaucoma does not correlate well with the amount of inflammation. Although heterochromia is an important diagnostic feature, the diagnosis can be made without heterochromia if other features are present.

4. Interstitial Keratitis Associated with Glaucoma

Interstitial keratitis causes angle closure glaucoma both from synechiae causing pupillary block and from synechiae in the angle, which may be due to chronic corneal-scleral inflammation. The chronic inflammation may be low grade.

Low Tension Glaucoma

Low tension glaucoma is defined as glaucomatous optic nerve head excavation and classic nerve fiber visual field defects in the paracentral or arcuate scotoma area without high intraocular pressures. Often no cause is evident; however, other possibilities should be considered.

Three possibilities are previous glaucoma, steroid glaucoma, and pigmentary glaucoma. Normal glaucoma may have previously been present but is not now present. Previous corticosteroid therapy may have increased the intraocular pressure and produced optic nerve damage that is not progressive because of discontinuance of the steroids. Also, patients with a pressure response to steroids that they are receiving may have masked pressures because of simultaneous use of systemic beta-blockers or digitalis-like compounds, which lower the intraocular pressure and mask a high tension glaucoma situation. Pigmentary glaucoma, which tends to occur intermittently in young patients, can leave residual nerve damage and present as low tension glaucoma.

There are additional nonocular causes of optic neuropathy that may masquerade as low tension glaucoma. Consider these two groups:

I. Neurologic
  A. Congenital colobomas and pits of the optic nerve
  B. Intracranial tumors
  C. Vascular anomalies
  D. Syphilitic optic neuropathy
  E. Opticochiasmatic arachnoiditis
II. Vascular
  A. Vasculopathies that occur with diabetes and periarteritis nodosa
  B. Anterior ischemic optic neuropathy
  C. Arteriolar sclerosis
  D. Internal choroid calcification and stenosis
  E. Major shock

After establishing the diagnosis of low tension glaucoma, there are important parameters to follow:

- Be sure that 24-hour diurnal pressure readings exclude an occult high tension glaucoma.
- Stereoscopic optic disc photography should carefully document the possibilities of progression.
- Sequential visual field examination should be done.

Pigmentary Glaucoma (Pigmentary Dispersion Syndrome and Glaucoma)

Characteristics

This type of glaucoma is not uncommon and usually appears in young men 20 to 40 years old who are nearsighted (myopic). There are wide swings in the intraocular pressure. The angle is open by gonioscopy; however, the angle is heavily pigmented with a characteristic pigment band. The pigment may also be liberated into the anterior chamber and may be floating in the aqueous as visualized with the slitlamp. The pigment collects on the inferior, posterior portion (endo-thelial) of the cornea in a triangular shape (Fig. 3.21). It is called Krukenberg's spindle (see color Fig. C.2).

Transillumination

There is characteristic pigment loss in the midperiphery of the posterior surface of the iris. These depigmented areas appear as linear slit-like defects that may later coalesce, causing general depigmentation. When the slit-like defects are present, transillumination shows a sunflower-like appearance, a diagnostic characteristic. Loss of pigment in this area is attributed to rubbing of the zonules of the lens against the pigment of the posterior portion of the iris as the iris dilates.

Lens-induced Glaucoma

Changes in the lens that can produce glaucoma are:

1. Cataract

Far-advanced cataracts may become swollen and liquified. These can cause the aqueous

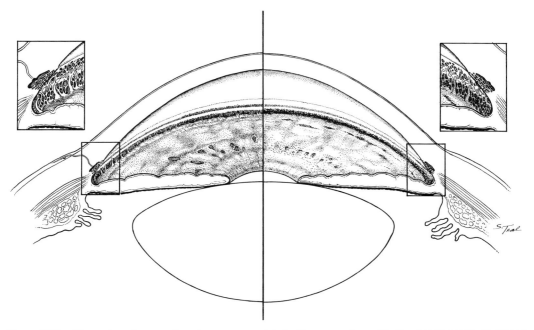

Figure 3.21.   Pigmentary glaucoma is a glaucoma associated with excess pigment in the chamber angle. Illustrated is a normal chamber angle on the *left* with excess pigment in the right angle. Pigmentary glaucoma is seen in young men and is associated also with myopia.

to be blocked from flow into the anterior chamber (pupillary block), and the angle where aqueous flows out may be closed, causing increased pressure.

2. Phacolytic Glaucoma

As the lens becomes cataractous and more mature, denatured lens proteins leak through the intact lens capsule. These proteins attract cells (macrophages) to the anterior chamber. These macrophages, because they are large, clog the trabecular meshwork and cause an increase in intraocular pressure. The pressure may be very high and cause corneal edema.

The diagnosis can be made by performing an anterior chamber tap (removing aqueous and cells from the anterior chamber with a needle and syringe) and observing under the microscope the macrophages loaded with denatured proteins.

3. Microspherophakia

An abnormally small, round lens may hinder aqueous flow from the posterior chamber to the anterior chamber. This pupillary block causes the iris to be pushed up against the trabecular meshwork (angle closure glaucoma), and high pressure ensues.

4. Ectopia Lentis

Dislocation of the lens (ectopia lentis) from its normal position behind the pupil may be associated with glaucoma (see page 286). Common causes of dislocated lenses are trauma, Marfan's syndrome, and hemocystinuria.

Exfoliation Glaucoma

Other Names

Pseudoexfoliation of the lens capsule; glaucoma capsular

Clinical Signs

The condition is characterized by the deposition of a fluffy, grayish white material throughout the anterior structures of the eye. Abnormal iris vessels may be present.

Lens Changes

Characteristically, there is a deposition of this fluffy material on the anterior lens surface. This gives a grayish appearance to the surface of the lens in the pupillary area. When the pupil is dilated, there is a clear zone where the pupil has rubbed the material from the lens. The periphery is again similar to the central lens disc-like deposition. Fluffy, dandruff-like material is found also at the edge of the pupillary margins, on the iris, on the zonules, and in the chamber angle (Fig. 3.22).

Transillumination

Transillumination of the iris will show a loss of pigment from the posterior portion of the iris in the area immediately adjacent to the pupil.

Pigment Deposition—Sampaolesi's Line

There is frequently heavy pigment deposition in the chamber angle and in a line above (anterior to) Schwalbe's line. This is called Sampaolesi's line.

Glaucoma and Exfoliation

Glaucoma may or may not be associated with the exfoliation syndrome (Fig. 3.23). If glaucoma is present, it is treated as an open angle glaucoma. Medical treatment with miotics, beta-blockers, or epinephrine compound is frequently not as effective as in regular open angle glaucoma. Patients may need laser trabeculoplasty or filtering procedures.

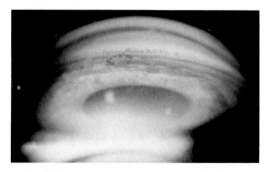

Figure 3.22. Chamber angle pseudoexfoliation. Pseudoexfoliation is a dandruff-like material in the eye and is associated with glaucoma. This is a gonioscopic (page 44) view of the chamber angle showing fluffy pseudoexfoliation material. (Credit: George Waring, M.D.)

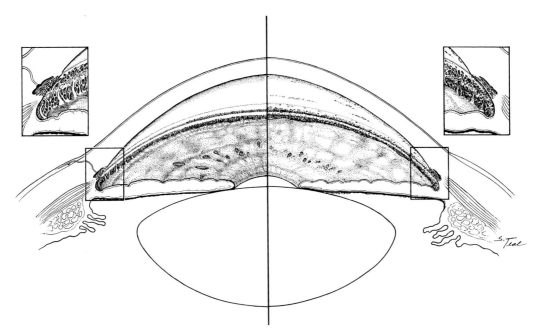

Figure 3.23.   Exfoliation is the presence of a fluffy, dandruff-like material in the anterior chamber. This material collects in and around the trabeculum and results in glaucoma. Typical lens changes of exfoliation are illustrated in color Fig. C.3. *Left,* normal; *right,* exfoliation.

Removal of the lens has no effect on the prognosis or development of glaucoma.

Characteristics of Exfoliation

A fairly common condition, exfoliation is found in elderly people, usually over the age of 65. There is a high association with primary open angle glaucoma. The source of the fluffy material is unknown. The condition often occurs in one eye only (monocular).

4

Retina

INTRODUCTION

In this chapter, a number of essential diseases of the retina and macula are described. Conditions that can be diagnosed as active inflammation of the retina or as postinflammation atrophic lesions are also included. For the most part, diseases that are diagnostically important as active inflammation and involve more than the retina are covered in Chapter 9, Ocular Inflammation. Interesting concepts, even if encountered rarely, are included if they have experimental or therapeutic implications.

ANATOMY

The retina is a transparent cellular layer that lines the interior eye posteriorly. With the ophthalmoscope, the yellow-red color observed—and frequently called the retina—is a result of the retinal pigment epithelium and the blood in the choroid. Anatomical landmarks help orient the observer viewing with the ophthalmoscope (Fig. 4.1).

The macula is located between the superior and inferior temporal blood vessels in the ret-ina. In young patients, the macula gives a bright and shiny reflex. It can easily be seen if you ask the patient to look at the light of your direct ophthalmoscope. The light of the ophthalmoscope is reflected as a pinpoint of light from the central depression of the fovea—the foveola.

HISTOLOGY

Macula

In evaluating the retina with the ophthalmoscope, the macula appears darker than the surrounding retina.[a] The center of the macula lies 3.5 mm lateral and 1 mm inferior to the temporal edge of the optic disc. The macula itself is 5.5 mm across, and it has a central area called the fovea, which is a pit 1.9 mm in diameter. The floor of the fovea is called the

---

[a]This increase in coloration is due to two factors: (a) increase in yellow xanthophyll pigment in the neuroretina in the region and (b) smaller size of the underlying retinal pigment epithelial cells, which are therefore more densely packed with more concentrated pigment.

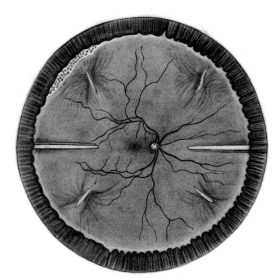

Figure 4.1. Anatomy of the full retina. This is a representation of the full retina of the right eye. By direct ophthalmoscopy or photography, only the posterior portion of this can be seen. Entire visualization requires specialized techniques with the indirect ophthalmoscope and scleral indentation. For orientation, the disc is at the center of the drawing with the retinal vessels, the arterioles and the veins, coursing out. The arcades are seen to course temporally (to the *left* of the drawing). There is a central macular region temporal to the disc. In the four quadrants are illustrated the four vortex veins, easily seen with direct ophthalmoscopy. Horizontally, the posterior ciliary arteries are illustrated. In the periphery are the scalloped borders, the ora serrata. At the *superior left portion* near the scalloped margin of the ora serrata, peripheral cystoid degeneration is noted.

foveola. The foveola has no rods, and the cones are found here in greatest density (15,000 per mm^2 in contrast to 4,000 to 5,000 per mm^2 in the outer portions of the fovea).

In the fovea, the neuroretina is about 90 μm thick compared to 350 μm in the surrounding fovea. The fovea is the only portion of the inner retina supplied by the choroidal circulation. Although the photoreceptor cells, the rods and cones, are supplied by the choroidal circulation, the inner portions of the retina are supplied by the central retinal artery except in the fovea.

The fovea is unique because the neurons of the inner retina together with the ganglion cells are displaced radially and outward (Fig. 4.2A). This allows light to fall unhindered on the foveal-concentrated cones. Interconnecting fibers of the cones become elongated to allow central thinning of the fovea. Those elongated fibers are known as the fiber layer of Henle.

Full-Thickness Retina

The full-thickness retina consists of ten layers (Fig. 4.3). Those layers from outer to inner are:

- Retinal pigment epithelium;
- Rods and cones;
- External (outer) limiting membrane;
- Receptor (outer) nuclear layer;
- Outer plexiform (molecular) layer;
- Inner nuclear layer;
- Inner plexiform (molecular) layer;
- Ganglion cell layer;
- Nerve fiber layer;
- Inner limiting membrane.

Cellular Anatomy

In general, the photoreceptors of the retina detect light. The retinal pigment epithelial cells provide metabolic support for the photoreceptors. The inner retinal structures are supported by Müller cells.

The photoreceptor cells are the rods and cones. In the young adult retina, there are 120 million rods and 6 million cones. The rods and cones, although they have distinctly different functions, show the same basic structural organization.

The photoreceptor cell transmits light through visual pigment absorption of photons in the outer segments. The outer segment of the photoreceptor cell is a light-sensitive portion. The cell has a constricted portion next to the outer segment, which is called the cilium and contains microtubules. The inner segment of the cell contains mitochondria, which provide energy for the processing in the outer segment. Additional anatomical features are an outer connecting fiber, an inner connecting fiber, a nucleus, and a synaptic region.

The two limiting membranes that have been described histologically are actually components of the Müller cells. The Müller cell is a retinal glial cell with processes that extend across the retinal layers between the external and internal limiting membranes. The nuclei of Müller cells are found in the inner nuclear layer.

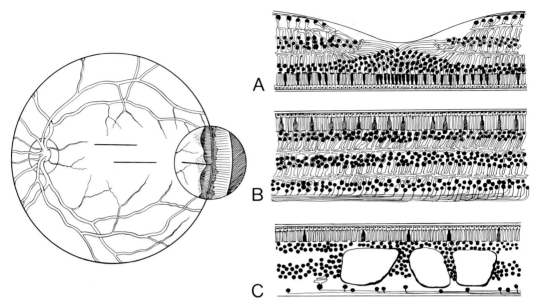

Figure 4.2. Retinal histology in fovea, macula, and periphery. In the general drawing of the retina showing the disc, the vascular arcades, the macula, and a magnified insert of the retinal periphery, there are three lines. These lines correspond to the cross-sections of the central fovea (*lower central line* and *A*), the macular region outside the fovea (*upper central line* and *B*), and the retinal periphery (*peripheral line* and *C*).

A, This represents the central fovea. In this area, the elements of the inner retina are displaced outward, causing retinal thinning over a concentrated area of pure cones. This is the area of central visual acuity. Elongated fibers necessitated by this radial displacement are called the fibers of Henle.

B, Full-thickness retina, illustrated in the macular region just outside the fovea, shows the major aspects of the retina including photoreceptors and layers formed by the horizontal cells, amacrine cells, bipolar cells, and Müller cells.

C, Peripheral retina is thinner than central retina. The ganglion cell layer becomes sparsely populated. Near the ora serrata, the peripheral retina may show cystic spaces, especially in the elderly. The inner layers are also lost, and the photoreceptors in the periphery become shorter and fewer. Some portions of the retina are lost where fusion of the unpigmented layer of the pars plana runs forward to the ciliary processes.

The inner retina contains the inner nuclear layer, cell bodies of the bipolar cells, horizontal cells, amacrine cells, and Müller cells (Fig. 4.4). The horizontal cells connect groups of photoreceptor cells. This connection allows variations of the group output signal. In the inner plexiform layer, the bipolar cells commonly synapse with the amacrine cells, which in turn modify the signal before passing it to the ganglion cells.

Müller cells, because they are specialized glial cells that form a scaffolding of the retina, expand in the inner retina as they approach the vitreous. With this expansion, they form a large end known as the footplate. These footplates can be seen clinically in the posterior pole as tiny reflecting dots. The term Gunn's dots (see page 297) has been given to these spots.

The ganglion cell layer, along with the nerve fiber layer, forms the innermost layer of the retina. The neuronal signal being passed to the ganglion cell layer has received considerable coding. Ganglion cell layers will have, because of this intergraded coding, a receptive field. The average ganglion cell services approximately 130 photoreceptors. In the macular region, however, the ganglion cell probably controls receptor fields with considerably fewer photoreceptors.

The ganglion cells that are receptive to a field have been determined to have a number of varied but specific functions. Some ganglion cells are turned on and off by bright light; others respond to patterns such as white on black or black on white. Some ganglion cells discharge to moving edges, while others respond only if a sustained discharge of light is projected onto the photoreceptors. Numerous other complex responses have been re-

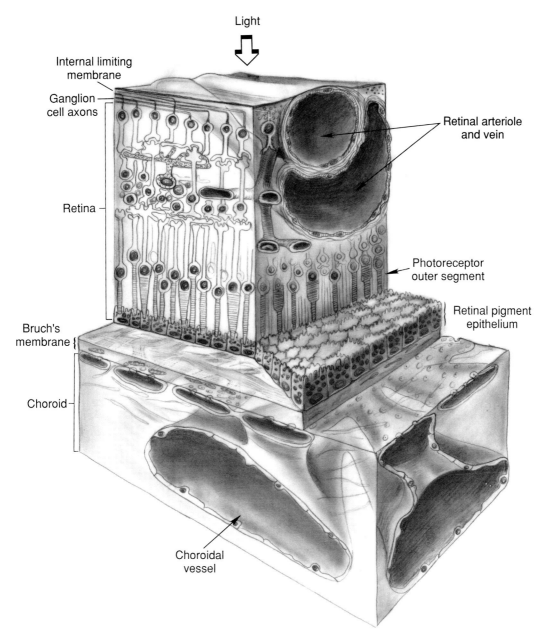

Light

Internal limiting
membrane

Ganglion
cell axons

Retinal arteriole
and vein

Retina

Photoreceptor
outer segment

Retinal pigment
epithelium

Bruch's
membrane

Choroid

Choroidal
vessel

Figure 4.3. Retina—anatomy and histology. Layered drawing represents the retina and adjacent structures both anatomically and diagrammatically. Above the retina would be the vitreous. Below would be the sclera. Neither are drawn. The bottom layer is the choriocapillaris. The layer above the choriocapillaris is Bruch's membrane. Above Bruch's membrane is the retinal pigment epithelium, which serves a barrier function to the choriocapillaris and selectively allows metabolic products to reach the photoreceptor cells. The outer portions of the photoreceptor cells (rods and cones) abut the retinal pigment epithelium. The retinal pigment epithelium actually phagocytoses parts of the photoreceptor cells shed as they are replaced. The inner retina consists of Müller cells, amacrine cells, bipolar cells, and horizontal cells. These connect to the ganglion cells, the most inner layer of cells, which contribute to the nerve fiber layer. The retinal arterioles and veins, just under the internal limiting membrane, course through the inner retina. Further differentiation of inner retinal cell function can be found in Fig. 4.4 on page 63.

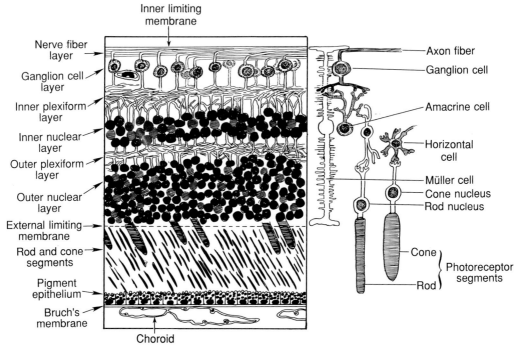

Figure 4.4. This diagrammatic representation of the retina compares histologic orientation *(left)* to actual cell function and position *(right)*. The vitreous (not drawn) would be at the top and the sclera below.

lated to specific ganglion cell discharges, suggesting the complexity of the transmission of a visual image.

The photoreceptor cells replace their visual components. New discs are formed in the cilium at a rate of about one to five an hour. As new discs are formed in the cilium, older ones are displaced toward the pigment epithelium and are shed from the tips of the outer segment in packets of about 30. The rod outer segment, for example, is entirely replaced every 8 to 14 days. The cone replacement is much slower than that of the rod, taking 9 months to a year to replace an outer segment fully. The rod discs are shed in light primarily after a prolonged darkness whereas the cone discs are shed at night.

The retinal pigment epithelium performs five major functions. It absorbs stray light and protects the photoreceptor cells, provides active transport of metabolites to the photoreceptor cells, establishes a blood-retina barrier, regenerates visual pigments, and phagocytoses shed disc from the outer segment of the photoreceptor cells.

The blood-retina barrier, maintained by the retinal pigment epithelium, is important in the conceptualization and diagnostic effectiveness of fluorescein angiography, as well as in understanding a number of disease processes. Free diffusion from the choriocapillaris into the neuroretinal area is prevented by the retinal pigment epithelium. Tight junctions, or zonular occludens, exist between the retinal pigment epithelial cells, forming a tightly binding cell membrane and providing the effective blood-retina barrier, which selectively transports only required substances to the photoreceptor cells.

BLOOD SUPPLY OF THE RETINA

The retina has two circulations: the central retinal artery and the choroidal circulation—the choriocapillaris. The central retinal artery is a true artery and is subject to the changes of antherosclerosis. The central retinal artery divides at the level of the optic disc into arterioles with a media of smooth muscles seven to eight cells thick. The arterioles are subjected to arteriolar sclerosis (hypertensive changes) but are not involved in the atherosclerotic process. These are end arterioles. The arteriole branches run in the nerve fiber layer below the internal membrane (Fig. 4.3).

The central retinal artery and the arteriolar system support the inner retina with the exception of the photoreceptor cells and the central fovea. Photoreceptor cells and the central fovea are nourished by the choriocapillaris, which provides metabolites to these areas through the retinal pigment epithelial barrier.

The choriocapillaris supplies photoreceptor cells and the area of the capillary free zone (400 μm across the foveola). The foveola, which has no blood vessels, is therefore saved from vessels obscuring visual acuity. Because it is a capillary-free zone, it receives its blood supply from the choroid.

Cilioretinal arteries from the ciliary circulation are seen in about 20% of patients and account for the blood supply to the macular region in these patients. These are important only with occlusion of the central retinal artery, when the cilioretinal artery may provide continued nourishment to the macular region and protect central acuity.

DIABETIC RETINOPATHY

Diabetic retinopathy is a general term given to the collective retinovascular complications

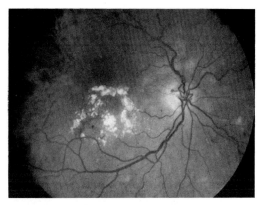

Figure 4.6. Background diabetic retinopathy with microaneurysms and perimacular exudates, frequently referred to as circinate retinopathy. Approximately 20% of diabetics will have diabetic retinopathy. (Credit: Paul Sternberg, M.D.) (See also color Fig. C.10.)

that occur with diabetes mellitus. There are three general classifications:

- *Background diabetic retinopathy* characterized by microaneurysms, macular edema, lipid exudates, and intraretinal hemorrhages (Figs. 4.5 and 4.6);
- *Preproliferative diabetic retinopathy* characterized by evidence of retinal hypoxia, that is, nerve fiber layer infarctions and intraretinal microvascular abnormality (IRMA);
- *Proliferative diabetic retinopathy* characterized by new blood vessel growth on the retinal surface (Fig. 4.7).

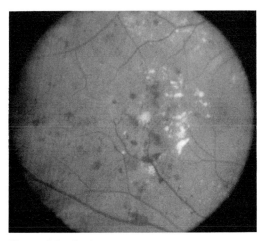

Figure 4.5. Background diabetic retinopathy. Small dark dots (representing microaneurysms) as well as white exudates are seen in the perimacular region. These findings are easily detected with the direct ophthalmoscope. (See also color Fig. C.9.)

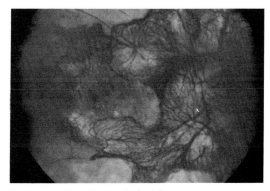

Figure 4.7. Proliferative diabetic retinopathy is a stage of diabetic retinopathy in which new vessel response to ischemia occurs. It is the most destructive type of diabetic retinopathy. Approximately 5% of diabetics will have proliferative changes. (Credit: Paul Sternberg, M.D.) (See also color Fig. C.11.)

Cause

The cause of diabetic retinopathy is unknown. However, there are a number of observed facts that have been variously correlated with the presence of diabetic retinopathy and provide a basis for understanding the complexities of the process.

Platelet Abnormalities

In diabetics, platelets adhere to various substances (e.g., damaged endothelial cells, collagen), and this has been attributed to an elevation in the levels of factor VIII (von Willebrand) in diabetics. Platelets are also found to have increased adherence to each other. It is thought that platelet adhesion and aggregation abnormalities may contribute to the focal capillary occlusions, which result in ischemia in diabetic retinopathy, the major feature of the subsequent severe disease changes.

Blood Vessel Abnormalities

An early change in the capillaries of diabetics is thickening of the basement membrane and loss of vessel-supporting elements, the pericytes. The ratio of pericyte to endothelial cell on the vessel wall in normal subjects is usually about 1/1. In diabetics, this ratio shifts significantly because of pericyte dropout.

Red Blood Cell Abnormalities

In diabetics, red blood cells have a tendency, like platelets, to aggregate. In addition, the red cell, which is normally pliable and capable of significant deformation while squeezing through very small openings, loses its pliability. This lack of deformability in diabetic red blood cells is thought to contribute to the inability of the cells to pass through capillaries.

Vasoproliferative Factors

The ischemic and hypoxic retina is thought to produce or release a vasoproliferative factor. This factor induces neovascularization.

Growth Hormone

The presence of growth hormone seems to play a supportive role in the development of diabetic retinopathy. Reversal of diabetic retinopathy has been seen in a woman with postpartum hemorrhagic necrosis of the pituitary gland (Sheehan's syndrome). Also, dwarfs with diabetes, who lack growth hormone, have shown no evidence of retinopathy.

Ophthalmoscopic Characteristics

Microaneurysms

Histologically, the first changes seen are increased thickness of the capillary basement membrane and pericyte dropout, but the first change detectable by the ophthalmoscope is the formation of a microaneurysm. Microaneurysms are dilations in the capillary wall in areas where pericytes are absent. An early microaneurysm is thin-walled but, later, endothelial cells proliferate and lay a basement membrane material around the microaneurysm. Fibrin and erythrocytes may occlude the lumen of the microaneurysm. In early cases, the microaneurysms are seen on the venous side of the capillaries but later they are seen on the arteriolar side.

Hemorrhages

When a capillary wall is weakened sufficiently, it ruptures. This causes an intraretinal hemorrhage. Two forms of hemorrhage may be seen with the ophthalmoscope: (a) a dot or blot hemorrhage, which is round or oval and occurs in the inner nuclear layer or outer plexiform layer, (b) flame- or splinter-shaped hemorrhages, which are superficial and occur in the nerve fiber bundles.

Venous Abnormalities

The veins can become dilated and may show irregular thickness, sometimes called "beading." Also, venous loops are seen, horseshoe-shaped deviations of the normal venous pathway.

Large Hemorrhage

Large, superficial hemorrhages may separate the internal limiting membrane from the retina. These hemorrhages may remain confined for weeks or months in this position or may break through into the vitreous (vitreous hemorrhage).

Macular Edema

When the blood-retina barrier is damaged by diabetes, fluid leaks into the retina and accumulates, especially in the macular outer plexiform layer. This retinal edema that occurs in the macula is seen as a thickening of the retina. It is best observed with the aid of binocular vision using a Hruby lens or a fundus contact lens. Macular edema causes a decrease in visual acuity, changes in color discrimination, and slow dark adaptation.

Lipid Accumulations

When leakage of fluid becomes severe, lipid accumulates in the retina. It is most often seen in the outer plexiform layer. These yellow deposits, also called hard exudates, may be scattered throughout the macula and may also accumulate in a ring around a group of leaking microaneurysms (circinate retinopathy).

Choriocapillaris Changes

The choriocapillaris may also be affected. Thickening of the basement membrane of the choriocapillaris occurs, and the lumina of the choriocapillaries may be occluded.

Preproliferative and Proliferative Retinopathy

Preproliferative diabetic retinopathy shows evidence of retinal hypoxia. Nerve fiber layer infarction and intraretinal microvascular abnormality (IRMA) are seen. Proliferative retinopathy is the onset of new vessel growth on the retinal surface.

Retinal hypoxia precedes new vessel formation. The most important sign is nerve fiber layer infarction caused by occlusion of the precapillary arterioles. Infarctions are seen with the ophthalmoscope as white, fluffy, superficial lesions. These have been termed cotton-wool spots or "soft exudates" (although they are not exudates). Additional signs of hypoxia are venous beading and IRMA. IRMA (dilated, irregular retinal vessels) may be difficult to differentiate from new vessel formation. (With fluorescein angiography (see Fig. C.16), however, the new vessels leak fluorescein, and the vessels of IRMA do not).

In proliferative retinopathy, vessels usually arise from the veins and begin as a collection of naked vessels. The new vessels grow on the retina or on the optic nerve head. Neovascularization on and around the nerve head is designated NVD (neovascularization of the disc). Neovascularization farther than one disc diameter away from the optic nerve is called NVE (neovascularization elsewhere).

As new vessels grow, they take the path of least resistance or grow along preformed connective tissue and move toward zones of retinal ischemia. In later stages, regression of the vascular system is associated with contracture of connective tissue components. This contraction results in both dense bands and thickening along the posterior vitreous face, which may result in retinal detachment and retinal tears. With progression of retinopathy, proliferative fibrovascular tissue appears. Fibrotic proliferation can lead to traction on the retina and may result in retinal detachment or tears.

New vessels are pulled forward into the vitreous cavity by contraction of the vitreous. Contraction of the vitreous is a significant cause of hemorrhage within the vitreous, breaks in the retina, and retinal detachment. When hemorrhage breaks into the vitreous, it may take months or years to clear.

Risk Factors

Genetics

HLA-B7 antigen is found in fewer patients with proliferative retinopathy than in controls. Patients with this antigen are 4 times less likely to develop proliferative retinopathy than those who do not inherit it. Also, diabetic patients with HLA-B15 are more likely to develop proliferative retinopathy.

Time from Onset of Diabetes

Patients who have long-standing diabetes have a greater incidence of diabetic retinopathy. Juvenile diabetics who have had diabetes for 5 years or less show no evidence of diabetic retinopathy. However, if diabetes has been present for 5 to 10 years, more than 25% have diabetic retinopathy. Of patients who have had diabetes for longer than 10 years, 71% will have diabetic retinopathy. After 30 years, 90% will have diabetic retinopathy and one-third of these will have changes of proliferative retinopathy.

Hypertension

The prevalence of exudates in early diabetic retinopathy is increased in patients with hypertension. An increase in hemorrhages is not associated with hypertension, however. Patients with proliferative diabetic retinopathy have systemic hypertension more often than patients with only background retinopathy.

Pregnancy

There is a clinical impression that pregnancy accelerates the changes of diabetic retinopathy.

Racial Factors

Blacks have a 20% higher risk of blindness than whites.

Sex

Woman have a 23% higher risk of blindness than do men.

Hyperglycemia

There are strong suggestions that hyperglycemia causes or at lease predisposes patients to retinopathy. Much of the evidence is experimental. There is a general feeling that lack of metabolic control of the diabetes predisposes to more severe retinopathy; however, there is no conclusive evidence that strict control of blood sugar will prevent diabetic retinopathy.

High Risk Characteristics in Proliferative Diabetic Retinopathy

High risk characteristics that predict a poor outcome in a diabetic retinopathy have been identified. These are based on the severity and location of new vessels and the presence of vitreous or preretinal hemorrhages. These characteristics include:

- Presence of NVD (new vessels disc) equaling or exceeding one-quarter to one-third of the disc area in extent, with or without vitreous or preretinal hemorrhage;
- Presence of either NVD or NVE (new vessels elsewhere) in one-half or more of the disc area and associated with vitreous or preretinal hemorrhages.

The extent of new vessel proliferation, the position of new vessel proliferation, and the association with preretinal or vitreous hemorrhages are important risk factors in deter-

mining the potential outcome of proliferative diabetic retinopathy.

Epidemiologic Importance

Diabetic retinopathy in the United States is one of the leading causes of legal blindness. [The primary cause is aging macular degeneration (page 130), which causes approximately 10% of the new cases of blindness each year.] Because the onset of diabetic retinopathy correlates with the length of time since the diagnosis of systemic diabetes and because improved techniques for diabetic management have prolonged life, diabetic retinopathy has become a significant economic and social factor in care of diabetic patients.

RETINAL DETACHMENT

Definition

Retinal detachment occurs when the neurosensory retina is separated from the retinal pigment epithelium (Fig. 4.8). Rhegmatogenous retinal detachment is associated with a break in the retina. Other causes of detachment are exudation, where fluid collects beneath the neurosensory retina, and traction from fibrovascular elements in conditions such as diabetic retinopathy and trauma.

Key Words

A *break* is any full-thickness retinal defect (Fig. 4.9). A *hole* is a round, atrophic break. A *tear* is a break caused by vitreous retracting.

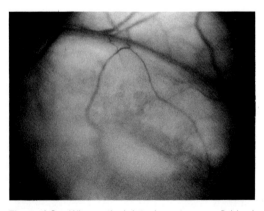

Figure 4.8. When retinal detachment occurs, fluid collects in the space behind the retina. Folds in the retina may occur, as illustrated in this photograph.

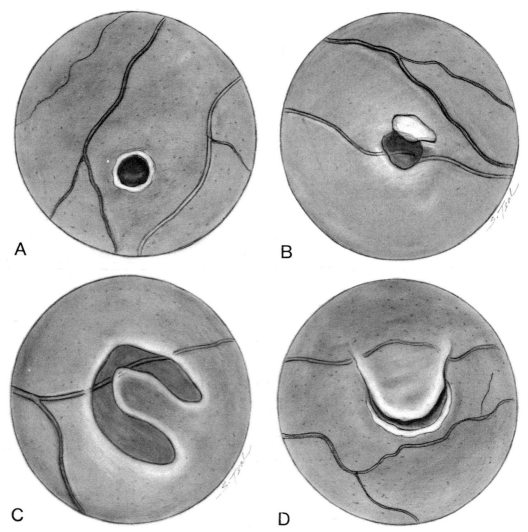

Figure 4.9. A break in the retina is usually in the periphery and is associated with vitreous abnormalities. Four different presentations are illustrated: **A**, round hole; **B**, operculum; **C**, horseshoe; **D**, flap. **A**, An atrophic retinal hole is a common type of retinal break. Atrophic holes may be seen with lattice degeneration (page 76). **B**, An operculated tear is a complete tear with the small, detached piece of retina floating in the vitreous above the hole. **C** and **D**, Illustrated is a type of retinal tear known as a horseshoe tear (**C**) or a retinal flap (**D**).

A *flap,* or horseshoe tear, is a tear in which a strip of retina is pulled by the vitreous. An *operculated tear* is when a piece of retina is torn completely free of the retinal surface and can be seen floating in the vitreous.

Rhegmatogenous Retinal Detachment

Clinical Appearance

In rhegmatogenous retinal detachment (a retinal detachment associated with a break in

the retina), a break can be found in 97% of the cases. In the other 3%, the break is assumed to be present.

Clinical diagnostic features are:

- The detached retina has a wrinkled appearance.
- The detached retina undulates with eye movements.
- Fixed folds in the retina may be present.

- Shifting fluid is almost never present (important in differential diagnosis).
- Small clumps of pigmented cells, frequently called "tobacco dust," may be present on the vitreous or in the anterior segment.
- The intraocular pressure is usually lower in the affected eye.
- About 50% of patients with rhegmatogenous retinal detachment will have flashes of light (photopsia) or floaters (entopsia).

Pathogenesis

Rhegmatogenous retinal detachment results from a complex interaction among the vitreous, the retinal pigment epithelium, and the retina. Numerous factors have been pinpointed to predispose to or cause retinal detachments. These factors are important to the ophthalmologist in determining patients at higher risk as well as in making a diagnosis of rhegmatogenous retinal detachment.

Essential Components

Retinal Pigment Epithelium. This single layer of hexagonal cells attaches to a thin basement membrane, which forms the innermost part of Bruch's membrane. Retinal pigment epithelial (RPE) cells have processes that extend into the spaces between the outer segments of the rods and cones. The RPE cells do not directly contact the photoreceptors, however, because a mucopolysaccharide fills the spaces between the RPE cells and the photoreceptors. This mucopolysaccharide forms a weak bond between the pigment epithelium and the sensory retina. When the bond is broken, as when fluid passes through a full-thickness retinal break or there is traction of the vitreous on the retina, the sensory retina separates from the pigment epithelium, causing retinal detachment.

Sensory Retina. Many features of the sensory retina have been associated with rhegmatogenous retinal detachment. The morphology of the retina, developmental variations in the retina, and degenerations of the peripheral retina all contribute to the retinal changes that result in rhegmatogenous retinal detachment.

The sensory retina is thin and weak in the periphery. It is here that the retina is predisposed to full-thickness retinal breaks. These full-thickness retinal breaks may be trophic holes, tractional tears, or a combination of both.

Developmental variations of the retinal periphery also can be associated with rhegmatogenous retinal detachments. These include enclosed ora bays, meridional folds, meridional complexes, and peripheral retinal excavations.

Degenerations of the peripheral retina may be trophic or tractional in origin. Trophic degenerations are associated with conditions such as typical degenerative retinoschisis (see page 79), reticular degenerative retinoschisis (see page 78), and primary retinal holes.

Lattice degeneration (see page 76) has both trophic and tractional components. Primary tractional degenerations associated with full-thickness tears include cystic retinal tuft, zonular traction retinal tuft, and retinal tears related to exaggerated vitreoretinal detachments.

The Vitreous Body.

Characteristics. The vitreous is a transparent, jell-like substance. Its volume is 4 to 5 cm^3 in the adult. Although the vitreous touches or attaches to a variety of structures within the eye, the firm attachment is the vitreous base, a band that straddles the ora serrata and extends around the circumference of the eye. The anterior portion of the vitreous base is thinner (about 0.25 mm) in the nasal horizontal portion than in the temporal horizontal portion (1.3 mm). The vitreous base itself measures approximately 3.2 mm in the anterior-posterior diameter. Examination by scleral depression shows that it has an undulating posterior border. The vitreous also attaches at the optic disc.

Posterior to the vitreous base, vitreoretinal adhesions are generally weaker. There may be, however, focal exaggerations in the vitreoretinal attachments in specifically identifiable sites: cystic retinal tufts, zonular traction retinal tufts, and certain areas around blood vessels.

Vitreous Degeneration and Detachment. With advancing age, the vitreous degenerates, becoming more liquid. With the

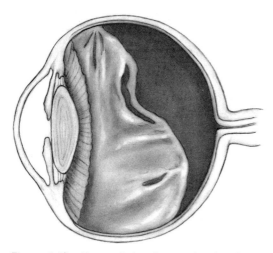

Figure 4.10. The posterior vitreous detaches in almost all persons as they age. The vitreous comes forward, leaving an optically clear space between the posterior part of the vitreous and the retina. Floaters and flashing lights (photopsia) may be associated with posterior vitreous detachment.

aid of a slitlamp, liquid cavities can be seen in the central and superior vitreous.

Degeneration may cause detachment of the vitreous from the optic disc. This is called posterior vitreous detachment (Fig. 4.10) and starts posteriorly and extends anteriorly, separating the vitreous from the optic disc, the retina, and the area posterior to the vitreous base.

The vitreous base is not involved in posterior vitreous detachment. However, the movement caused by the detached vitreous exerts traction on the vitreous base, which may result in retinal detachment.

In an aphakic eye, an eye without a lens, the vitreous movement may be increased because of lack of support by the lens. This excess movement of the vitreous and the resultant tugging on the retina is thought to be the cause of the increased incidence of retinal detachment in aphakic eyes.

In essence, the pathogenesis of rhegmatogenous retinal detachment is related to three major features: *(a)* the weakness of the bond between the retinal pigment epithelium and the sensory retina, *(b)* characteristic changes in retinal anatomy due to developmental variations or degeneration producing full-thickness retinal holes or a predilection to full-thickness retinal tears, and *(c)* vitreoretinal attachments and vitreous degeneration producing traction and secondary retinal tears.

Additional Risk Factors

Patients with myopia and Marfan's syndrome, which influence the size and shape of the eye, have an increased incidence of rhegmatogenous retinal detachment. Coloboma, vitreoretinal dysplasias, retinal vascular disorders such as sickle cell disease, metabolic diseases such as diabetic retinopathy, inflammations, neoplasms, degenerations, and injuries all may predispose to rhegmatogenous retinal detachment.

Incidence

The incidence of rhegmatogenous retinal detachment is approximately 0.01% per year. Some groups are more vulnerable than others. Aphakic patients (lens removed), for example, have an incidence of 1 to 3%. (About 50% of aphakic detachments occur 1 year after cataract extraction.)

Differential Diagnosis of Rhegmatogenous Retinal Detachment

1. Retinoschisis. Retinoschisis (see page 79) is a split in the retina in the outer plexiform layer. It occurs most often inferotemporally but also superotemporally. The footplates of Müller cells can occasionally be seen as "snowflakes," and the retinal vessels appear sclerotic. The outer layer of the schisis appears pock-marked on scleral depression. The inner layer is oval and smooth. A typical peripheral cystoid degeneration (see page 78) can be found anterior to the schisis cavity in all cases. Retinoschisis is bilateral in 50 to 80% of patients. Seventy per cent of patients with retinoschisis are hyperopic.

Retinoschisis can cause a full-thickness retinal detachment. Three per cent of patients with retinal detachment have retinoschisis. (For more detail, see page 79.)

2. Exudative Retinal Detachment. An exudative detachment results from fluid passing into the subretinal space, detaching the retina. A subretinal ocular condition damages the retinal pigment epithelium, allowing the choroidal fluid to pass across the retinal pigment epithelium into the subretinal space. Two leading causes are tumors and inflammation.

Shifting fluid is a subretinal fluid response to gravity. When the patient is moved from a sitting position to a lying position, the fluid shifts. Exudative detachments also have a smooth surface in contrast to the wrinkled surface of a rhegmatogenous retinal detachment. Fixed folds are usually not seen in exudative detachments.

3. Traction Retinal Detachment. Vitreous membranes can pull the retina and produce detachment. The most common causes are proliferative retinopathies, such as diabetic retinopathy (see page 65), or penetrating injuries. The retina in these detachments is smooth on the surface and without fluid movement, in contrast to the shifting fluid of exudative detachments. The detachment is concave toward the front of the eye, whereas rhegmatogenous retinal detachments are convex.

4. Choroidal Detachment. In this condition, the retina is elevated but not separated from the pigment epithelium. The separation may be caused by serous fluid or hemorrhage. It occurs after operation and in eyes with sustained low intraocular pressure.

Peripheral Lesions Not Associated with Retinal Detachment

These lesions are usually not seen with routine direct or indirect ophthalmoscopy. Scleral depression is needed to reveal these lesions.

Peripheral Retinal Excavation. Small oval depressions align with the meridional folds. Peripheral retinal excavation is seen in 10% of all autopsy eyes. There is a predilection for the superior temporal quadrant. This lesion is caused by loss of inner retinal layers.

Peripheral Chorioretinal Atrophy. See Paving Stone Degeneration (page 78).

Retinal Pigment Epithelial Hyperplasia. The retinal pigment epithelial cells can proliferate when stimulated by chronic, low grade traction. The result is a diffuse retinal pigment epithelial hyperplasia. This is seen as dark black flecks strattling the ora serrata. It is demarcated roughly by the vitreous base,

pars plana, and peripheral retina. Retinal pigment epithelial hyperplasia is also seen in areas of focal traction—lattice degeneration, postinflammation, and trauma.

Retinal Pigment Epithelial (RPE) Hypertrophy. This is an aging change seen at the periphery just posterior to the ora serrata. Histopathologically, large cells have melanin granules that are larger and more spherical than the smaller and lancet-shaped granules seen in hyperplasia and normal RPE cells.

Lesions That May Precede Retinal Detachment

Lattice Degeneration. See page 76.

Vitreoretinal Tufts (Tags). These are small, peripheral elevations of the retina. They are caused by traction of the vitreous or the lens zonules. Pigment epithelial hyperplasia may surround the area. The detachment results from a retinal tear when the vitreous detaches (see Posterior Vitreous Detachment, Fig. 4.10).

Meridional Folds. These are redundant folds in the retina most often seen superonasally. They are associated with dentate processes in the periphery or extend from ora bays. Retinal tears occasionally occur at the posterior limit of the meridional fold.

VASCULAR OCCLUSIONS

Arteriolar Occlusive Disease

Central Retinal Artery Occlusion (CRAO) (Fig. 4.11)

Symptoms. Patients have a sudden onset of severe visual loss in one eye. There is no associated pain.

Cause. CRAO is due to an arteriosclerosis plaque lodging at the level of the lamina cribrosa. Embolization from a distant site may be a contributing factor in some cases.

Ophthalmoscopy Findings. After a few hours, the retina becomes edematous and appears *white* or *opaque*. There is a reddish orange reflex from the intact choroidal vasculature under the intact foveola. The red spot contrasts with the surrounding white retina and is known as a *cherry red spot*.

Course. With time, the retinal artery re-

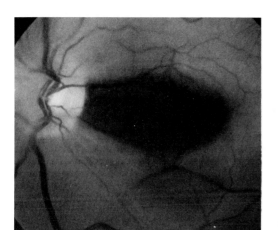

Figure 4.11. Retinal artery occlusion produces retinal edema. The retina becomes white a few hours after total occlusion. In this photograph, the optic disc is seen on the *left*. The dark area in the *center* is actually normal retina supplied by a cilioretinal artery from the choroidal circulation. Around the normal dark area is the characteristic whitish, opaque discoloration of the retina caused by ischemia due to arterial occlusion.

opens and the retinal edema clears. However, a severe effect on visual acuity persists.

Branch Retinal Artery Occlusion (BRAO)

BRAO causes edema and an opaque, white retina due to infarction. This is limited to the area of distribution of the vessel involved. The edema resolves as the vessel recanalizes. A permanent field defect results.

Causes

Occlusion of central and branch retinal arteries is due to embolization and thrombosis of affected vessels. The emboli may be:

- Cholesterol emboli from carotid arteries;
- Calcific emboli from cardiac valves;
- Platelet-fibrin emboli.

Unusual causes are:

- Talc in drug abusers;
- Fat from fractures and trauma (Purtscher's retinopathy, Fig. C.15);
- Septic emboli from endocarditis.

Venous Occlusive Disease
Branch Retinal Vein Occlusion (BRVO)

Cause. Retinal veins share a common adventitia with the arteries and arterioles. This common adventitia binds the artery and vein together so that the arteriole wall presses on the vein, resulting in a turbulent flow, endothelial cell damage, and eventually thrombotic occlusion. Arteriolar diseases predisposing to BRVO include systemic hypertension (about 70%), diabetes (about 10%), and arteriolar sclerosis.

Ophthalmic Findings. Branch vein occlusion will affect the retina in the area supplied by the vein. Ophthalmic findings are:

- Superficial hemorrhages;
- Retinal edema;
- Cotton-wool spots (nerve fiber layer infarcts) (see page 279).

The superotemporal quadrant of the retina is the most commonly affected (63%). Nasal occlusions are rare.

Prognosis. Approximately 50 to 60% of patients will maintain 20/40 or better visual acuity. It takes approximately 6 months to have maximal spontaneous resolution. The outcome relates to the extent of capillary damage and to the degree of retinal ischemia. Macular edema, when present, may reduce vision.

Extensive retinal ischemia may result in *neovascularization* from the retina or from the optic nerve. This occurs in 22% of temporal branch vein occlusions. Visual loss from vitreous hemorrhage secondary to neovascularization can also decrease vision. Permanent visual loss from BRVO is due to cystoid macular edema, lipid exudates with prolonged edema, subretinal fibrosis, or epiretinal membrane formation.

Central Retinal Vein Occlusion (CRVO) (Fig. 4.12)

Occlusion of the central retinal vein is divided into two types: *(a)* partial occlusion, a milder form, and *(b)* a complete or ischemic form, the more severe form.

Figure 4.12. Photograph of central retinal vein occlusion (**A**) with an example of fluorescein angiographic findings (**B**). Venous occlusions may be associated with ischemia and neovascular changes. (Credit: Louis Antonucci, M.D.)

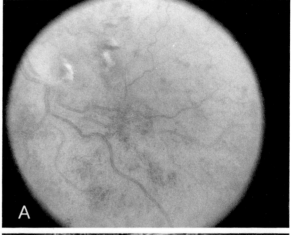

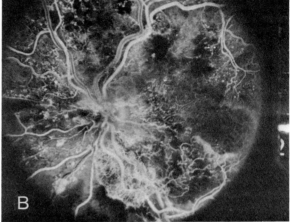

Mechanism. Both types of CRVO have a common mechanism—thrombosis of the central retinal vein at the level of the lamina cribrosa.

Partial CRVO has the following characteristics:

- Optic disc swelling;
- Tortuosity and dilation of branches of the central retinal vein;
- Dot- and flame-shaped hemorrhages in the retina;
- Macular edema (with loss of visual acuity), a variable finding;
- Fluorescein angiography (p. 87) showing minimal areas of nonperfusion.

Prognosis.

Partial occlusion. Complete resolution will be seen in almost one-half of the cases. Approximately one-quarter will progress to complete occlusion, and another quarter will show partial resolution. The visual prognosis is directly related to the initial vision after CRVO. Immediate severe visual loss indicates a poor prognosis. Anterior segment neovascularization is a rare finding in partial CRVO.

Complete Occlusion. Complete CRVO is characterized by extensive retinal edema and hemorrhage in all four quadrants. The ophthalmoscopic findings have been termed "blood and thunder" retinopathy. The veins are dilated and tortuous. Cotton-wool spots (see page 279) are seen, evidence of ischemia. Fluorescein angiography shows widespread areas of capillary nonperfusion.

The visual prognosis is poor. Only 10% of eyes will achieve vision better than 20/400.

There is a high incidence of anterior segment neovascularization with CRVO (as high as 60%), which results in severe glaucoma. When it does occur, neovascularization is seen within 6 months of onset. Most neovascularization is seen during the first 3 months and is termed *90-day glaucoma*.

Associations. Commonly associated with CRVO are cardiovascular disease, hypertension, and diabetes. Less common associations are blood dyscrasias, dysproteinemias, and vasculitis. Open angle glaucoma is present in one-fifth of patients with CRVO.

RETINITIS PIGMENTOSA (FIG. 4.13)

Definition and Associations

Retinitis pigmentosa is a term for a number of retinal dystrophies that are inherited and that may be associated with a variety of systemic problems. For example, the Laurence-Moon-Biedl syndrome presents with obesity, mental retardation, polydactyly, and hypogo-

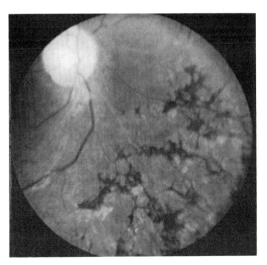

Figure 4.13. Retinitis pigmentosa. The pigmentary changes seen in the retina can be variable. Illustrated are changes frequently described as "bone spicule." Note also the disc, which is atrophic, and the retinal arterioles, which are attenuated. These changes are all consistent with the diagnosis.

nadism with retinitis pigmentosa. Usher's syndrome (see page 76) is associated with deafness.

Bassen-Kornzweig syndrome is of interest because it can be arrested in the early stages with high doses of vitamin A. Affected patients have steatorrhea and ataxia associated with retinitis pigmentosa.

Pathology

In retinitis pigmentosa, the rods of the retina degenerate. There is atrophy of both the remaining retina and the pigment epithelium.

The typical clinical appearance of retinitis pigmentosa is due to migration of epithelial cells that contain pigment. These cells eventually collect along retinal vessels.

Clinical Signs

Night Blindness as an Early Clinical Symptom

Night blindness may occur before signs of the disease are seen. Night blindness usually occurs in youth.

Later Abnormalities

The visual fields constrict from the periphery. Macular vision is usually spared until late in the course of the disease.

Appearance

The appearance of the fundi can be dramatic. The collection of retinal pigment tends to form clumps that are pointed and are descriptively called *bone spicules.* This is most often seen both in the periphery and at the equator of the eye. Pigment collects around retinal vessels.

Although almost always a bilateral disease involving all of the retina, on occasion the disease can be limited to one eye or sectors of the retina. The retinal arteries are narrowed and, later in the disease, the optic disc shows a waxy pallor.

Diagnosis

- Visual fields: Constriction of the visual fields and the presence of ring scotoma can be seen.
- Clinical fundus appearance: Bone spicule pigment clumping, collection of

pigment around arterioles, narrowing of the retinal vessels, and waxy pallor of the optic disc are seen.

- Electrooculogram (EOG): Abnormal findings are seen.
- Electroretinogram (ERG): The electroretinogram that tests rod function (scotopic) is abnormal. The electroretinogram that tests cone function (photopic) is normal.

Differential Diagnosis of Syndromes Associated with Retinitis Pigmentosa

I. Bassen-Kornzweig syndrome
   A. Autosomal recessive
   B. Crenated red cells
   C. Serum abetalipoproteinemia with steaborrhea
   D. Spinocerebellar degeneration with ataxia
   E. Treated with vitamin A
II. Alström's syndrome
   A. Autosomal recessive
   B. Childhood blindness
   C. Obesity
   D. Diabetes mellitus
   E. Neurosensory deafness
   F. Chronic renal disease (in late stages)
III. Bardet-Biedl syndrome
   A. Autosomal recessive
   B. Polydactyly
   C. Obesity
   D. Mental retardation
   E. Hypogonadism
IV. Cockayne's syndrome
   A. Autosomal dominant
   B. Premature senile appearance
   C. Mental retardation
   D. Deafness
   E. Peripheral neuropathy
   F. Dermatitis
V. Friedreich's syndrome
   A. Recessive
   B. Deafness
   C. Mental retardation
   D. Spinocerebellar ataxia
VI. Kearns-Sayre syndrome
   A. External ophthalmoplegia (see page 116)
   B. Cardiac conduction defects with heart block
   C. Hearing loss
VII. Leber's congenital amaurosis
   A. Autosomal recessive
   B. Severe visual loss at birth or within the 1-year of life
VIII. Mucopolysaccharidosis
   A. Hunter's disease (type II), which has manifestations of gargoylism, mental retardation, enlarged spleen and liver
   B. Sanfilippo's disease (type III), which has manifestations of deafness, mental retardation, and seizures
IX. Refsum's disease
   A. Recessive
   B. Peripheral neuropathy
   C. Cerebellar ataxia
   D. Deafness
   E. Increased blood levels of phytanic acid
X. Syphilis—Congenital and acquired syphilis can cause pigmentary disturbances that may be confused with retinitis pigmentosa. Although the fundus appearance of syphilis is called "salt and pepper," changes do occur that may be indistinguishable from a classic retinitis pigmentosa.
XI. Usher's syndrome
   A. Autosomal recessive
   B. Deafness—The association of deafness with retinitis pigmentosa is common to a number of syndromes. In Usher's syndrome, this association is so common that, in childhood, severe deafness is due to Usher's syndrome in about 5% of cases. Of those cases where children are both deaf and blind, approximately 50% are secondary to Usher's syndrome.

PERIPHERAL RETINAL DEGENERATIONS (FIG. 4.14)

Lattice Degeneration

Appearance

Lattice degeneration is a trophic retinal degeneration occurring primarily at the equator.

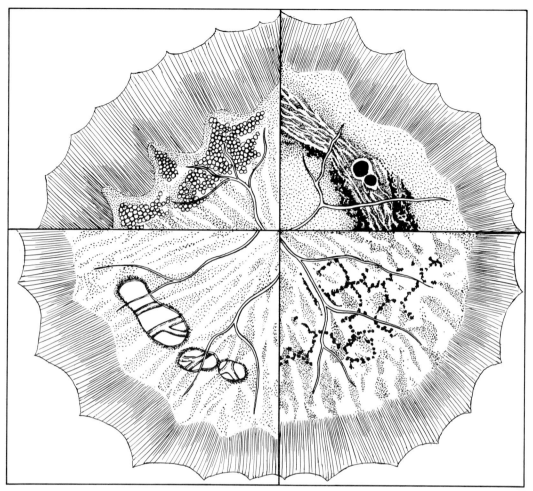

Figure 4.14. Four types of peripheral retinal degeneration: peripheral cystoid degeneration *(top left)*, lattice degeneration *(top right)*, paving stone degeneration *(bottom left)*, and reticular degeneration *(bottom right)*. Most important is lattice degeneration, which may precede retinal detachment. Lattice degeneration is most often seen near the equator. The other degenerations are seen in the far periphery.

It is often associated with retinal tears along the posterior and lateral margins of the lesions.

Lesions may be single or multiple. When there are multiple lesions, they may be arranged in two, three, or even four rows. These rows are parallel to the equator.

A typical lesion shows a sharply demarcated retinal thinning located circumferentially with altered retinal pigment accumulating along interlacing white lines. The white lines appear as a network and are a distinguishing feature. Round, punched-out areas

of retinal thinning or hole formation may occur.

In adjacent areas, the vitreous loses its gel-like characteristic and becomes liquified. Small, yellow-white particles at the margin of the lesion adjacent to the vitreous are noted. Vitreoretinal attachments, which are exaggerated, are seen at the margin of the lesion.

Sclerotic retinal blood vessels are seen in areas of the lesion. Loss of retinal neurons, accumulations of extracellular material in the degenerative retina of the lesion, and alterations of the internal limiting layer of the retina are also seen.

Prevalence

Lattice degeneration is present in 1 of 10 patients. It is bilateral in almost half and it is commonly seen in myopia.

Lattice degeneration may be responsible for retinal detachment (rhegmatogenous) when the retinal hole allows passage of fluid behind the retina. Even though 1 of 10 people have lattice degeneration, the incidence of retinal detachment is less than 0.005 to 0.01% per year. It is obvious that most patients with lattice degeneration do not develop retinal detachment.

Paving Stone Degeneration

Other Names

Cobblestone degeneration, peripheral chorioretinal atrophy

Description

Paving stone lesions are in the periphery of the retina between the ora serrata and the equator (see Fig. 4.14). They are separated from the ora serrata by normal retina. They are raised, sharply demarcated, and white or yellow-white. The lesions may be single or multiple. At times, they may become confluent, but most often they are separate. Prominent choroidal vessels are seen at the base of the lesions.

Position

The lesions of paving stone degeneration are found in the *inferior temporal quadrant* in about three-quarters of the cases. The next most frequent site is the inferior nasal quadrant.

Histology

The histologic characteristics are:

- Retinal thinning;
- No retinal pigment epithelium;
- Intact Bruch's membrane (with sensory retina closely applied to it);
- Absent choriocapillaris;
- Hypertrophy and hyperplasia of the pigment epithelium at the margin.

Frequency

These lesions are commonly seen and can be found at autopsy in 25% of cases. They are most often unilateral but may be bilateral in about one-third of cases.

Peripheral Cystoid Degeneration (Cystoid Degeneration)

Characteristics

Peripheral cystoid degeneration is seen in the area of the ora serrata extending posteriorly for 2 to 3 mm. The specialized viewing techniques of indirect ophthalmoscopy, usually with scleral depression or with a fundus contact lens, are needed to see these lesions. Peripheral cystoid degeneration appears as small bubbles.

Histology

Peripheral cystoid degeneration is caused by spaces that develop in the outer plexiform and inner nuclear layers. These spaces coalesce to form interlacing tunnels separated by pillars that extend from the inner to the outer retinal layers. The cystoid spaces cause a bubbly appearance with stippled depressions between the bubbles formed by the retinal pillars.

Position

The degeneration begins at the ora serrata. Cystoid degeneration is most extensive in the *superior and temporal quadrants*. It may extend posteriorly and may encircle the globe. At times, it may reach from the ora to the equator.

Incidence

This degenerative process may be seen in infants only 1 year old. All adult eyes will have some evidence of cystoid degeneration.

Complication

The only complication of typical cystoid degeneration is when the spaces coalesce and the cavities extend to develop into a degenerative retinoschisis (see page 79).

Reticular Degeneration

Other Names

Reticular cystoid degeneration, reticular peripheral cystoid degeneration

Characteristics

Reticular degeneration shows a prominent linear, reticular pattern that corresponds to the retinal vessels. The lesions are often demarcated by retinal blood vessels posteriorly. There is a finely stippled internal surface to the lesion, which may occur in the shape of an irregular angle. The lesion may be single or multiple.

Histology

Spaces that develop in the nerve fiber layer are divided by delicate retinal pillars. Reticular degeneration is almost always continuous with peripheral cystoid degeneration and is almost always located posterior to this cystoid degeneration.

Incidence

Reticular cystoid degeneration is present in approximately one-fifth of all adult patients and is bilateral in more than 40% of these patients. The process is most prevalent in the *inferior temporal quadrant*.

Progression

Reticular degeneration may progress to reticular degenerative retinoschisis (bullous retinoschisis) (see below).

RETINOSCHISIS
Definition

Retinoschisis is a splitting of the retina into layers. Retinoschisis should be differentiated from retinal detachment, in which the retina retains its full thickness but is separated from the pigment epithelium. In retinoschisis, the inner retinal layer (outer plexiform) is separated from the outer retinal layer.

Other Terms

Senile retinoschisis, macrocyst, giant cyst of the retina

Various Forms of the Process

I. Most commonly associated with aging
II. Other less common forms of retinoschisis
  A. Juvenile retinoschisis (X-linked inheritance)
  B. Retinoschisis secondary to vitreous traction as a part of proliferative retinopathy

Histopathology

In the early stages of the separation, the inner layer consists of the ganglion cell and nerve fiber layers, which contain arteries, veins, and superficial capillaries. In later stages, as the inner layer atrophies, the retinal blood vessels may become fragile and rupture, causing hemorrhage into the cavity. Atrophy can also produce multiple round or oval holes in the inner layers.

The outer layer is less atrophied as time progresses. The photoreceptor outer segments, which are in the outer layer, are well preserved. Holes in this outer layer are rare.

The cyst that forms is frequently filled with mucopolysaccharide. Accumulation of mucopolysaccharide is not the cause but rather the result of the splitting.

Retinoschisis is due to the coalescence of multiple smaller Blessig-Ivanov microcysts (see Fig. 4.2.C) of the peripheral retina. This microcystic peripheral degeneration is common. In its early development, tunnels form between the microcysts in the outer plexiform layer. A second system of spaces in the internal portion of the retina at the level of the inner nuclear layer then develops.

Clinical Appearance

The following features of retinoschisis differentiate it from retinal detachment.

- There is no shifting fluid or change in shape with movement of the eye or when placing the patient in different positions so that gravity variously affects the eye.
- Shadows are cast by vessels on the inner layer. On the inner surface, the retinal vessels may have a normal red coloration but, as time progresses, they can become attenuated and assume a white coloration. The shadows cast by these vessels are a hallmark of retinoschisis.
- On the inner surface, it is also possible to distinguish white spots or "snowflakes" (insertions onto the internal limiting membrane of the footplates of residual Müller cells).
- The outer layer has a mottled appearance in contrast to the inner layer, which is smooth.
- Demarcation of pigment lines is not as-

sociated with retinoschisis (unless there is also a retinal detachment).

- The outer layer when submitted to pressure by scleral depression, shows "white with pressure."
- Of all cases, 75% are located in the inferior temporal quadrant and 25% are in the superior temporal quadrant. Retinoschisis rarely occurs in nasal quadrants. Almost all retinoschisis cavities extend to the ora serrata.
- The visual field scotomas caused by retinoschisis have a sharp border. In cases of retinal detachment, visual field defects have a graduated border.

Symptoms

Of all patients with retinoschisis, one-quarter have no symptoms. Forty per cent of patients will have floaters or photopsia (flashing lights).

Refractive Error

Retinoschisis may occur with any refractive error, but there is a higher proportion of patients with hyperopia (farsightedness). Central visual acuity is rarely affected because less than 1% of patients have involvement of the macula.

Clinical Course

There will be no progression of the retinoschisis after diagnosis in 85% of patients. The risk of retinal detachment is low.

TOXOPLASMOSIS

Definition

Ocular toxoplasmosis is caused by *Toxoplasma gondii*. This organism is a common cause of inflammation in the posterior portion of the eye (posterior uveitis).

Nature of the Infection

The initial infection with *Toxoplasma gondii* is usually subclinical. This primary infection affects lung, heart, and brain (pneumonia, myocarditis, or encephalitis). After the initial infection, the organism remains encapsulated in large cysts. The organism is extremely common, and 50% of the adult population have positive antibodies to *T. gondii*.

Congenital Infection

Toxoplasmosis can be transmitted to the unborn child during acute infection in the mother. Congenital passage of the disease to the fetus occurs only during acute infection. Acute infection occurs only once. Therefore, those who are antibody-positive or who have had one child with congenital toxoplasmosis will not give birth to a child with congenital toxoplasmosis.

Association with Immunosuppression

Once the body accommodates to the organism, the immune response usually controls the parasite and there is no dissemination or proliferation. However, when the immune system is compromised (as in immunosuppression from disease or from drug therapy), patients previously infected with *T. gondii* are at considerable risk of developing serious ocular complications of the disease.

Pathology

Toxoplasma gondii organisms have been found only in the retina. These organisms cause retinitis associated with cells in the vitreous. The posterior vitreous base may detach, and cellular precipitates on the posterior face of the vitreous may cause a decrease in vision.

Establishing the Diagnosis

Antibody Titers

The positive antibody test to *Toxoplasma gondii* is only suggestive of a possible diagnosis of invasion in the retina causing posterior uveitis. As 50% of the population have a positive antibody test, the presence of antibody titers is not pathognomonic. Changing antibody titers also are not helpful because ocular lesions alone do not affect, in most circumstances, systemic titers.

Clinical Appearance

In the acute stage of toxoplasmosis, a focal lesion involving the retina causes necrosis. It is usually a circumscribed, white or slightly *yellowish white lesion* that has indistinct or fluffy borders. Lesions vary in size from a few millimeters to 5 to 6 disc diameters. The overall appearance of the lesion is constant in color and consistency. *Exudative cells in the overlying vitreous are common* in toxoplasmosis and are a key diagnostic feature when the differential diagnosis of presumed ocular histoplasmosis syndrome is considered. *Satellite scars,* small scars close to or in the area of the active lesion, are highly suggestive of an active toxoplasmic retinitis. Inactive satellite scars are frequently seen in congenital toxoplasmosis.

Diagnosis is based on a combination of clinical appearance and antibody testing. A positive antibody titer (even a 1/1 dilution) is considered significant but frequently not conclusive.

*Additional Laboratory Tests for
Toxoplasmic Disease*

- Indirect fluorescent antibody test
- Indirect hemagglutination
- Enzyme-linked immunosorbent essay (ELISA)
- Fluoroimmunoassay (FIAX)

These tests are used to reassess a negative antibody titer in a patient who has a lesion consistent with toxoplasmosis.

FREQUENTLY ENCOUNTERED CONCEPTS AND DISEASES
Acute Retinal Necrosis Syndrome (ARN)

Characteristics

ARN occurs in healthy patients at any age. The onset is variable and may be rapid or slow. The condition can be unilateral or bilateral (BARN). When bilateral, the second eye may be involved months after the first eye.

Diagnosis

Multifocal patches that may coalesce are seen as white areas in the peripheral retina and are associated with vascular occlusive hemorrhage and prominent vasculitis. Both arteries and veins are affected. Inflammation and uveitis are also present. The vitreous becomes hazy from the inflammation.

Course

With resolution of the acute lesions, a diffuse pigment stippling occurs in the involved areas of the retina. The involved areas show sharp demarcation from the normal areas. Poor vision often results.

Complications

Extensive retinal atrophy, optic nerve atrophy, retinal detachment, and changes in the macular region secondary to edema and macular pucker are possible complications.

Cause

A viral cause is presumed.

Cytomegalovirus Retinitis
Cause

This retinitis is caused by the cytomegalic virus, a DNA virus of the herpes group.

Characteristics

Ophthalmoscopy shows a clear separation between involved and uninvolved areas of the retina. Involved areas are opaque and white with multiple intraretinal hemorrhages. After the acute phase, a diffuse atrophy occurs.

Prognosis

Loss of vision results from retinal degeneration and macular changes. Retinal breaks occur, and retinal detachment may result.

Laboratory Diagnosis

The virus can be cultured from urine, serum, and tears. It can also be cultured from intraocular specimens—aqueous and subretinal fluid.

Epiretinal Membranes
Definition

Epiretinal membranes are changes in the internal limiting membrane (see Figs. 4.2 and 4.3). These changes are without blood vessels and are due to cellular proliferation and eventual fibrosis.

Causes

- Idiopathic
- Inflammation
- Anterior segment surgery
- Retinal detachment (rhegmatogenous)
- Penetrating injury

Pathology

The most common form, a simple epiretinal membrane, causes the least visual disturbance. Glial cells and collagen form a thin membrane over the macular area.

Surface wrinkling, or cellophane retinopathy, occurs when the glial membranes wrinkle the retinal surface and distort the internal limiting membrane. This clinical sign is associated with a mild decrease in visual acuity.

In the most severe form of epiretinal membrane, macular pucker occurs. A thick membrane covers the surface of the retina. Visual reduction is due to poor light transmission through the membrane, distortion of the retinal architecture, and cystoid macular edema.

Fluorescein Angiography

Characteristics shown are tortuosity of retinal vessels, diffuse macular hyperfluorescence, and, in late stages, diffuse mild leakage of the dye.

Choroideremia

Definition

Choroideremia is a retinal degeneration.

Heredity

Choroideremia has an X-linked recessive inheritance; therefore, males are affected and females are carriers.

Affected Males. Affected males show loss of both the retinal pigment epithelium and the underlying choriocapillaris. This retinal pigment epithelial loss starts in the midperipheral fundus and then progresses toward the anterior portion of the eye and toward the posterior pole. The progression is slow, and central vision is not lost until late in the disease.

The electroretinogram indicates rod/cone degeneration. The electrooculogram is abnormal, and dark adaptation is abnormal. Fluorescein angiography shows distinctive findings and can confirm the diagnosis of choroideremia. The onset is usually in patients 4 to 20 years old.

The symptoms are peripheral visual loss and night blindness, with progression to central visual loss.

Female Carriers. Female carriers will develop milder symptoms and may have retinal degeneration on ophthalmoscopic examination. The fundus signs seen in many female carriers include pigment clumping in the subretinal areas and a granular appearance of the retinal pigment epithelium. Electrophysiologic tests, such as the electroretinogram, dark adaptation, and visual field examinations, are usually normal. There is rarely any functional defect in carriers.

Differential Diagnosis of Choroideremia.

1. Retinitis Pigmentosa. Patients with retinitis pigmentosa usually have bone spicule formation in the equatorial regions, may have choroidal sclerosis, and have a relative preservation of the retina pigment epithelium anteriorly; all of these structures are lost in choroideremia.

2. Gyrate Atrophy. Gyrate atrophy is autosomal recessive. The inheritance pattern can help to distinguish it from choroideremia. Also, the pigment epithelium appears darker than when compared to the lighter fundus appearance of choroideremia.

Acute Posterior Multifocal Placoid Pigment Epitheliopathy (AMPPE)

Characteristics

AMPPE starts as a rapidly progressive bilateral visual loss, which often follows a preceding virus-like systemic illness. It usually affects young people.

Diagnosis

By ophthalmoscopy, multifocal, yellowish white lesions are seen. These lesions are deep at the level of the retinal pigment epithelium and choriocapillaris.

Fluorescein Angiography

Acutely, the lesions block choroidal fluorescence. After resolution, hyperfluorescence or *window defects* occur in the areas of retinal pigment epithelial atrophy.

Associated Conditions

Vitreous inflammation, nongranulomatous uveitis, and inflammation of the sclera (scleritis) or of the optic disc (optic neuritis) may be associated with APMPPE.

Prognosis

After varying periods, the visual recovery is good.

Complications

Although unusual, a subretinal neovascular membrane may complicate vision recovery.

Cause

The cause of this acute inflammatory condition is not known. It is not known whether this is a vasculitis or a direct pigment epithelial disorder. Pleocytosis and elevated cerebrospinal fluid protein can be seen in the cerebrospinal fluid. A viral (herpes virus) hypersensitivity reaction, especially as APMPPE is frequently associated with viral syndromes, is a possibility.

Gyrate Atrophy

Characteristics

This is an autosomal recessive disease that starts in early childhood.

Ophthalmologic Findings

There is loss of the pigment epithelium and choriocapillaris in scalloped configurations. The remaining retinal pigment epithelium appears hyperpigmented. Myopia and cataracts are common.

Diagnosis

The diagnosis can be confirmed by testing the serum ornithine levels. Diagnostic levels are 6 to 10 times normal.

Electroretinography

The electroretinogram is abnormal. Progressive visual field loss and night blindness are seen.

Treatment

Patients are placed on ornithine-restricted diets supplemented with oral vitamin B_6. This treatment is thought to stop the progression of the retinal degenerative changes.

Sickle Cell Retinopathy

Hematologic Considerations

Normal adult hemoglobin is called hemoglobin A. A red blood cell with hemoglobin A has certain characteristics: it is a biconcave disc, is pliable and flexible, delivers oxygen to surrounding tissue, and flows easily through capillaries.

Sickle cell hemoglobin is referred to as hemoglobin S. Red blood cells containing hemoglobin S have abnormal characteristics: they tend to have elongated shapes resembling sickles, they are more rigid, they have difficulty flowing through the lumina of small blood vessels, and they create ischemic areas because of these obstructive characteristics. Hemoglobin S is formed because mutation causes substitution of the amino acid valine for glutamic acid.

An additional abnormal hemoglobin is created by the substitution of lysine for glutamic acid. This is known as hemoglobin C.

Basics of Hemoglobin Combinations.

Normal. Normal adult hemoglobin is hemoglobin A.

Abnormal Hemoglobins. Hemoglobin S and hemoglobin C are abnormal. Patients can be homozygous or heterozygous for the form of hemoglobin. Various combinations result in different clinical presentations.

Sickle Cell Anemia (SS Disease). Homozygous SS

Sickle Cell C Disease (SC Disease). Heterozygous, hemoglobin S and hemoglobin C

Sickle Cell Trait (AS Hemoglobin). Heterozygous, hemoglobin S and hemoglobin A

Thalassemia

Thalassemia (also called Mediterranean anemia) may produce a heterozygous disease known as *sickle cell thalassemia* (hemoglobin thalassemia and hemoglobin S). In this condition, the sickle cell gene is inherited from one parent, and thalassemia is inherited from the other.

Clinical Considerations

The SS combination, or sickle cell anemia, results in severe systemic symptoms. Recurrent hemolysis, chronic anemia, and sickle cell "crises" from hypoxia and infarction occur. Sickle cell anemia (SS) causes death during the first few decades of life.

Sickle cell C disease (SC disease) and sickle cell thalassemia (S-thal) produce milder anemias and less severe systemic symptoms. The sickle cell trait (AS hemoglobin) is the mildest form of all.

Ocular complications of sickle cell hemoglobinopathies are most severe in sickle cell C disease and in sickle cell thalassemia. Ocular complications are retinal neovascularization, hemorrhage in the vitreous, and retinal detachment, all of which are characteristic of sickle cell C disease and sickle cell thalassemia hemoglobinopathies.

Clinical Ocular Features

Nonproliferative Sickle Retinopathy.
Asymptomatic Changes.
Black Sunburst. Black sunbursts are fundus lesions characteristic of sickling. They are circumscribed, are one-half to two disc diameters in size, are ovoid, have stellate or spiculate borders, and are located in the equatorial region. They are frequently associated with refractile, yellowish granules.

Black sunburst lesions rarely affect vision and are most often seen in patients with sickle cell thalassemia, sickle cell anemia, and sickle cell C disease (in that order). They are rarely seen in patients with the sickle cell trait.

Venous Tortuosity. This is a common characteristic of sickle cell retinopathy, occurring in one-half of the patients with sickle cell anemia and about one-third of the patients with sickle cell C disease. This is an uncommon finding in patients with sickle cell trait or sickle cell thalassemia.

Refractile Deposits. Refractile deposits are glistening and granular. They are characteristic of sickling and are seen in patients with sickle cell anemia, sickle cell C disease, and sickle thalassemia. They are infrequent in patients with the sickle cell trait.

Refractile deposits are like cholesterol crystals, but they are not lipid. They are probably hemosiderin that has been sequestered in intraretinal cavities. Vision is not affected by these deposits.

Silver Wire Arterioles. Occlusions of the peripheral arterioles, which are common in sickling, may take on a chalky white or *silver wire* appearance. True sheathing of the peripheral vasculature is uncommon in sickling.

Salmon Patch Hemorrhage. When peripheral arteriolar obstruction occurs, a hemorrhage may occur at the point of occlusion. Hemorrhages are confined to substance of the retina or may break into the subhyloid space. They are small, ovoid, and about one-quarter to one disc diameter in size. They start out red but later progress through a series of color changes from pink to orange and then finally to white. The salmon patch hemorrhages may disappear as hemolysis occurs. If hemosiderin remains, they may result in glistening refractile deposits.

Symptomatic Lesions.
Central Retinal Artery Occlusions (see page 72). Although rare, central retinal artery occlusion has a devastating effect on vision. Because it affects young people, it is all the more dramatic.

Macular Arteriole Occlusions. Also rare, occlusion of macular branch arterioles results in significant visual defects. Vasoproliferation in the region of the macula, however, rarely occurs.

Retinal Venous Occlusions. Retinal venous occlusions are rare. Central vein occlusions and branch vein occlusions have been observed in young patients.

Choroidal Vascular Occlusions. Occlusion of the choroidal vasculature can be extensive.

Angioid Streaks. Angioid streaks (see page 248) have been reported in all of the major sickle cell hemoglobin combinations. Angioid streaks, however, are infrequent complications of sickling. Visual disability from the streaks is uncommon in patients with sickle cell hemoglobinopathy but does occur in patients with pseudoxanthoma elasticum (see Fig. 16.3).

Proliferative Sickle Cell Retinopathy.
Proliferative sickle cell retinopathy is classified into five stages that reflect the increasing severity of the retinopathy as well as the sequence of events.

Stage 1: Proliferative Arteriolar Occlusions. The first ophthalmoscopic abnormality is proliferative arteriolar occlusion. The arteriolar capillary bed fails to fill, and the veins that drain the affected portion do not fill in the peripheral fundus. It is presumed that sickle cell erythrocytes, which have lost their pliable, flexible nature, act either as microemboli or to increase blood viscosity so that thrombosis occurs.

The peripheral nonperfusion of the retina that results from the occlusion is easily demonstrated by fluorescein angiography (page 87). With the ophthalmoscope, the interface between the nonperfused retina and the perfused retina, approximately at the equator of the globe, can be seen as a contrast between the orange-brown normal fundus and the abnormal grayish brown of the ischemic fundus just anterior to it. Clearly defined fundus markings are absent in the ischemic area and chalky white (silver wire) arter-ioles are seen in the ischemic area. True sheathing of the vessels is rare in sickle cell patients.

Stage 2: Peripheral Arteriolar-Venular Anastomoses. Peripheral arteriolar-venular anastomoses follow the occlusions. The anastomoses shunt blood from the occluded arterioles to adjacent venules. These anastomoses are not seen easily on ophthalmoscopy and usually require fluorescein angiography for visualization.

Stage 3: Neovascular Proliferation. Neovascular capillary buds sprout at sites of previous arteriolar occlusions and arteriolar-venular anastomoses. The growth is inward toward the ora serrata, that is, from the perfused retina to the nonperfused retina. New capillaries often sprout into fan-shaped configurations. These have been called *sea fans.*

The neovascular lesions most often affect the superior temporal quadrant of the eye. Other retinal quadrants affected with neovascular lesions, in decreasing order of presentation, are inferotemporal, superonasal, and inferonasal.

Sea fans occasionally undergo spontaneous resolution. They are most commonly observed in patients with sickle cell C disease and sickle thalassemia. They are uncommon in patients with other sickle cell hemoglobinopathies. It is thought that the chronic anemia in sickle cell disease is a protective factor against retinal ischemia and secondary neovascularization.

Stage 4: Vitreous Hemorrhage. Vitreous hemorrhage is a frequent complication of retinal neovascularization in sickle cell retinopathy. Vitreous hemorrhages are rare in sickle cell anemia but occur in more than one-fifth of patients with sickle cell C disease. They are also seen in sickle cell thalassemia. Because retinal neovascularization is rare in patients with the sickle cell trait, vitreous hemorrhage is also rare. Sea fans are composed of weak or friable tissues; therefore, minor ocular trauma or vitreous traction can lead to rupture of these vessels and subsequent vitreous hemorrhage.

Stage 5: Retinal Detachment. Retinal detachment may occur and may be rhegmatogenous (see page 69) or nonrhegmatogenous. Tears in the retina can usually be found in patients with retinal detachment due to sickle cell retinopathy. However, the tears may be difficult to see because they are obscured by fibrovascular tissue. Most cases of retinal detachment have been reported in patients with sickle cell C disease.

Retinopathy of Prematurity

Another Name

Retrolental fibroplasia—In the past, retrolental fibroplasia was a term in common use for the retinopathy of prematurity. The term is generally reserved now for nonacute, late scarring changes that occur in very severely affected infants.

Definition

Retinopathy of prematurity occurs in low birth weight infants and refers to changes of ischemia, blood vessel growth, and fibrosis (proliferative retinopathy) that occur because of inadequate oxygen delivery to the peripheral retina.

Prevalence

The prevalence is best correlated with birth weight. With less than 1501-g birth weight, the prevalence, depending upon the study, ranges from 4 to 65%. In infants of less than 1001-g birth weight, the prevalence ranges from 40 to 77%. Scarring (cicatricial) sequelae are most common in lower birth weight infants. Cicatricial sequelae may occur in as many as 20 to 40% of affected infants. Blindness occurs in approximately 5% of infants with active retinopathy of prematurity. At a minimum, 500 infants are blinded by retinopathy of prematurity each year.

Background

Vascularization of the human retina is unique among organs in that no blood vessels are present before the 4th month of gestation. After the 4th month, mesenchymal cells sprout from the hyaloid vessels at the disc. These cells move through the inner layers of the retina, developing the retinal vascularization. The retinal vessels reach the ora serrata nasally at about 8 months of gestation but do not completely vascularize the temporal retinal periphery until after the birth of a full-term infant.

The retina is susceptible to the changes of retinopathy of prematurity only before complete normal vascularization has occurred. The *temporal retina* is frequently involved in retinopathy of prematurity because the vasculature there develops last.

The incompletely vascularized retina is affected by oxygen. Oxygen causes vasoconstriction followed by vascular closure. Hypoxia results. Sustained hypoxia causes endothelial proliferation from vascular complexes adjacent to the retinal capillaries closed during hypoxia. New vessels are formed and grow onto the surface of the retina and into the vitreous. Vitreoretinal adhesions develop, and hemorrhages occur. Fibrous and glial tissue ingrowth occurs. Vitreoretinal traction is the final result.

The newly formed vessels are exquisitely sensitive to oxygen and constrict easily. This hypersensitivity results in eventual hypoxia. It is generally thought that ischemic retina due to hypoxia produces a factor that induces vasoproliferation. The presence of the immature retina is essential to the fundamental response to oxygen.

Clinical Classifications

Retinopathy of prematurity is divided into two general classifications, acute and cicatri-cial. The acute phase is when active new vessels respond to hypoxia. The cicatricial phase refers to fibrosis, contracture of proliferative tissue, vitreous and retinal traction, retinal distortion, and detachment.

Acute Retinopathy of Prematurity. Acute retinopathy of prematurity is divided into four stages: *Stage 1:* A demarcation line is seen between vascularized and nonvascularized retina. A translucent, normal, vascularized retina contrasts with the gray, nonvascularized retina. *Stage 2:* The demarcation line in stage 1 now has height, width, and volume (a ridge). *Stage 3:* The ridge is associated with extraretinal fibrovascular proliferation. *Stage 4:* Stage 3 findings are associated with serous retinal detachment. *Plus Disease:* In any of the stages of acute retinopathy of prematurity, aggressive changes may occur that are called *plus disease.* Plus disease is identified by retinal vascular dilation and tortuosity, vitreous haze, pupillary rigidity, and iris vascular dilation.

The locations of acute retinopathy of prematurity are divided into three zones: *Zone 1* is a posterior retina within 60° of the optic nerve. *Zone 2* is a larger circle around zone 1, with the edge touching the nasal ora anteriorly. This leaves some retina peripherally. *Zone 3* is the temporal peripheral retina that is not included in the circle formed in zone 2.

Cicatricial Retinopathy of Prematurity. Cicatricial retinopathy of prematurity is divided into five stages: *Stage 1:* Minor peripheral changes with retinal pigmentation and vitreous opacification. *Stage 2:* Temporal vitreoretinal fibrosis with dragging of the posterior retina. *Stage 3:* Additional peripheral fibrosis with contracture and retinal fold. *Stage 4:* Partial ring of retrolental fibrovascular tissue and partial retinal detachment. *Stage 5:* Complete ring of retrolental fibrovascular tissue with total retinal detachment.

Myopia of greater than 6 diopters is associated with later cicatricial changes. Also with the cicatricial changes are retinal pigmentation, microvascular abnormalities, and vitreous membranes. The retina can be dragged temporally with heterotopia of the fovea, which may be associated with strabismus, amblyopia, and pseudoexotropia. Retinoschisis and localized detachments may also be seen.

Guidelines in Diagnosing and Monitoring Retinopathy of Prematurity

- Examination of all high risk infants— those born at less than 36 weeks of gestation or with a birth weight of less than 2000 g who have received oxygen therapy (*a*) at the time of discharge and (*b*) again at 3 to 6 months of age (often at 7 to 9 weeks)
- Special attention to infants with birth weight of less than 1000 g

If early disease is detected, examination at 2- to 3-month intervals during the active phase is generally recommended.

Risk Factors in Retinopathy of Prematurity

- Mechanical ventilation
  —Length of time infant is receiving oxygen
  —Oxygen concentration
- Low birth weight
- Gestational age
- Occurrence of apnea requiring bag or mask resuscitation
- Intraventricular hemorrhage
- Septicemia
- Blood transfusion
- Severity of illness

FLUORESCEIN ANGIOGRAPHY

Fluorescein is a unique and safe injectable drug. When stimulated by blue light of wavelength 490 nm fluorescein emits a longer wavelength of yellow green light at 530 nm. Fluorescein is also selectively distributed in the eye where it is supplied by two circulations to the eye, choroidal and retinal. Choroidal vessels pass fluorescein dye freely through endothelial capillary junctions and the dye is rapidly distributed in the choroid.

Fluorescein does not pass into the retinal capillary bed from the choroid due to the tight junctions between the retinal pigment epithelial cells. The retinal arterioles, veins, and capillaries also do not allow fluorescein through the intracellular tight junctions (see Fig. 4.3). Therefore in the normal eye, fluorescein courses through the retinal vascular system but does not permeate vessel walls.

These features have allowed development of fluorescein as a significant diagnostic technique in ophthalmology. The drug is injected into an arm vein and within a few seconds fills the choroidal circulation first with easy access to the choroid. This is represented as a back ground flush of fluorescence. It then courses through the arterioles and veins. Rapid photography, using a blue (filtered) light to augment the fluorescence, provides a pictorial record of these rapid filling phases.

Diagnostically, abnormalities of the normal fluorescent patterns are broken down into hypofluorescence and patterns. *Hypofluorescence* is caused when visualization of the normal choroidal pattern is blocked by pigment or blood or if there is improper filling of vessels. *Hyperfluorescence* occurs when fluorescein: 1) leaks from retinal vessels as seen in macular edema or in neovascularization of the retina, 2) leaks through the normally impenetrable retinal pigment epithelium from the choroidal circulation, 3) pools in actual or created spaces, 4) is more easily seen through the retinal pigment epithelium which lacks pigment (window defect).

For examples see:

Purtcher's retinopathy Figure C.16 pg. xvi
Central vein occlusion Figure 4.12 pg. 74
Central serous choroidopathy Figure 16.14 pg. 268

5

Neuroophthalmology

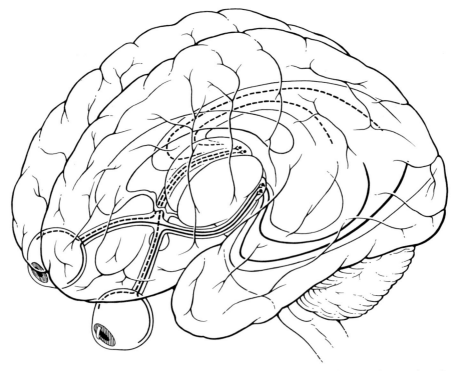

Figure 5.1. The visual pathways include the retina, optic disc, optic nerve, chiasm, optic tract, lateral geniculate body, optic radiations, and occipital cortex.

THE PUPIL

To read this section, you need:

- Basic understanding of neurosensory and neuromotor transmission;
- Knowledge of the anatomy of the iris (see page 306);
- Basic knowledge of the functions of the parasympathetic and sympathetic nervous systems (see Figs. 5.2 & 5.3).

What you will learn in this section:

- Pathways of pupillary reflex;
- Pharmacologic testing of pupillary function;
- Disease processes that cause pupillary dysfunction;
- Evaluation of pupillary function.

Definition

The pupil is the aperture of the eye that is formed by the iris. The changing size of the pupil regulates the amount of light that reaches the retina.

Pupillary Terminology

Frequently Used Terms

Mydriasis—a dilated pupil (greater than 6 mm)
Miosis—a constricted pupil (less than 2 mm)
Pinpoint pupil—a maximally constricted pupil
Fixed pupil—a pupil that does not move with light stimulation to the retina
Relative afferent pupillary defect (Marcus Gunn)—altered pupillary reaction caused by decreased transmission through the reflex arc of pupillary constriction, specifically in that area that runs from the eye to the brain
Irregular pupil—any pupil that loses its normal round configuration

Infrequently Used Terms

Keyhole pupil—a pupil that appears as an inverted keyhole usually due to a cut in the upper portion of the iris during a surgical procedure
Iridoplegia—paralysis of the pupil (a fixed pupil)
Hippus—a rarely used term for wide swings in size of the pupil; not a disease process and not caused by disease, hippus has been loosely associated with tense, nervous people

How Light Changes Pupillary Size

Pupil size is determined by two opposing forces—the sphincter (constrictor) muscle and the dilator muscles. The sphincter muscle of the iris, a muscle that circles the pupillary border, constricts the pupil. The sphincter muscle is under the control of the parasympathetic nervous system. The dilator fibers of the iris radiate out from the pupil in the stroma of the iris. These fibers are under sympathetic nervous system control. This sympathetic action opposes the parasympathetic action. Understanding these constricting and dilating forces and their separate parasympathetic and sympathetic control systems forms the basis for understanding the pupil, pupil abnormalities, and the drugs used in testing the pupil.

Pupil size is regulated by light. Light passes into the eye and activates sensory responses in the retina. The result is a visual response. In addition to vision, there are pupillary fibers in the retina that respond to light intensity. As everyone knows, light causes pupillary constriction; dark results in pupillary dilation.

The pupil constricts through stimulation of the parasympathetic nervous system (Fig. 5.2). The pupil dilates with stimulation of the sympathetic nervous system (Fig. 5.3).

How to Test for Pupillary Abnormalities

1. Direct Pupillary Response

Shine a bright light directly into the pupil. The pupil should constrict briskly. Remove the light. The pupil should dilate briskly.

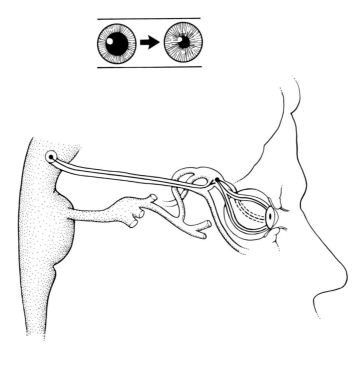

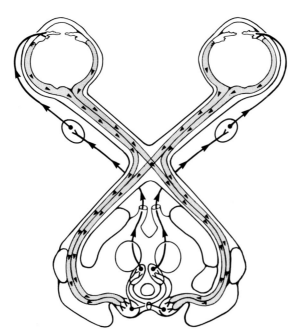

Figure 5.2. Parasympathetic pathway. Parasympathetic stimulation causes constriction of the pupil. The course of the parasympathetic nerve is shown in the *top diagram,* from the central nervous system to the periphery. *Below* is a diagram of the pathway of the light reflex to the optic nerve and to the brain stem through the Edinger-Westphal nucleus to the ciliary ganglion to the pupil. The cross-over of fibers results in consensual pupillary response—when a light is shown in one eye, the fellow eye also constricts.

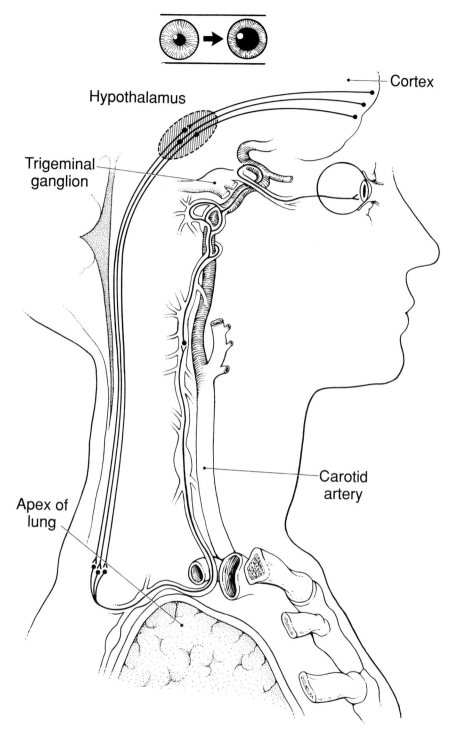

Figure 5.3. Sympathetic pathway for pupillary dilation. The long course of sympathetic innervation to the pupil allows active conditions to affect sympathetic stimulation. Sympathetic stimulation produces pupillary enlargement. Loss of this sympathetic influence to the pupil results in constriction. Particularly note the relationships of the axons to the superior apex of the lung and the carotid artery. Also note the course of the trigeminal ganglion and the hypothalamic cortical connections.

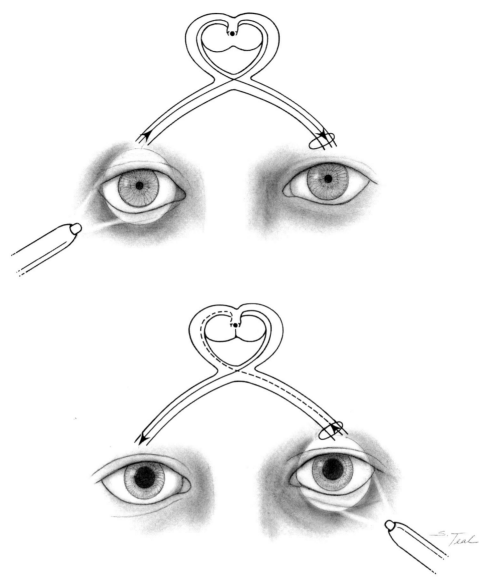

Figure 5.4. Swinging flashlight test for relative afferent pupillary defect. The circle represents the position of a lesion in the left optic nerve. The pupil changes because of impaired transmission in the left optic nerve.

2. Consensual Pupillary Response

Both pupils react together. When one eye is stimulated with a direct light, the opposite eye also responds. The consensual pupillary response is the confirmation of brisk constriction and dilation in the eye opposite the eye in which the light is directed.

3. Changing Illumination

This test uses a difference in background illumination to check changes while observing both pupils at the same time. Usually a change in room illumination is used. In a bright room, both pupils should be equally constricted. In a dark room, both pupils should be equally dilated.

4. Swinging Flashlight Test [Test for Relative Afferent Pupillary Defect (also called Marcus Gunn pupil)] (Fig. 5.4)

In normal pupillary responses, if a light is moved about every second back and forth be-

Horner's syndrome–a lack of sympathetic innervation causes a miotic pupil on the involved side.

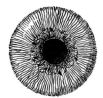

Third nerve paralysis causes a dilated pupil on the involved side.

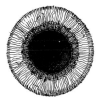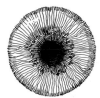

Adie syndrome causes a dilated pupil on the involved side due to ciliary ganglion interruption of parasympathetic stimulus.

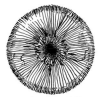

Argyll Robertson pupil, pathognomonic of syphilis, causes bilateral miotic pupils.

Figure 5.5. Pupil diagnosis. A comparison of pupils with different sizes.

Important Clinical Pupil Abnormalities (Fig. 5.5)

Horner's Syndrome

The Clinical Appearance. On the involved side, the Horner's syndrome pupil remains small. The opposite eye reacts normally. Therefore, in dim illumination, pupillary difference will be accented as the involved side remains constricted and the normal side dilates. In bright illumination, however, because the normal pupil is also constricted, the difference between pupils is little or none.

Cause for Horner's Syndrome. Horner's syndrome is due to a disruption of sympathetic innervation. The disruption can be anywhere along the sympathetic path, either peripheral or central (Fig. 5.6).

tween the two pupils, both pupils remain constricted, with a slight dilation between swings. If, however, there is a blockage to neural transmission in one eye, usually from optic nerve dysfunction, the pupillary response will become unequal. In essence, there is dilation when the involved eye is stimulated (a phenomenon known as pupillary escape). When unequal responses are present, a Marcus Gunn pupil is diagnosed (see page 101). The Marcus Gunn pupil is also called relative afferent pupillary defect.

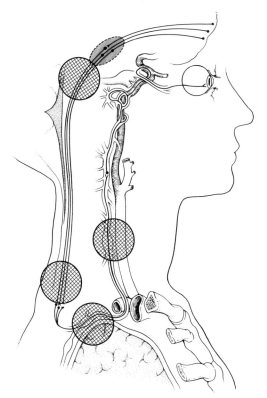

Figure 5.6. Horner's syndrome is produced by lesions at various points of the sympathetic pathway *(crosshatched circles).*

Associated Findings. Horner's syndrome is associated with lid droop (ptosis) of the involved side as well as abnormal sweating. Horner's syndrome can present as a congenital abnormality. In these cases, there is hypopigmentation of the iris on the involved side. [Horner's syndrome is one diagnosis in the differential for unequal iris color between eyes (heterochromia)].

Importance. Horner's syndrome in adults may indicate malignancy. A complete workup, especially for tumors near the apex of the lung (Pancoast's tumor), should be considered.

Approximately one-third of all Horner's syndromes are caused by neoplasms, either bronchiogenic carcinomas or metastatic carcinomas. In patients over 50, neoplasm is the most common cause of Horner's syndrome.

Tonic Pupil (Adie's Pupil) (Fig. 5.5)

Clinical Findings. Tonic pupil is usually dilated or mid-dilated. The reaction to light, with a cursory examination, will not be present. If light is shown in the pupil for a number of minutes, however, slow constriction occurs. Tonic pupil is usually unilateral; if it is bilateral, the onset is at different times and responses in both eyes tend to be asymmetrical. Accommodation (see Fig. 7.5A), that is, the near focus mechanism, is decreased and patients will have difficulty seeing clearly at near.

Cause. Tonic pupil is caused by interruption of the parasympathetic system, thought to be in the ciliary ganglion. The specific agent or event is unknown.

Argyll Robertson Pupil (Fig. 5.5)

Clinical Presentation. Argyll-Robertson pupils react poorly to light and are miotic. The condition is bilateral.

Dissociation of Near Response. The near response is the association of pupillary constriction with change of gaze focus from distance to near. When the near response is tested, the pupils become smaller. Because the pupils are already miotic, it takes careful observation to confirm this response.

Significance. Argyll-Robertson pupil is associated with syphilis. Any patient showing this pupillary abnormality should have an FTA-ABS serum evaluation.

Pharmacologic Considerations of Horner's Syndrome

The diagnosis of Horner's syndrome can be confirmed by the topical use of 1% Paredrine or 1% Neo-Synephrine (both stimulators of the sympathetic system, i.e., sympathomimetics). These drugs at low concentrations will dilate the denervated Horner's pupil, but they will have no effect on the normal pupil. The denervated pupil dilates because it becomes hypersensitive to sympathomimetic drugs.

Two per cent cocaine is also used for diagnosis of Horner's syndrome, but the action of cocaine is different from that of the sympathomimetic drugs, Paredrine and Neo-Synephrine, which stimulate directly. Cocaine blocks the nerve terminal uptake of norepinephrine, which causes dilation and acts only on the pupil with intact sympathetic innervation.

Because the blockage of norepinephrine action is different from hypersensitive stimulation, cocaine is used to determine the location of the lesion. By the use of both cocaine and a sympathomimetic drug, the origin of the lesion can be determined to be either first neuron (central) or second or third order neuron (peripheral). This is important not only for diagnosis but also for prognosis. Generally, central lesions are more serious and peripheral lesions are more benign.

When Horner's syndrome is a result of a first order neuron interruption, norepinephrine will be present, and the blockage of norepinephrine uptake by cocaine will not increase norepinephrine and will not cause pupillary dilation. The response of the pupil to sympathomimetics will be the same in both the first neuron and the second and third neuron because of denervation hypersensitivity. Only cocaine and its special action can help differentiate the site of the lesion.

In summary:

- *First neuron:* involved pupil dilates to Paredrine 1% or Neo-Synephrine 1% and dilates to 2% cocaine.
  Paredrine YES; cocaine YES

- *Second and third neuron:* involved pupil dilates to Paredrine 1% or Neo-Synephrine 1% but does not dilate to 2% cocaine.
  Paredrine YES; cocaine NO
- *Normal:* pupil will not dilate to Paredrine 1% or Neo-Synephrine 1% but will dilate to 2% cocaine.
  Paredrine NO; cocaine YES

Two additional points should be remembered about pharmacologic testing. First, in both sympathomimetic and cocaine testing, drops should be instilled in *both eyes* and the reactions of the involved and the normal pupil should be compared. Second, after the use of cocaine, the use of the sympathomimetics (Paredrine or Neo-Synephrine) for testing is *invalidated for 48 hours.*

Location of the lesion can help determine the cause of Horner's syndrome. Remember that the first neuron runs from the hypothalamus to the spinal cord, the second runs from the spinal cord to the superior cervical ganglion, and the third runs to the peripheral innervation of the ocular structures. This course provides an opportunity for a number of lesions in a variety of positions along the pathway to cause Horner's syndrome (see Fig. 5.6):

- Central lesions cause Wallenberg's lateral medullary syndrome (posterior inferior cerebellar artery syndrome).
- Cervical cord lesions (one-half of all Horner's syndrome patients have these lesions) can be due to trauma, syringomyelia, tumor, and, rarely, demyelinating disease.
- Chest lesions of the apex and superior mediastinum are usually due to bronchiogenic carcinoma (Pancoast superior sulcus syndrome).
- Neck lesions (fibers here are within the carotid sheath) can cause Horner's syndrome due to enlarged lymph nodes, tumor abscess, trauma, surgery, or acute carotid thrombosis.
- Brachial plexus level lesions are usually caused by birth trauma (may be associated with Klumpke's paralysis of the ipsilateral arm).

Important Clinical Aspects of Pupillary Responses

1. Why the Pupil Remains Constricted during Sleep or under Anesthesia

The sympathetic system, which controls dilation, is under a cortical influence. Under sleep or anesthesia, this cortical influence is lost and the normal sympathetic dilator tone to the pupils is decreased. With this decrease in force for dilation, the pupil becomes constricted because of uninhibited parasympathetic stimulation. Therefore, the pupils will remain miotic during sleep or during deep anesthesia.

2. Importance of Pupillary Responses with Third Nerve Palsies and Diabetes

When the third nerve is affected (ptosis, globe down and out, vision unchanged), the presence or absence of a pupillary response is important. Preservation of pupillary response indicates a diabetic origin of the third nerve palsy. However, absence of the pupillary response suggests neurologic conditions such as aneurysm.

Pharmacologic Considerations in Adie Syndrome

Adie syndrome, caused by a lesion of the ciliary ganglion frequently of unknown cause, is due to disruption of parasympathetic stimulation. The pupil develops a denervation hypersensitivity. As a result, the pupil will constrict to ⅛% pilocarpine if Adie pupil is present, but little or no constriction will occur in the normal pupil. (The reaction with 2.5% methacholine is the same as that to pilocarpine.) This differential pharmacologic test is important because Adie pupil is a benign condition. Appropriate diagnosis may avoid extensive neurologic workup for more serious conditions.

The characteristics of tonic pupil (Adie syndrome) are a dilated pupil with:

- Absent or markedly decreased reaction to light;
- Slow constriction to near and slow redilation;
- Sector palsies of the pupillary sphincter (vermiform movements); and

- Supersensitivity to methacholine 2.5% and pilocarpine ⅛%, causing constriction.

VISUAL PATHWAYS

Anatomy

Cranial Nerves III, IV, and VI

Eye movements are under the control of three major cranial nerves: the oculomotor (III), trochlear (IV), and abducens (VI) nerves. Nuclei for the oculomotor and trochlear nerves are in the midbrain, and that for the abducens nerve is located in the pons. All three nerve nuclei have paramedian locations.

Oculomotor Nerve. The oculomotor efferent fibers pass ventrally in the midbrain through the red nucleus and exit in the subarachnoid space ventrally. The nerve then passes under the origin of the posterior cerebral artery and lateral to the posterior communicating artery, an important relationship because a third nerve palsy is frequently associated with aneurysm.

The third nerve runs in the cavernous sinus. It lies inferior and medial to the trochlear and abducens nerves in the anterior part of the sinus. In certain conditions, the pupillomotor fibers of the third nerve in the sinus may be preferentially spared so that eye movements may be restricted and the pupil may be normal.

As the third nerve enters the orbit, it divides into two branches:

1. Superior Branch.   The superior branch innervates the superior rectus muscle and the levator palpebrae superioris.

2. Inferior Branch.   The inferior branch gives off twigs to the inferior and medial rectus muscles and a long twig to the inferior oblique muscle. From the twig to the inferior oblique, a division passes through the ciliary ganglion, which supplies the sphincter of the pupil and the ciliary body by way of the short ciliary nerves.

The most common conditions that affect the third nerve are aneurysm, tumor, inflammation, and vascular disease.

Abducens Nerve.   The abducens nerve nucleus is located caudal in the paramedian pontine tegmentum. Efferent fibers of the abducens oculomotor nucleus course to the lateral rectus muscle and pass ventrally. The nucleus of the sixth nerve is frequently involved in brain stem vascular disease. The sixth nerve passes through the superior orbital fissure (annular segment) to supply the lateral rectus muscle.

The most common conditions affecting the sixth nerve are tumor, vascular disease, multiple sclerosis, infection, diabetes, and trauma.

Trochlear Nerve.   The trochlear nerve is the only cranial nerve that exits the brain stem dorsally and *crosses* to supply the contralateral superior oblique muscle. The trochlear nerve passes through the cavernous sinus, traveling with the other oculomotor nerves, and enters the orbit through the superior orbital fissure. It supplies the superior oblique muscle.

The most common condition to affect the fourth nerve is *trauma*. Contrecoup contusions occur because the nerve exits dorsally and passes around the midbrain. Trochlear nerve palsies are significantly less common than abducens or oculomotor palsies.

The Retina

The impulses from the retina are collected by the ganglion cell. Each ganglion cell sends a single nerve fiber to the central nervous system. A single nerve fiber courses through the optic disc, optic nerve, optic chiasm, and optic tract to synapse in the lateral geniculate body. Ganglion cells responsible for transmitting central vision send axons from the foveal area to the temporal aspect of the optic disc. These fibers are known as the *papillomacular bundle.*

Optic Disc

The optic disc is the point at which all ganglion cell axons exit from the eye. The optic disc is 3 or 4 mm nasal to the fovea and is 1.5 mm in diameter. There are no photoreceptors overlying the disc. This creates an area in the field of vision of the eye, representing 5° to 7° of the visual space, that is a blind spot (or absolute scotoma). It is in the temporal visual field and is called the blind spot of Mariotte.

The intraocular portion of the optic nerve (represented by the optic disc is only 1 mm long. Optic nerve fibers at the disc are non-myelinated in most individuals. The blood supply to the optic disc is not totally understood but is important in certain visual field abnormalities due to disease processes such as glaucoma. It is thought that the optic disc receives its blood supply either from choroidal vessels or from branches of the short posterior ciliary arteries.

Optic Nerve (Orbit)

The optic nerve within the orbit is 20 to 30 mm long and 3 to 4 mm in diameter. Fibers within the optic nerve are myelinated. The optic nerve is surrounded by three layers of meninges—dura mater, arachnoid, and pia mater.

The optic nerve enters the optic canal at the apex of the orbit. Within the canal the nerve measures 4 to 9 mm in length and 4 to 6 mm in width. After entering the optic canal, the nerve runs posteriorly and medially forming an angle of 30° with an imaginary line in the midsagittal plane.

The optic nerves leave the canals and converge on the optic chiasm. To reach the chiasm, the optic nerves extend posteriorly and medially and ascend at a 45° angle. The intracranial portion of the optic nerve is 10 to 16 mm long.

Optic Chiasm

Nerve fibers, representing retinal points and transmitted in the two optic nerves, join in the optic chiasm. In the optic chiasm, some fibers pass uncrossed whereas others cross (see page 103).

Macular fibers form a large portion of the chiasm. Nasal, crossed macular fibers decussate in the posterior portion of the chiasm, whereas nasal retinal ganglion cells form ventral fibers that cross interiorly within the chiasm. These fibers loop into the terminal portion of the opposite optic nerve, a loop that has been called Willebrandt's knee.

The optic chiasm has significant contiguous structures lying close to the third ventricle and above the pituitary gland.

Optic Tracts

The optic tracts begin at the posterior of the chiasm. Each tract diverges and continues posteriorly to end in the lateral geniculate body. The tracts contain visual and pupillomotor fibers. They also contain crossed nasal retinal fibers from the opposite eye and uncrossed temporal retinal fibers from the eye on the same side. All visual fibers in the optic tract synapse in the geniculate body; however, the pupillomotor fibers project through the geniculate body.

The Lateral Geniculate Body

The termination of all visual pathway fibers separates into six layers in the lateral geniculate body. Retinal ganglion cells from the eye on the same side synapse in layers II, III, and V, whereas cells from the opposite side synapse in layers I, IV, and VI. In the lateral geniculate body, a 90° rotation occurs so that the nerve fibers from the superior retina lie medially (not superiorly) in the lateral geniculate body and fibers from the inferior retina lie laterally. As fibers leave the lateral geniculate body, retinal fibers lie superiorly and inferior retinal fibers lie inferiorly in the optic radiation and cerebral cortex.

Optic Radiations

From the optic tracts, the visual fibers pass into the optic radiations. Superior fibers leave the lateral geniculate body and proceed directly to the occipital cortex. Inferior fibers loop around the ventricular system into the temporal lobe; this is known as Meyer's loop.

The optic radiations contain three main groups of fibers: the superior portion contains fibers from the inferior visual field, the inferior portion contains fibers from the superior visual field, and the central portion contains fibers of central vision from the macula.

Occipital Cortex

Occipital cortex is also called the striate cortex or area 17. This area is situated along the superior and inferior lips of the calcarine fissure.

Macular fibers make up the majority of the occipital cortex. Macular fibers lie at the occipital tip of the lobe. More peripheral visual field fibers project to the visual cortex and lie more anteriorly along the medial side of the hemisphere.

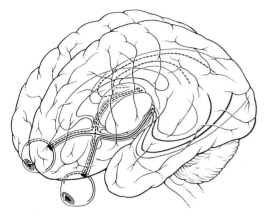

Figure 5.7. The optic disc is the point at which all ganglion cell fibers leave the eye to enter the optic nerve. The optic disc is 1 mm in depth and approximately 1.5 mm across.

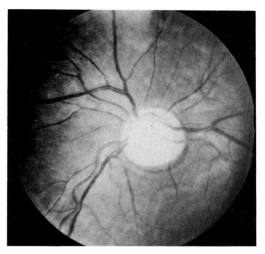

Figure 5.8. Optic nerve atrophy. The optic nerve appears pale and white in contrast to the normal nerve, which has a pinkish coloration. There is a large cup in the optic nerve. The edge of the cup can be estimated to be where the arteries and veins on the nerve head dip posteriorly.

Optic Disc (Fig. 5.7)

In the region of the optic disc, we can see ophthalmoscopic changes that are significant. The most frequent clinical sign is disc swelling or, later, pallor (Fig. 5.8); the vision may or may not be affected. In this section of the text, common changes of the optic disc are discussed.

Papilledema

Papilledema (Fig. 5.9) is passive swelling of the optic disc. It is caused by increased intracranial pressure and is usually not associated with central visual loss.

Clinical Correlations. Infratentorial tumors that arise from the cerbellum and fourth ventricle tend to increase intracranial pressure *early* by obstruction of flow. Tumors at the base of the skull and in the brain stem, such as pontine glioma, however, cause increased intracranial pressure *late*. Supratentorial tumors and third ventricular tumors frequently cause papilledema. Papilledema is rarely seen with pituitary adenomas. The incidence of papilledema is low in parasagittal and parietooccipital tumors. Of patients with cerebral tumors, 60% will have papilledema at some time during the course of the disease.

Papilledema is uncommon in infants because the fontanels are not closed and the cranial sutures are not fused. The fontanels will bulge with an enlarging tumor mass and surrounding edema. Papilledema will not usually occur until the age of 2 to 10 years.

As a rule, papilledema is bilateral. Unilateral papilledema may be encountered in special circumstances.

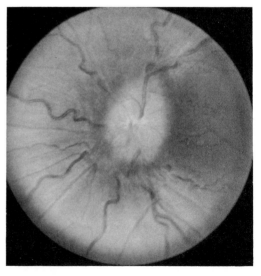

Figure 5.9. Papilledema is a blurred disc margin secondary to increased intracranial pressure. Its characteristics are a reddish discoloration of the disc (hyperemia) engorgement and tortuosity of the retinal vessels, a blurred disc margin, obscuration of the small marginal vessels along the optic disc, and loss of the normal central physiologic cup.

- A frontal lobe tumor may compress the optic nerve on the side of the tumor, causing optic atrophy while simultaneously increasing the intracranial pressure and producing papilledema in the other eye (called Foster Kennedy's syndrome).
- There may be preexisting unilateral optic disc anomaly or optic atrophy preventing swelling.
- When the perioptic meningeal space is interrupted by compression or obliteration due to congenital anomalies or tumors, only one side may show papilledema.

Cause of Papilledema. Increased pressure of the blood supply to the optic nerve produces axoplasmic transport obstruction. Intraaxonal swelling occurs because the axoplasm cannot flow down the axon.

Features of Papilledema by Ophthalmoscopy (Fully Developed Edema)

- Blurred disc margins;
- Elevation of the disc margins;
- Edema most evident in inferior and superior margins;
- Optic nerve fibers appearing striated;
- Small vessels at the disc margin that are obscured as they cross the margin;
- Hyperemic disc;
- Capillary and venous dilation;
- Hemorrhages at the disc and peripapillary retina (flame shape);
- Absent spontaneous venous pulsations (may be variable);
- Obliterated central cup (may not occur until the late stages).

Symptoms of Papilledema. The majority of patients do not lose vision. Only in the late stages is vision lost. This *preservation of central vision* is a differential diagnostic point between papilledema and disc swelling due to inflammation (papillitis, neuritis).

Recurrent transient obscuration of vision in one or both eyes, which may alternate between the two eyes, may help to establish the diagnosis. This transient obscuration lasts usually about 5 seconds and rarely more than 30 seconds. The obscuration of vision starts and ends abruptly. Vision is restored to normal at the end of the attack. Attacks occur frequently during the day and may be precipitated or aggravated by a sitting position, by stooping, or by turning the head abruptly.

Anterior Ischemic Optic Neuropathy (AION)

Clinical Presentation.

Onset. The onset is usually in middle age or later (aged 50 years and older).

Visual Loss. There is usually a rapid, painless loss of vision in one eye. Patients may characteristically notice the visual loss on awakening in the morning. In up to one-quarter of patients, visual loss may occur in a series of steps over days to weeks. This has been likened to a "stuttering" downhill course. The amount of visual loss is variable.

The visual field loss is unique. An *altitudinal* or broad arcuate visual field defect is present in 70 to 80% of patients with AION. The altitudinal defect is most commonly *inferior.* A visual field defect is less common in the central or nerve fiber bundle area. Altered color vision (dyschromatopsia) usually parallels the acuity loss.

Afferent Pupillary Defect. Afferent pupillary defect (see page 92) will be present unless there has been contralateral optic neuropathy, which would mask the decreased conduction defect.

Optic Disc Changes. Optic disc swelling is present at the onset of the visual loss but may on occasion precede the visual loss. The disc usually appears pale, although occasionally it may be hyperemic. Only portions of the disc may be involved. Very commonly, there are hemorrhages in the adjacent nerve fiber layers. Focal peripapillary arteriole narrowing is seen in 50% of the patients with AION and is more common in hypertensive patients. Optic atrophy appears as early as 1 week after the onset of symptoms but usually takes 3 weeks to appear.

Prognosis. Visual improvement is rare after the lowest level of visual acuity has been reached.

Causes of Anterior Ischemic Optic Neuropathy. By far the most common cause is giant cell arteritis. There is also a nonarteritic cause of AION. Other disorders much less frequently present as AION.

Giant Cell Arteritis (Also Discussed on Page 166). Giant cell arteritis is caused by inflammatory thickening and thrombosis within the microvascular circulation around the optic nerve head. (This circulation comes from short posterior ciliary arteries.) Giant cell arteritis occurs in older individuals (mean age, 70 years). Visual loss is severe, and vision is less than 20/200 in three-quarters of the patients.

If untreated, the second eye becomes affected in 65% of patients, usually within a few weeks. Therefore, establishment of the diagnosis is important.

Associated Systemic Symptoms. The most reliable and consistent symptoms are

- Headache;
- Temporal artery tenderness;
- Pain on chewing (jaw claudication).

Giant cell arteritis may also be associated with polymyalgia rheumatica, which presents with malaise, anorexia, weight loss, fever, and joint and muscle pain (arthralgias, myalgias). About 40% of patients with polymyalgia rheumatica will have fully developed giant cell arteritis, 16% with permanent visual loss. Many more will develop more benign forms of giant cell arteritis.

It is not uncommon for giant cell arteritis to present without symptoms. Giant cell arteritis should be looked for when evaluating an older patient with visual loss, either uniocular or biocular.

Diagnosis.

1. Erythrocyte sedimentation rate. A Westergren sedimentation rate of greater than 70 mm per hour is suggestive of diagnosis. In giant cell arteritis, values of greater than 100 mm per hour are often found. This test is extremely useful but is nonspecific for giant cell arteritis. Also, a few patients with giant cell arteritis will not have positive erythrocyte sedimentation rates.

2. Temporal artery biopsy. There is a 5 to 10% false-negative biopsy rate in giant cell arteritis. The biopsy is taken from the temporal artery. There are involved areas interspersed with normal areas. Because of these "skip areas," a biopsy of 3 to 6 cm of arterial specimen is advised.

Unilateral temporal artery involvement may also occur. If giant cell arteritis is suspected and one temporal biopsy is negative, a biopsy on the opposite side may be considered.

Important Clinical Point. If giant cell arteritis is suspected clinically, steroids should be started immediately. The results of the biopsy can be used to confirm the diagnosis. Steroids are effective in treatment, and there is rarely justification for waiting for a biopsy report when the diagnosis is suspected. Prompt treatment is especially important because steroids reduce the chance of involvement of the second eye, reduce systemic complications, and improve symptoms dramatically within a few hours to days. The response to steroids may also help establish the diagnosis.

Nonarteritic Anterior Ischemic Optic Neuropathy. The mean age of onset for this group is 60 years. When compared to giant cell arteritis, the visual loss is not as severe, being worse than 20/200 in 42% of patients. Usually, there are no associated symptoms. The second eye is affected in 40% of patients; in a large majority, this occurs within 1 year of onset in the first eye. Repeated attacks in the same eye are extremely rare. The erythrocyte sedimentation rate (ESR) in these patients is usually consistent with age, which is not true in giant cell arteritis. (The ESR normally rises with advancing age.)

Nonarteritic anterior ischemic optic neuropathy is associated with the following conditions:

- Hypertension—36 to 45%;
- Diabetes—10 to 20% [high association (50%) of diabetes with anterior ischemic optic neuropathy in patients under the age of 40];
- Carotid disease—rare cause;
- Cardiovascular disease—a questionable association.

The cause of nonarteritic anterior ischemic optic neuropathy is probably widespread occlusive disease within the microvascular supply to the optic nerve head. There is an *association in this condition with a small cup/disc ratio in the fellow eye.* It is probable that alterations in the disc relate to mechanical causes: axoplasmic flow stasis and axonal swelling. Axonal swelling leads to microvascular compression and further ischemia. The whole process results in necrosis and loss of nerve fibers.

In contrast to giant cell arteritis, the use of steroids in this condition is questionably effective and controversial. Other forms of therapy have also proved nonproductive in preventing visual loss in this disease.

Other Disorders Causing AION.

1. Non-giant cell vasculitis is caused by systemic lupus erythematosus, unspecified connective tissue disease, or periarteritis nodosa.

2. Migraine can cause AION. This is in a *younger age group,* usually under 30. Migraine has usually been previously diagnosed at the onset of AION. AION occurs immediately after a typical migraine attack and is usually *unilateral.*

3. Severe blood loss anemia usually occurs in debilitated patients in the 40- to 60-year-old age group. Visual loss occurs within 48 hours. Involvement is usually bilateral and may be symmetrical.

4. Cataract extraction can precede AION by a few weeks. The cause is unknown. However, the diagnosis is important because AION tends to occur after operation in the fellow eye.

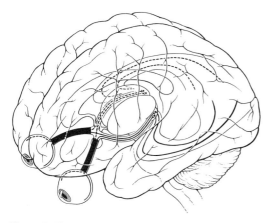

Figure 5.10. The optic nerve courses from the globe to the optic chiasm.

Optic Nerve (Fig. 5.10)

Optic Neuritis

Clinical Features of Optic Nerve Involvement.

- Visual acuity normal or reduced
- Color vision normal or reduced
- Visual field—central scotoma
- Relative afferent pupillary defect
- Possible disc pallor or swelling

Clinical Characteristics. Optic neuritis occurs in younger patients (20 to 50 years) and more often affects women than men. It is typically monocular. The visual loss occurs over a few hours to many days and is extremely variable. Visual field loss includes a central scotoma (page 357) in more than 90% of cases. Less frequent are arcuate or altitudinal defects. Altered color vision (dyschromatopsia), worse for red, occurs out of proportion to the acuity loss.

Pain. Periocular pain usually precedes the visual loss and is characteristically worse with movements of the eyes. Pain is present in more than 80% of patients.

Pupillary Defect. An afferent relative pupillary defect is caused by decreased conduction (see page 92).

Optic Disc Swelling (Papillitis) (Fig. 5.11). Papillitis is present in less than one-half of the cases. Optic disc swelling has no correlation with visual loss or the prognosis for visual recovery.

Course. Most cases spontaneously improve. The improvement starts within a few weeks and continues for weeks to months. Visual recovery to the 20/30 to 20/40 range occurs in 50 to 80% of patients.

Causes of Optic Neuritis.
- Idiopathic (may be a forme fruste of multiple sclerosis)
- Multiple sclerosis. The risk of developing multiple sclerosis after an isolated single episode of optic neuritis has been reported to be up to 85%. A prospective study has shown that, within a 7-year follow-up period, 35% develop definite or probable multiple

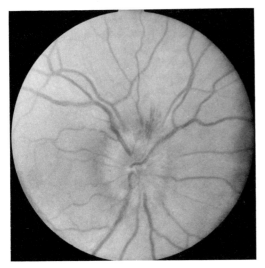

Figure 5.11. Optic neuritis is an inflammatory condition of the optic disc. When compared to papilledema, optic neuritis characteristically causes decrease in vision, whereas papilledema is not associated with a visual loss until later. Optic neuritis is localized inflammation of the optic nerve; papilledema is swelling around the optic nerve secondary to increased intracranial pressure.

sclerosis. The risk of developing multiple sclerosis is higher in women than in men and is higher in the younger age group (from 21 to 40 years) than in the older age group.

- After viral infection. Optic neuritis after viral infection is usually bilateral and occurs in children or young adults. Vision usually returns to normal. The association with multiple sclerosis is extremely low. When the diagnosis can be made, postinfection neuritis usually follows measles, mumps, or herpes zoster.
- Granulomatous inflammations: syphilis, sarcoidosis
- Other causes: sinusitis, tuberculosis, paralytic disease

Differential Diagnosis of Optic Neuritis.
1. Anterior Ischemic Optic Neuropathy (AION). See Table 5.1
2. Hereditary: Leber's Optic Neuropathy. Leber's optic neuropathy occurs in young persons and most often occurs in males. After one eye is affected, the second eye is affected within a few weeks. There is severe visual loss unassociated with pain in most cases. There is pathognomonic fundus change. Peripapillary telangiectatic vessels occur within the peripapillary nerve fiber layer, which swells. These are shunt vessels and do not leak fluorescein.

3. Compression of the Optic Nerve. When compression causes decreased vision, the course is usually slowly downhill. There may also be orbital changes such as proptosis, eyelid signs, and limitation of ocular motility. If there is intracranial compression, it may affect the other eye. A junctional scotoma (see page 310) may be present.

4. Other Rare Causes: Toxic or nutritional deficiencies; infiltration from carcinoma, leukemia, or granulomatous disease processes.

Table 5.1.
Differential Diagnosis of Neuritis and Ischemic Optic Neuropathy

Optic Neuritis	Anterior Ischemic Optic Neuropathy
Young patient, most often female	Usually older than 50
Monocular	Starts monocular; high percentage become binocular
Altitudinal or arcuate visual field defect (see page 106)	Central scotoma (see page 357) characteristic
Color vision disturbance out of proportion to visual loss	Color vision disturbance proportional to visual loss
Typical pain with motion of the globe	Usually painless
Afferent pupillary defect present	Afferent pupillary defect present
Visual improvement common	Visual improvement rare
Questionable response or no response to steroids	Steroids reduce symptoms, decrease incidence of opposite eye involvement, may decrease recurrence
Erythrocyte sedimentation rate (ESR) normal	ESR abnormal if giant cell arteritis is the cause

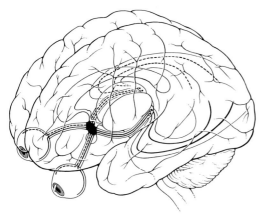

Figure 5.12. The optic chiasm is where the optic nerves meet and the optic tracts diverge. The optic chiasm is where some nerve fibers cross and others pass uncrossed.

The Chiasm

The chiasm (Fig. 5.12) is important in differential diagnosis because it produces characteristic symptoms and signs. The visual fields in patients with chiasmal lesions most often show the highly specific bitemporal hemianopsia, which is so characteristic as to be diagnostic.

Awareness of chiasmal lesions that produce visual loss and optic atrophy is also important when following patients with glaucoma. Optic atrophy atypical in either appearance or progression in a glaucoma patient should make the ophthalmologist suspect a chiasmal lesion.

Chiasmal Syndromes

The optic nerves meet in the chiasm, where some visual fibers cross to the opposite side while others pass through without crossing. Fibers then course into the optic tracts from the chiasm. Because of the anatomical distribution of crossed and uncrossed fibers in the chiasm, characteristic visual field changes occur—*bitemporal hemianopic defects.*

To understand the localizing visual field changes of chiasmal lesions, think of nerve fiber crossing. One-half of the nerve fibers in the chiasm are crossed; that is, the right eye fibers go to the left brain and the left eye fibers go to the right brain. The temporal field of vision is served by axons from the retinal elements nasal to the fovea, and these are exclu-

sively crossing fibers. Macula fibers are crossed and clustered in the posterior chiasm. Crossed fibers in the temporal visual fields tend to cross anterior in the chiasm and sweep briefly into the contralateral optic nerve (Willebrandt's knee) before going on into the chiasm.

The result of a chiasmal lesion is a bitemporal defect of the visual field. In a bitemporal defect, the temporal portion of the left field and the temporal portion of the right field are affected. Because of the nerve fiber distribution, the vertical meridian is not crossed by the defect, an important diagnostic point.

Other causes of bitemporal defects are congenital tilted optic disc, papilledema with enlarged blind spots, and nasal sector retinal lesions bilaterally. Although these lesions may produce bitemporal defects, differential diagnosis from a chiasmal syndrome is not difficult because the vertical meridian is usually not respected except in chiasmal involvement.

Signs and Symptoms

Of all brain tumors, 25% occur in the chiasm. Approximately half of these will present with ophthalmic symptoms. This makes the physician's awareness of chiasmal symptoms all the more important.

Symptoms associated with a chiasmal syndrome may include headaches, fatigue, impotence, menorrhagia, and signs of gonadal, thyroid, or adrenal insufficiency. Classical signs and symptoms of chiasmal syndromes are:

- Bitemporal visual field defects that respect the vertical meridian;
- Endocrine dysfunction;
- Normal or reduced vision;
- Normal pupils unless visual field involvement is asymmetrical (optic atrophy may be present if long-standing);
- Papilledema rarely;
- See-saw nystagmus as a good localizing sign, although it is unusual.

Additional Important Points about the Chiasmal Syndrome

- Chiasmal syndrome may be related to a failure to thrive in children; think craniopharyngioma.

- Small pituitary tumors may not produce visual defects early.
- Lesions of the posterior chiasm tend to produce small paracentral bitemporal defects.
- Lesions of the posterior optic portion of the chiasm may produce blindness on one side with a temporal field defect in the upper quadrant of the opposite side (due to Willebrandt's knee) (see Fig. 16.43).
- Visual field defects with chiasmal syndrome may be extremely variable, and classical bitemporal hemianopsia may not be present.
- Decompression of a chiasmal lesion that is causing compression chiasmal dysfunction may result in visual return.

Causes of Chiasmal Dysfunction

Common Causes of Chiasmal Dysfunction.
1. Pituitary Adenomas. These tumors tend to be small with symptoms related to hormonal dysfunction. Adenomas do not affect visual acuity and visual fields unless they have grown very large.

Pituitary tumors that involve the chiasm are divided into nonsecreting and secreting types. Secreting types produce Cushing's syndrome or acromegaly. The most common nonsecreting tumor type is pituitary adenoma.

2. Craniopharyngioma. These are common tumors in children. They are often associated with growth delay and failure to thrive.

3. Sphenoid Meningiomas. These are predominantly seen in middle-aged women. Patients may remain remarkably free of symptoms until the disease process has progressed.

4. Intracranial Gliomas. These are most often found in children who may or may not have manifestations of neurofibromatosis (see page 168).

Less Common Causes of Chiasmal Dysfunction.
1. Sinus Mucoceles. There is usually a long-standing history of recurrent sinus infection when mucoceles are present.

2. Suprasellar Aneurysms. In these cases, visual fields tend to be high and asymmetrical. Patients may have episodes of severe pain.

3. Compression by a Dilated Anterior Third Ventricle. Tumors, such a pineal tumor, may produce obstructive hydrocephalus, which in turn causes a falsely localizing bitemporal hemianopsia.

4. Empty Sella Syndrome. This is usually associated with pseudotumor cerebri but may follow surgical treatment for pituitary tumor.

Causes of Chiasmal Dysfunction Not Related to Compression.
1. Demyelination. Demyelination is a rare cause of bitemporal hemianopsia and multiple sclerosis. The chiasm is known to be frequently involved in multiple sclerosis, however, as evidenced on postmortem examinations.

2. Optochiasmic Arachnoiditis. This is a rare cause.

3. Trauma. This is usually from frontal impact on the skull, which may disrupt the chiasm.

4. Occlusive Vascular Disease. This is rare because of the multiple sources of blood supply to the chiasm.

5. Aneurysms of the Internal Carotid or Anterior Cerebral Arteries. These may present as a chiasmal syndrome.

A Rare Cause of Chiasmal Dysfunction. Posterior fossa lesions may cause hydrocephalus with dilation of the third ventricle, which exerts pressure on the chiasm. This may present with visual field defects suggestive of a chiasmal lesion. Patients with posterior fossa lesions will also have papilledema.

Posterior Pathways: Optic Tract (Fig. 5.13), Radiations (Fig. 5.14), and Occipital Lobe (Fig. 5.15)

Important Diagnostic Features

- Visual acuity may be normal or reduced.
- Color vision may be normal or reduced.
- Visual field—homonymous defect, incongruous.
- Relative afferent pupillary defect may be present.
- Disc pallor may be present.

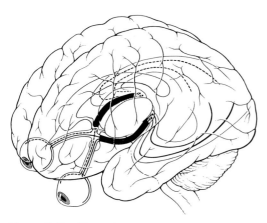

Figure 5.13. The optic tract is that portion of the visual fibers that leaves the optic chiasm and extends back to the geniculate body.

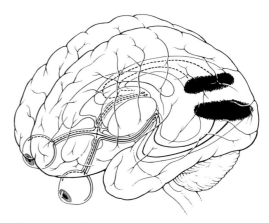

Figure 5.15. Visual fibers terminate in the visual cortex. The macula is represented by those visual fibers most posterior in the occipital cortex. Temporal fibers are more anterior.

In addition to visual field changes, other characteristics may help localize lesions within the visual pathways.

All lesions anterior to the optic radiations (and the geniculate) will interrupt nerve fibers whose cell bodies connect with retinal ganglion cells. With lesions anterior to the optic radiations, therefore, characteristic patterns of nerve fiber layer dropout and optic nerve atrophy will occur.

Of retrogeniculate lesions, temporal lobe lesions often cause seizures and formed visual hallucinations. Parietal lobe lesions may cause visual perceptual difficulties, agnosias, acalculia, and left/right confusion.

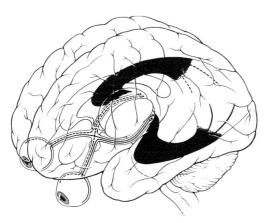

Figure 5.14. Optic radiation. Nerve visual fibers synapse in the geniculate bodies. After that synapse, visual fibers radiate posteriorly to terminate eventually in the occipital cortex.

Abnormalities in optokinetic nystagmus (see page 112) are most often associated with parietal lobe lesions. The optokinetic nystagmus will be abnormal when targets are rotated toward the lesion. This will be opposite to the side of the hemianopsia. A combination of a homonymous hemianopsia and abnormal optokinetic nystagmus suggests a parietal lobe lesion, most often a neoplasm.

In the occipital lobe, where congruous homonymous hemianopsia and sparing of the macula occur, unformed visual hallucinations may also occur. It is very unusual for occipital lobe lesions to cause abnormalities in optokinetic nystagmus.

Optic Tract Syndrome

Description. Optic tract syndrome is characterized by incongruous homonymous hemianopsia, reduced central visual acuity, and a relative afferent pupillary defect. Optic atrophy (Fig. 5.8) may or may not be present. Disturbances of visual function are often described vaguely. A washout of colors and fine detail or a description of glare may be initial signs.

The relative afferent pupillary defect is seen in 80% of patients with optic tract syndrome. The defect is usually present in the eye on the same side as the lesion (but occasionally it is on the opposite side).

Causes. The most common causes are craniopharyngioma, pituitary tumor, aneurysm, and demyelinating disease.

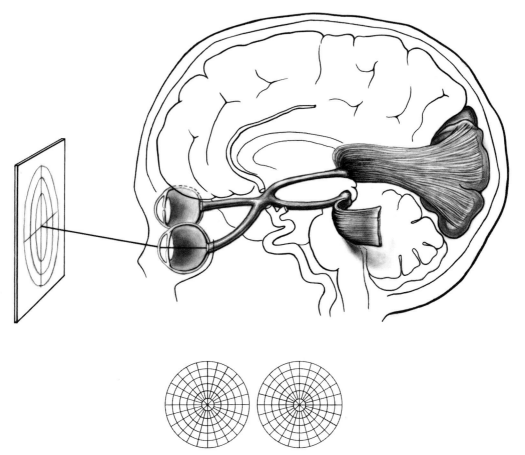

Figure 5.16. Visual fields—basics. Illustrated are the visual field screen and the direction of light. The left eye is being tested. The optic pathways, including the optic nerves, the optic chiasm, the optic tracts, and the optic radiations, are shown. Below are two diagrammatic representations of the visual field used for mapping visual field defects. Visual field testing is done one eye at a time, as illustrated. Recording outlines are presented for the left eye and the right eye.

Visual Field Defects (Fig. 5.16)

Optic Nerve (Fig. 5.17)

Visual field defects due to optic nerve lesions generally show a loss of field in the central visual area. This is because 25% of all fibers in the optic nerve subserve the central 5° of the visual field. Optic nerve defects cause:

1. Central Scotoma. This is a blind spot in the center of vision that is characteristic of optic neuritis but may also be caused by compression of the optic nerve.

2. Cecocentral Scotoma. These are blind spots around the area of central vision that are associated with toxic optic neuropathies.

Cecocentral scotoma is also associated with both Leber's optic neuropathy and optic pit with serous retinal detachment.

3. Arcuate Scotoma. These are arc-like defects in the visual field either above or below the area of fixation. Arcuate scotomas are caused by damage to superior and inferior quadrant nerve fiber bundles. They are seen with optic neuritis and ischemic optic neuropathies. However, arcuate scotomas are classically associated with open angle glaucoma (see page 48).

4. Altitudinal Field Defect. This is a field defect in either the lower half or, at times, the upper half of the visual field. The defect crosses the midline and is associated with ischemic optic neuropathy. Compression of an intracranial portion of the optic nerve can also produce an altitudinal defect.

Optic Chiasm (Fig. 5.18)

The classic sign of chiasmal visual field involvement is bitemporal hemianopsia. These defects do not cross the vertical midline.

Fiber damage at the anterior angle of the chiasm may produce a *junctional scotoma* (see page 310), which is loss of visual acuity and a central scotoma in one eye with a superior temporal field defect in the opposite eye. Lesions damaging the chiasm produce bitemporal hemianopsia with a field defect without loss of central visual acuity. Characteristically, posterior angle chiasmal defects produce *bitemporal hemianopic scotomas.*

Optic Tract

Visual field defects of the optic tract are homonymous (that is, they occur in each eye on the same side of the visual space). Optic tract field defects respect the vertical midline. In optic tract defects, there may be incongruity (that is, a lack of similarity of the homonymous defects between the right and the left field).

Retrogeniculate Lesions (Fig. 5.19)

The homonymous hemianopsias that are produced by lesions in the temporal lobe tend to have an incongruous appearance (that is, lack of similarity between the eyes) and tend also to be denser in the superior field areas. Homonymous hemianopsias produced by parietal lobe lesions tend to be relatively more congruous than those due to temporal lesions and have either complete or denser inferior field defects.

Occipital Cortex

Visual fields in patients with occipital cortex lesions show homonymous hemianopsias (Fig. 5.20) that are similar or extremely congruous (Fig. 5.21). Sparing of the macula occurs with occipital lesions. In addition to homonymous hemianopsias, other visual field defects may be classically associated with occipital lobe lesions.

1. Checkerboard Field. This is a bilateral, incomplete homonymous hemianopsia that is superior on one side and inferior on the other side.

2. Bilateral Homonymous Hemianopsia with Macular Sparing—Keyhole Field. This usually presents as a tubular field. With careful field analysis, however, vertical meridian can be found, which shows the characteristics of bilateral homonymous hemianopsia.

3. Cortical Blindness. This is a rare syndrome of complete blindness associated with normal pupillary responses.

4. Bilateral Homonymous Altitudinal Defects. These are most often inferior and are caused by infarction or trauma to both occipital lobes.

Homonymous Hemianopsias (Fig. 5.20)

Of all homonymous hemianopsias, 90% are due to stroke. Occipital lobe homonymous hemianopsia is associated with macular sparing. Parietal lobe hemianopsias are associated with asymmetrical optokinetic nystagmus responses. Visual acuity is never reduced by a homonymous hemianopsia, even when the macula is involved, because 20/20 vision is possible with only half of the macular area functioning. In homonymous defects of the temporal lobe, the upper field is denser and, in parietal lesions, the lower field is denser.

Binasal Field Defects. Binasal defects are caused by bilateral retinal or optic nerve lesions. They are not due to compression of the optic chiasm. Only bitemporal hemianopsias are produced by lesions of the chiasm.

Monocular Field Defects. Field defects from retinal and optic nerve lesions produce monocular field defects. These do not, in general, respect the vertical meridian.

A monocular field defect may be caused by a posterior brain (retrogeniculate) lesion. The visual fields of the two eyes do not completely overlap in the occipital cortex. In each temporal field, there is 30° in the peripheral region that is monocular in each eye. The nerve fibers corresponding to this monocular retinal region are located in the most anterior portion of the visual cortex. Lesions that affect this anterior visual cortex may produce a purely monocular visual field defect in spite of being posterior to the chiasm. This field defect is called the *temporal crescent syndrome.*

Figure 5.17. Visual field—optic nerve lesion. A transection of the left optic nerve produces complete blindness in the left visual field.

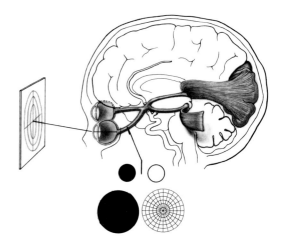

Figure 5.18. Visual fields—bitemporal hemianopsia. In the chiasmal regions, visual fibers from both eyes cross while others from both eyes remain on the same side as their origination in the eye. This combination of crossing and noncrossing produces characteristic field defects within the chiasm. Illustrated are the crossing and noncrossing fibers in the chiasm. A lesion at the chiasm is diagrammatically represented as loss of vision on the temporal side of both eyes. Actual visual field representation is noted *below*. This is called bitemporal hemianopsia.

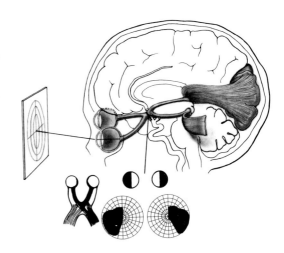

Figure 5.19. Visual field—homonymous quadrantanopsia. Illustrated is a lesion in the optic radiations. A lesion anterior in the optic radiation produces homonymous quadrantanopsia. This is involvement on the same side of both visual fields in only the involved quadrant. Illustrated is a superior right homonymous quadrantanopsia. These may be irregular when comparing one side to the other (incongruity).

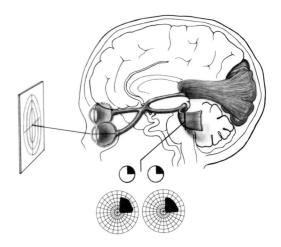

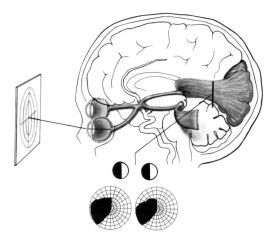

Figure 5.20. Visual field—homonymous hemianopsia. Illustrated is a lesion in the posterior portion of the optic tract. The visual field defect as measured in both eyes will be on the same side (homonymous), and half of the visual field is involved (hemianopsia). The diagram of homonymous hemianopsia and the appearance of a field defect on the visual field screen are illustrated. There is a distinct vertical line. This distinct vertical line should be sought in a neurologic field when hemianopsia is suspected. Illustrated is a left homonymous hemianopsia.

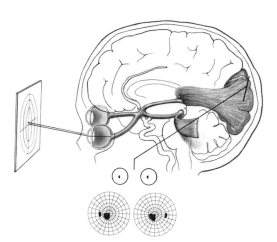

Figure 5.21. Visual field—occipital lobe lesion. Illustrated is a lesion in the posterior portion of the brain near the macular region, which produces sharp visual defects that are almost exactly alike (congruous). The diagrammatic representation and the appearance on visual field charting are both shown. The vertical line is carefully respected, a typical feature of neurologic fields. The reproducibility between the left eye and the right eye is more exact the more posterior the lesion. This type of posterior lesion is most often vascular in origin.

CRANIAL NERVE PALSIES

The causes of isolated third nerve, isolated fourth nerve, or isolated sixth nerve palsies are 30% undetermined, 20% microvascular (diabetes, hypertension), 15% traumatic (except in fourth nerve palsy, with 30% due to trauma), 15% due to tumor in third nerve and sixth nerve palsies, and 15% due to aneuryism in third nerve palsy.

Sixth Nerve Palsies

Congenital sixth nerve isolated palsies are rare.

Acquired Sixth Nerve Palsies

1. Nuclear. This is an inability of the eye to move (a horizontal conjugate gaze palsy) to the same side as the lesion. There is an associated facial nerve (VII) palsy. This palsy is most often caused by ischemia, infiltration, trauma, inflammation, or compression.

2. Vascular. A cause of Foville's syndrome (see page 294) and Millard-Gubler syndrome (see page 321). The causes are ischemia, tumor infiltration or compression, infection, or inflammation, particularly demyelination.

3. Subarachnoid. Caused by increased intracranial pressure. Can be due to basilar artery aneurysm, tumor, or meningitis. It can also be seen after shunting for hydrocephalus or after lumbar puncture. Brain stem herniation can cause traction on the nerve and present with palsy of the sixth nerve.

4. Cavernous Sinus. Check for a sixth nerve palsy and a Horner's syndrome on the same side as the lesion. This may also be associated with Gradenigo's syndrome (page 297).

5. Orbit. Restriction of the rectus muscle causing poor out-turning of the eye (abduction) may simulate palsy.

Third Nerve Palsies

Congenital Third Nerve Abnormalities

Congenital third nerve palsy is unilateral and presents with lid droop (ptosis) and loss of ocular movements (ophthalmoplegia) to varying degrees.

Acquired Third Nerve Palsies

1. Nuclear. This is extremely rare. It presents with bilaterial ptosis when ptosis is present. There is bilateral limitation of upgaze.

2. Fascicular. This presents as ophthalmoplegia on the same side as the lesion with pupillary involvement. There are a number of associated signs:

A. Nothnagel's Syndrome. Third nerve involvement on the same side as the lesion with cerebellar ataxia, dysmetria, and dysdiadochokinesia.

B. Benedikt's Syndrome. This is third nerve involvement on the same side as the lesion with contralateral involuntary movements of choreoathetosis, Parkinson's tremor and hemiballismus. There is involvement of the red nucleus.

C. Claude's Syndrome. This is a combination of Nothnagel's and Benedikt's syndromes.

D. Weber's Syndrome. This involves the third nerve on the same side as the lesion with a contralateral hemiparesis.

All of these syndromes are associated with ischemia or infiltration and other less common causes.

3. Subarachnoid. This may present as a possible pupil-sparing third nerve palsy. It can be caused by trauma, ischemia, aneurysm, or meningitis.

4. Cavernous Sinus. This is usually associated with other cranial nerve palsies. The sphenocavernous syndrome involves the cavernous sinus, third nerve, fourth nerve, sixth nerve, and the first and second branches of the fifth nerve. The superior orbital fissure syndrome involves the third nerve, the fourth nerve, the sixth nerve, and the first branch of the fifth nerve.

5. Orbital Apex Syndrome. This involves the third, fourth, and sixth nerves and the first branch of the fifth nerve, as well as the optic nerve, with proptosis of the globe and chemosis of the orbit. It is caused by a mass within the orbit, which originates in the orbit, the paranasal sinuses, or the intracranial cavity.

Trochlear Palsy (IV)

Palsies of the trochlear nerve (cranial nerve IV) are most frequently due to trauma. Closed head trauma is due to contrecoup forces transmitted to the brain stem by the free tentorial edge. Bilateral traumatic trochlear palsies occur where the nerves emerge together. The second most common cause of trochlear palsies is diabetes mellitus. A less common cause is pressure on the nerve due to hydrocephalus, vascular loops, or tumors. Aneurysm is a very rare cause of an isolated trochlear palsy.

Congenital fourth nerve paralysis, which is not uncommon, may present as a long-standing head tilt. The head tilt is used to maintain binocular vision.

Diagnosis

The three-step test (see page 153) is used to diagnose trochlear nerve palsy.

How to Distinguish between a Unilateral and a Bilateral Superior Oblique Paralysis (Fourth Nerve)

In bilateral superior oblique palsy, one finds:

- Right hypertropia in left gaze and left hypertropia in right gaze;
- A positive Bielschowsky head tilt test (see page 260) to each shoulder;
- A small vertical deviation in the primary position and V-pattern esotropia (see page 258) in downgaze;
- Underaction of both superior oblique muscles with no or only mild overaction of inferior oblique muscles;
- Greater than 6° of ocular torsion by the double Maddox rod;
- A history of severe head trauma with coma.

FACIAL NERVE (SEVENTH NERVE)

Clinical Evaluation of Facial Nerve Function

The facial nerve is responsible for movements of the face and blink. Normally, movements of the face and blink are symmetrical. An asymmetry indicates lack of facial nerve function.

Various muscle groups are tested by asking the patient (*a*) to smile, (*b*) to close the lids forcibly, and (*c*) to wrinkle the forehead.

The corneal blink reflex is tested by touching the cornea and observing the blink. This tests not only facial nerve function (blink), but also trigeminal nerve function (sensory from the cornea).

The sensory portion of the facial nerve can also be tested. Taste on the anterior two-thirds of the tongue and cutaneous sensation along the external auditory canal can be tested. Autonomic functions such as salivation and lacrimation can also be tested.

Lesions of the facial nerve from the cerebellopontine angle to the geniculate ganglion impair all functions of the nerve, whereas lesions distal to the geniculate ganglion affect only certain functions, depending upon location.

Common Facial Nerve Lesions

Bell's Palsy

This is the most common type of facial neuropathy. It occurs in adults.

Bell's palsy starts as a sudden onset of facial paralysis. Pain may precede the palsy. Facial numbness may also be reported. Decreased tearing and diminished taste may also be noted. The cause is unknown. It is associated, however, with diabetes mellitus, hypertension, and pregnancy.

Of all patients, 75% will have complete spontaneous recovery. Among the 25% of patients without total recovery, partial recovery may occur. Aberrant regeneration of the nerve is common.

The most serious complication is corneal exposure while blink remains inactive or diminished. Corneal exposure may be severe and may result in perforation. In mild cases, artificial tear preparations and lubricants are satisfactory. In more severe cases, the eyelid must be taped shut or closed with sutures (tarsorrhaphy).

Tumors of the Cerebellopontine Angle

Cerebellopontine angle tumors involve the facial nerve.

Sarcoidosis

Sarcoidosis involves the facial nerve more than any other cranial nerve. The point of involvement is usually the parotid gland. Facial nerve involvement is often bilateral and tends to be asymmetrical.

Others

See also Melkersson-Rosenthal syndrome (page 319), Ramsay Hunt's syndrome (page 348), and Fisher's syndrome (page 292) (facial diplegia may occur with Fisher's syndrome).

RECORDING OF NYSTAGMUS

Objective recording of eye movements may be performed by electronystagmography or movies.

Diagrammatic methods

1. 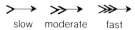 indicates direction of the fast phase.
2. ⌒↘ indicates rotary nystagmus.
3. Length of arrow shows excursion of beat or amplitude.
4. Number of barbs on the arrow indicates frequency.

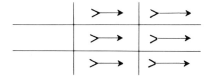

    slow   moderate   fast

5. This diagram shows slow frequency jerk nystagmus beating to the left, increasing on left gaze.

Figure 5.22. Nystagmus graphic representation. Nystagmus may be represented by a series of arrows. The length of the arrow, the number of barbs on the arrow, and the direction of the arrow all help show graphically the character of the nystagmus. (Credit: John Keltner, M.D.)

NYSTAGMUS

Definition

A nystagmus is a rhythmic oscillation of the eyes, that is, a back and forth movement. Usually, nystagmus is characterized by the equality or inequality of the back and forth movement. *Jerk nystagmus* is when the initial movement, or slow phase, is followed by a fast movement to the opposite side, a fast phase. The jerk nystagmus is named for the direction in which the fast phase occurs. *Pendular nystagmus* consists of a back and forth movement in which both phases, opposite in direction, are of equal velocity.

Recording of Nystagmus (Fig. 5.22)

The clinical recording of nystagmus can be enhanced with the following useful method. An arrow indicates the direction of the fast phase of the nystagmus. In rotary nystagmus, the arrow is curved. The length of the arrow determines the excursion of the beat or the amplitude of the beat. The number of barbs on the back end of the arrow indicates the relative frequency. Arrows are then diagramed in the nine positions of primary gaze and the cardinal positions of gaze.

Endpoint Nystagmus

Endpoint nystagmus is a jerk nystagmus of fine amplitudes and fairly moderate fre-

quency. It is found only at the extreme positions of gaze. The fast phase of endpoint nystagmus is in the direction of gaze. The amplitude of the nystagmus is often greater in the eye that is looking away from the nose (abducting eye). This nystagmus is physiologic.

Optokinetic Nystagmus

Optokinetic nystagmus is jerk nystagmus that is physiologic. It is elicited by moving a stimulus in front of the visual field. The slow phase is a pursuit movement of the target; the fast phase is a recovery (saccadic) movement in the opposite direction. The parietooccipital region controls the slow phase pursuit movement to the left, and the left frontal lobe controls the fast recovery phase to the right. Voluntary inhibition is difficult.

Two moving stimuli can be used to produce optokinetic nystagmus. (*a*) The optokinetic drum is a drum in the shape of an oversized coffee can painted with vertical alternating black and white stripes. The drum is mounted so it rotates (page 331). When the drum is held close to the eyes and rotated, nystagmus can be elicited. (*b*) A cloth tape a few inches high and a few feet long with alternating red and white squares can be moved horizontally in front of the eyes to cause optokinetic nystagmus.

Vestibular Jerk Nystagmus

This is the result of altering the input of the vestibular nuclei to the horizontal gaze centers. The slow phase is initiated by the vestibular nuclei, and the fast phase is initiated by the brain stem. Vestibular nystagmus can be horizontal, rotary, or vertical.

Sensory Deprivation Nystagmus

Sensory deprivation nystagmus occurs when afferent visual defects result in a loss of central vision. This is a pendular nystagmus. The eyes move slowly back and forth, somewhat like the pendulum of a grandfather's clock. Characteristically, this nystagmus is decreased by convergence. The severity of sensory deprivation nystagmus depends upon the severity of visual loss.

Latent Nystagmus

This nystagmus is elicited by covering the seeing eye. It occurs in the eye that is occluded. When the eye is again allowed to see, the nystagmus disappears.

Vestibular Nystagmus

This nystagmus is due to loss of vestibular function. The fast component is toward the normal side, and the slow component is toward the abnormal side. Vertigo is always associated with vestibular nystagmus.

Upbeat Nystagmus

This occurs in the primary position of gaze. It is associated with impaired upward pursuit movements. It is localized to lesions of the anterior vermis and lower brain stem. Upbeat nystagmus is caused by drug intoxication and Wernicke's encephalopathy.

See-Saw Nystagmus

One eye rises with an intorsion movement while the other eye falls with an extorsion movement. See-saw nystagmus is usually associated with bitemporal hemianopsia and third ventricular tumors.

Congenital Nystagmus

Congenital nystagmus varies with the position of gaze. In primary gaze, there is a pendular or equal excursion of the to-and-fro movements. In gaze away from the primary position, however, the nystagmus becomes the jerk type, with a fast component and a slow component.

The *null point* is the position in which the eyes are placed to minimize the nystagmus. When the head is turned, the patient utilizes the null point to maintain the best visual acuity. Convergence (page 150) will also decrease the amplitude of congenital nystagmus.

Patients with congenital nystagmus do not have oscillopsia (see page 333), nor do they have severe reduction in their visual acuity.

Gaze-evoked Nystagmus

This is a jerk nystagmus of slow frequency that resembles endpoint nystagmus. It occurs in gaze positions away from the primary and may be of considerable amplitude. It is often associated with cerebellar disease and may occur with hemispheric or brain stem lesions.

Rebound Nystagmus

This is a jerk type nystagmus. It has a rapid phase directed toward the position of gaze but reverses direction after several seconds of eccentric gaze. If the gaze returns to the primary position, a spontaneous nystagmus in the opposite direction occurs. Rebound nystagmus may occur on gaze to one or both sides. It is evoked by changing fixation and is inhibited by eye closure. Rebound nystagmus is associated with cerebellar parenchymal disease or lesions of the posterior fossa.

Downbeat Nystagmus

Ocular Characteristics

Both eyes move rapidly downward and slowly upward. The nystagmus can be present in all positions of gaze but is most frequently seen in *downgaze* and *lateral gaze.* In most patients, lateral gaze will increase the frequency or the amplitude of the nystagmus. The neutral zone, where the nystagmoid movements are least, is usually in upgaze.

Symptoms

Oscillopsia (see page 333) and blurred vision are common symptoms.

Causes

- Infarction
- Idiopathic cerebellar degeneration syndromes

- Multiple sclerosis
- Developmental abnormalities that affect the base of the skull, for example, Arnold-Chiari malformations
- Drugs such as phenytoin, carbamazepine, and lithium

Drug-induced Nystagmus

Drug-induced nystagmus can be seen with barbiturates, tranquilizers, phenothiazines, anticonvulsants (especially phenytoin and carbamazepine), and lithium carbonate. Drug-induced nystagmus is precipitated by movement of the eyes into certain fields of gaze, most often lateral and upgaze.

Periodic Alternating Nystagmus (PAN)

This type of jerk nystagmus has a spontaneous cycling. In the central gaze position, there is about a 10-second period during which no movement is seen, followed by a 90-second period of right-beating nystagmus of increasing and decreasing amplitude. After a second period of no movement lasting about 10 seconds, there is another 90-second period with increasing and decreasing amplitudes of a left-beating nystagmus. This cycling persists even though the eyes are fixated on the target and in the dark. PAN is frequently associated with the perception of a moving environment (oscillipsia). PAN is very rare, but is characteristic of damage to the midline cerebellum.

AMAUROSIS FUGAX

Definition

Amaurosis fugax is a term used for transient loss of vision. It is a common symptom and is frequently an important indication of the presence of a vascular abnormality. It is the most important symptom of impending stroke. Characteristically, it:

- Is transient;
- Is monocular;
- Occurs for less than 10 minutes; and
- Produces blindness or partial blindness.

Vascular Categories

Aortic Hypoperfusion

With aortic hypoperfusion, amaurosis fugax has a gradual onset and the visual loss presents as peripheral constriction. In other words, the patient indicates closure from the outside of vision like the shudder of a camera. This may happen with changes in posture; a direct relationship to a certain position may be recognized by the patient. The visual loss is transient, with the duration of lost vision varying from patient to patient.

Carotid Emboli

Abrupt, severe visual loss occurs with carotid emboli. The visual loss is usually associated with some sort of altitudinal visual field defect. It tends to last 1 to 5 minutes.

Vertebrobasilar Vascular Abnormalities

Vertebrobasilar abnormalities occur in older individuals.[a] In adults, the *bilateral* visual obstruction due to vertebrobasilar vascular abnormalities is usually vague and ill-defined. It is very poorly localized and lasts only seconds. It is frequently associated with other signs and symptoms such as vertigo, dizziness, numbness, and diplopia.

Steal Syndrome

Characteristics. Steal syndrome is transient blindness associated with vigorous use of the extremity on the side opposite the blindness.

Cardiac Sources of Emboli

- Atheromas
- Calcification from aortic valves
- Platelets (from atheromas)
- Systemic lupus erythematosis
- Myocardiac infarction
- Myxoma
- Arrhythmias, especially atrial fibrillation

Associated Hemologic Conditions

- Anemia
- Hypercoagulability
- Abnormal viscosity

Note the following additional causes of amaurosis fugax:

- Severe anemia, as in acute blood loss;
- Dysproteinemia;

---

[a]Young males may have amaurosis fugax with no known cause. This passes with age. It is most commonly seen in teenagers.

- Polycythemia;
- Altered coagulation, as with birth control pills;
- Systemic hypertension;
- Medical therapy for hypertension that lowers the systemic blood pressure.

Differential Diagnosis

Migraine (see page 129) may produce an amaurosis fugax type symptom; however, it is easily distinguished by the characteristics of migraine such as aura, family history, early age of onset, duration of 20 to 30 minutes, and a characteristic progression of the visual disturbance.

There are *ocular diseases* that can mimic amaurosis fugax:

- Refraction changes, as seen with diabetes mellitus;
- Keratoconus;
- Narrow angle glaucoma;
- Macular edema; and
- Others.

Evaluation of a Patient with Amaurosis Fugax

- Detailed ophthalmologic examination including visual field testing, intraocular pressure determinations, and slitlamp examination provide evidence of ischemia including anterior chamber reaction and rubeosis iridis.
- Detailed direct ophthalmoscopy should be performed to search for emboli.
- Ophthalmodynamometry determines arteriole perfusion pressure. References between eyes are most helpful in establishing the diagnosis of carotid artery disease.
- General examination with careful cardiac examination is necessary.
- Laboratory studies should be performed:
  —Complete blood count;
  —Sedimentation rate;
  —Screening test for diabetes mellitus;
  —Screening test for collagen vascular disease;
  —FTA-ABS;
  —Test for dysproteinemias;
  —Noninvasive flow studies.

ANEURYSM
Saccular (Berry) Aneurysms

These small aneurysms are outpouchings of the arteriole walls and look like a sac or a berry. These aneurysms are found in patients after puberty. They are rare during the first 2 decades of life. There is a slightly higher incidence in women than in men.

Ninety-five percent of saccular aneurysms are located in the carotid arteriole system. (The other 5% occur in the vertebrobasilar system.) Most aneurysms are asymptomatic throughout life. The highest risk of bleeding is between ages 40 and 64. Approximately one of five patients will have multiple aneurysms when one is discovered. Aneurysms less than 5 mm in size do not rupture. The mortality is 20% for the first hemorrhage of an aneurysm and 42% for a second hemorrhage.

The third nerve is involved in 68% of unruptured internal carotid artery aneurysms. Of unruptured posterior communicating aneurysms, 87% have third nerve involvement. Symptoms of unruptured aneurysms result from compression of the cranial nerves, especially II, III, IV, V, and VI, and include visual field defects (mostly chiasmal).

Fusiform Aneurysms

These aneurysms are mainly due to atherosclerosis. They are situated along the trunks of arteries. Rupture is unusual, and thrombosis is the most common complication.

CAROTID-CAVERNOUS SINUS FISTULA

Intercavernous carotid artery aneurysms are about 3% of all aneurysms. The most consistent sign is ophthalmoplegia, which frequently is a combination of a partial sixth and a total third nerve palsy. Anisocoria is common and can be due to either sympathetic or parasympathetic pupillomotor paresis. Pupillary sparing occurs with this syndrome. If diabetes, the most common cause of a third nerve palsy with pupillary sparing, has been previously excluded, intercavernous aneurysms should then be considered.

The onset of signs and symptoms of intercavernous carotid artery aneurysms is slow. Diplopia on lateral gaze is often the earliest symptom. Ptosis may also occur. Pain can be in the trigeminal region.

Carotid-cavernous fistulas form after the rupture of an intercavernous aneurysm. The rupture of an intercavernous aneurysm into the cavernous sinus establishes a direct communication between the arterial system and the venous system. Arterial pressure is then transmitted through the veins of the orbit.

Signs

The ophthalmic vein is enlarged. Conjunctival veins dilate, resulting in orbital venous congestion. Ocular bruits are common (heard by use of the stethoscope placed over the orbit). Proptosis is also common. Redness and swelling of the conjunctiva occurs. Double vision, blurred vision, and pain about the eye are of lesser frequency.

A fully developed syndrome of carotid-cavernous fistula is:

- Pulsating exophthalmus;
- Ocular bruit;
- Ophthalmoplegia;
- Conjunctival chemosis;
- Lid edema;
- Dilated conjunctival vessels;
- Visual loss;
- Raised intraocular pressure.

The characteristic bruit disappears on compression of the carotid artery in the neck. Symptoms are usually unilateral, although they may be bilateral. The diagnosis is made by carotid angiography. Carotid-cavernous sinus fistulas can occur spontaneously from the rupture of an aneurysm but are also associated with trauma to the orbit and cranium, blunt injuries to the head, atherosclerosis, and surgical procedures.

Prognosis

Spontaneous remission does occur, usually of the idiopathic types. These fistulas may remain stable for years.

Long-Term Sequelae

Visual loss, optic atrophy, proptosis, glaucoma, cataract, and ophthalmoplegia all result from the prolonged presence of a carotid-cavernous sinus fistula.

PROGRESSIVE EXTERNAL OPHTHALMOPLEGIA

Definition

The normal range of ocular motility is 50° in (adduction), 50° out (abduction), 50° down, and 40° up. With advancing age, the limitation of upgaze decreases to 20°. External ophthalmoplegia is a decrease in this range of motion. The ophthalmoplegia may be progressive or nonprogressive.

Differential Diagnosis

I. Nonprogressive ophthalmoplegia
   A. Congenital fibrosis syndrome
   B. Congenital myopathies
   C. Cranial nerve palsies
   D. Long-standing strabismus
   E. Orbital trauma
II. Progressive external ophthalmoplegia
   A. Supranuclear palsy
      1. Huntington's chorea
      2. Wilson's disease
      3. Lipid storage disease
      4. Ataxia telangiectasis
      5. Hereditary spinocerebellar disease
   B. Progressive supranuclear palsy
      1. Dorsal midbrain syndrome
      2. Mesodiencephalic junction tumor
      3. Progressive multifocal leukoencephalopathy
   C. Neuromuscular junction—myasthenia gravis
   D. Muscle problems
   E. Kearns-Sayer syndrome
   F. Oculopharyngeal muscular dystrophy
   G. Myotonic dystrophy
   H. Dysthyroid ophthalmopathy
   I. Inflammatory orbital pseudotumor with orbital myositis
   J. Carotid-cavernous fistula
   K. Neurodegenerative disorders
      1. Abetalipoproteinemia—Bassen-Kornzweig syndrome
      2. Vitamin E deficiency

CHRONIC PROGRESSIVE EXTERNAL OPHTHALMOPLEGIA (CPEO) (KEARNS-SAYRE SYNDROME)

This is a multisystem disease involving the nervous system, the visual system, the cardiac system, and the endocrine system.

Ocular Characteristics

Lid droop (ptosis), which is almost always bilateral, precedes the changes in ocular motility by months to years. As the ophthalmoplegia (loss of ocular movement) progresses, it is bilateral and symmetrical. Loss of ocular movement is less in downgaze than in other areas of gaze. In about one-quarter of the patients, other facial muscles such as the orbicularis oculi, the frontalis, and the muscles of chewing are involved.

There is a pigmentary retinopathy of the posterior pole. It is associated with optic atrophy and vascular attenuation. Visual field defects occur, and there are cataracts. There may be mild night blindness, and visual acuity may decrease.

Dark adoptometry and the electroretinogram (ERG) are often normal. If the ERG is abnormal, there is a decreased *B*-wave.

Involvement of the Neurologic System

Cerebellar ataxia, pendular nystagmus, hearing loss, and mental retardation all occur. There is an increase of cerebrospinal fluid protein. The basal ganglion may be calcified, and there may be a spongiform brain degeneration.

Cardiac System Involvement

This may occur months to years after the onset of the initial ocular ptosis. There is a conduction disturbance with heart block. Pacemakers may be necessary. Mitral valve prolapse and idiopathic hypertrophic subaortic stenosis occurs.

Endocrine System Involvement

Patients are of short stature. Hypoparathyroidism occurs in hypomagnesia.

Pathology

This is one of the many diseases classified under mitochondrial cytopathy. CPEO, however, is the only one of the mitochondrial cytopathies that includes progressive ophthalmoplegia.

INTERNUCLEAR OPHTHALMOPLEGIA (INO)

Ocular Signs

- Failure of, or abnormal, adduction of the eye on the side of the lesion
- A disassociated nystagmus on abduction of the eye opposite the lesion

Pathology

This is a lesion in the medial longitudinal fasciculus (MLF). It is in the MLF that internuclear ophthalmoplegia blocks the pathways that provide the gaze movements of both eyes.

The paramedian pontine reticular formation (PPRF) is thought to be the center of lateral gaze. The PPRF sends fibers to the sixth nerve nucleus on the same side and the third nerve nucleus on the opposite side. The medial longitudinal fasciculus is the pathway from the PPRF on the opposite side to the third nerve nucleus on the same side as the medial longitudinal fasciculus. It is here that internuclear ophthalmoplegia blocks gaze.

Classification of Internuclear Ophthalmoplegia

This finding may be unilateral or bilateral. Depending on severity, the lesion may produce asymmetry of bilateral clinical observations.

Internuclear ophthalmoplegia may occur anterior or posterior in the MLF. In the anterior connections, convergence is affected; in the posterior connections, convergence remains intact.

INO Plus

In patients with lesions in the medial longitudinal fasciculus, other eye movement disorders may occur. The one-and-a-half syndrome is internuclear ophthalmoplegia, in which the lesion of the PPRF on the same side results only in outward movement of the eye opposite to the lesion.

Cause

INO is most commonly associated with multiple sclerosis. It can also be seen with vascular disease and trauma.

MYASTHENIA GRAVIS

Ocular Symptoms

Ocular signs and symptoms are the initial manifestations of myasthenia gravis in more than 65% of patients. Eventually, regardless of the mode of onset, ocular manifestations will be present in about 90% of patients.

Various Historical Classifications

There are many forms of myasthenia gravis, including congenital, infantile, generalized, and ocular forms. It is convenient to divide the ocular forms and general forms into two distinct clinical groups. It is now believed, however, that most patients with ocular myasthenia, with careful clinical examination and single-fiber electromyogram studies, will be shown to have subclinical forms of a generalized disorder.

Cause

Myasthenia gravis is considered to be an autoimmune disorder. Autoantibodies to acetylcholine receptors in voluntary striated muscle are found in 80 to 90% of patients who have generalized symptoms and about 70% of patients who have ocular muscle signs and symptoms. There is also a high association of myasthenia gravis with other autoimmune disorders.

Autoimmune Disorders That Occur with Myasthenia Gravis

- Graves' disease
- Hashimoto's thyroiditis
- Rheumatoid arthritis
- Polymyositis
- Dermatomyositis
- Scleroderma
- Lupus erythematosus
- Idiopathic thrombocytopenic purpura
- Hemolytic anemia
- Multiple sclerosis
- Others

Ocular Signs

The two most common ocular signs are drooping eyelid *(ptosis)* and extraocular muscle weakness (causing *strabismus*). Characteristically, these show *variability* for short and extended periods and present as "fatigue" with spontaneous remission and then recurrence. Also there is *asymmetrical weakness* of the extraocular muscles, which is a characteristic feature. This presents as unilateral ptosis or asymmetrical limitation of duction. (Contrast the symmetrical weakness and absence of variability that are features of chronic progressive external ophthalmoplegia.)

The following are the most common and important signs:

- Ptosis;
- Strabismus;
- Fatigue of the lid levator;
- Lid twitch (Cogan's lid twitch);
- Limited duction;
- Quiver eye movements;
- Gaze-evoked nystagmus;
- Facial weakness (orbicularis oculi muscles).

Diagnosis

In Adults

Edrophonium (Tensilon) test is used. The new recommended dosage is 2-mg increments given i.v. gradually, as opposed to the larger doses previously recommended. Pretreatment with atropine reduces systemic side effects of edrophonium.

In Children

Prostigmin (neostigmine) is used in children to establish the diagnosis.

In Both Adults and Children

In both of these tests for children and adults, the ptosis and the limitations of gaze from strabismus are observed. If improvement is seen, the test is positive, an indication of myasthenia gravis.

Association with Thymic Hypoplasia and Thymoma

Thymic hypoplasia is common in younger patients. Thymoma occurs in about 15% of cases. When thymoma is present, it is invasive in about one-third of patients. For that reason, when myasthenia gravis is suspected, appropriate studies should be done to rule out thymic involvement. Thymus tumors are relatively uncommon in patients with ocular myasthenia gravis.

Additional Tests

Antiacetylcholine receptor antibodies can be used as a diagnostic test, which is positive in a majority of patients with generalized, nonocular myasthenia gravis. Electromyography to test single muscle fiber fatigue by repetitive stimulation can also be used. This is primarily used in generalized myasthenia gravis because electromyography of nonocular muscles is frequently normal in patients with ocular myasthenia gravis.

MYOTONIC DYSTROPHY

Ocular Characteristics

External ophthalmoplegia, bilateral *ptosis,* and *lid lag* are characteristic. There may be difficulty in closing the eyelids due to orbicularis oculi weakness. There is a decreased blink along with poor lid closure.

All of these patients have *cataracts* presenting as whorls and stellate opacities. Changes are commonly known as Christmas tree cataract. *Pigmentary retinopathy* occurs. Iris neovascular tufts and low intraocular pressure have been reported. The pupils are usually normal.

Systemic Characteristics

This is an autosomal dominant disorder. It affects muscle membranes and the conducting system. In general, the muscle weakness is worse in the morning, during excited states, in cold situations, and during pregnancy. Wasting of the facial muscles and dysfunction of the temporomandibular joint are common. Patients may have a monotonous voice because of facial muscle abnormalities. Other systems involved include the cardiac, the pulmonary, and the endocrine.

Skeletal thickening occurs, as in Padget's disease. Mental retardation, decreased hearing, and frontal baldness also occur.

PSEUDOTUMOR CEREBRI

Diagnostic Criteria

- Increased intracranial pressure with papilledema
- Normal computed tomographic (CT) scans
- Normal cerebrospinal fluid composition

Presenting Symptoms

Headache and disturbance of visual acuity are the most common symptoms. Diplopia, tinnitus, and dizziness, as well as nausea and vomiting, may occur.

Common Associations

- Obesity
- Pregnancy

Less Common Associations

- Middle ear disease
- Radical neck dissection
- Nonspecific infections
- Corticosteroid withdrawal
- Medications (vitamin A, tetracycline, others)

Cause

Unknown

Course

The course of pseudotumor is often self-limited, with the condition resolving within 3 to 9 months. The visual fields and the appearance of the optic disc by photography should be followed during the course of pseudotumor cerebri.

Onset

This is primarily seen in younger people, with a peak incidence in the third decade of life. There is a 2/1 female preponderance.

Symptoms

Papilledema is bilateral, although it may be asymmetrical. Serious visual loss may occur in as many as 25% of patients. Visual field defects are usually in the nerve fiber bundle distribution, and inferior nasal defects are most common. The central 5° of the field is usually not involved early. The visual acuity generally remains normal during the early stages, until optic nerve damage is extensive.

Diagnosis

CT scanning or magnetic resonance imaging can rule out a mass lesion. The ventricles in pseudotumor cerebri are normal or small-sized.

Lumbar Puncture

Intracranial pressure of less than 200 mm H_2O is normal. A pressure greater than 250 mm H_2O is abnormal. (Normal intracranial pressure by lumbar puncture does not rule out the possibility of pseudotumor cerebri because patients experience fluctuations in pressure.)

OPTIC NERVE GLIOMA

Clinical Presentation

Vision loss is the most common facial symptom. With visual loss, strabismus and nystagmus may result. Signs depend upon the position of the tumor. The tumor may be in the optic nerve or in the chiasm. Optic nerve tumors in the intraorbital region may produce proptosis. Edema of the optic nerve disc or optic atrophy may be present. Chiasmal tumors may produce endocrine dysfunction from hypothalamic involvement. Optociliary shunt vessels may occur at the optic disc with gliomas.

Onset

Of gliomas, 75% present in the first decade of life and 90% present within the first 20 years of life.

Pathology

Gliomas are benign astrocytic proliferations. They are very slow-growing.

Association with Neurofibromatosis

There is a high association of gliomas with neurofibromatosis. In patients with neurofi-

bromatosis, 10% will have radiographic findings of glioma. Bilateral gliomas are highly suggestive of neurofibromatosis. Café au lait spots should be sought because they are common in neurofibromatosis. Thickening of the optic nerve shown by x-ray film and enlargement of the optic foramen are common findings in patients with gliomas of the optic nerve.

MALIGNANT OPTIC GLIOMA

This is a tumor that occurs in adults (compare with benign tumors in children) and that originates in or near the anterior visual pathways. Signs and symptoms include visual loss with pain in one eye. Visual loss often progresses in the opposite eye, complete blindness occurs with 2 to 4 months, and death occurs within 6 to 9 months.

DORSAL MIDBRAIN SYNDROME (PARINAUD'S SYNDROME)

Ocular Abnormalities

The first abnormality noted is impairment of upgaze. Downgaze may also be affected. The downgaze is most often present.

With time, upgaze attempts are replaced by slow upward movements and then by retraction of the globe. A convergence retraction nystagmus is a result of a cocontraction of the extraocular muscles. This retraction nystagmus can be demonstrated by testing optokinetic nystagmus (see page 112).

Pupillary abnormality is light-near dissociation. Pupils are usually mid-dilated and may show some corectopia.

Lid retraction (Collier's sign) is easily seen because the lid is retracted, usually above the corneal-scleral junction, showing an area of white sclera.

Skew deviation (vertical divergence of the eyes) may be seen in supranuclear disturbances.

Differential Diagnosis

I. Neoplastic
   A. Pinealoma
   B. Posterior third ventricular tumor

C. Brain stem glioma
D. Metastatic tumor
II. Vascular
   A. Midbrain infarction or hemorrhage
   B. Arteriovenous malformation
   C. Angioma
III. Infective
   A. Syphilis
   B. Tuberculosis
   C. Poliomyelitis
   D. Viral encephalitis
IV. Degenerative
   A. Multiple sclerosis
   B. Lipid storage disease
   C. Kernicterus
   D. Olivopontocerebellar degeneration
V. Miscellaneous
   A. Congenital hydrocephalus
   B. Head trauma
   C. Neurofibromatosis
   D. Other

IMPORTANT POINTS IN NEUROOPHTHALMOLOGY

- *Sudden bilateral ptosis* in a woman: Think breast carcinoma metastatic to the caudal central nucleus.
- *Recurrent pupillary sparing* of the third nerve: Think either diabetes or sphenoid sinus mucocele.
- *Isolated pupillary dilation* (also known as internal ophthalmoplegia) in an alert patient without other signs or symptoms is most often due either to a topical drug such as atropine or tonic pupil (ciliary ganglion involvement).
- *Ophthalmoplegia with normal pupils:* Think neuromuscular junction disorder such as myasthenia gravis, myopathy such as chronic progressive external ophthalmoplegia, or thyroid disease.

6

Important Concepts

Cataract	Gonococcal Conjunctivitis	Functional Visual Loss
Headache	Ocular Syphilitic Disease	Ocular Injuries
Age-related Macular	Acquired Immune Deficiency	Traumatic Hyphema
Degeneration	Syndrome	Chemical Burns
Venereal Diseases and the Eye	Ultraviolet Light and Sunglasses	Corneal Scleral Lacerations
Chlamydia Conjunctivitis	Eye Disease among the Elderly	Rupture of Globe

CATARACT

Definition

A cataract is any opacity of the crystalline lens (Fig. 6.1) of the eye.

Classification

General

The classification of cataracts is confusing even to the experienced ophthalmologist. The

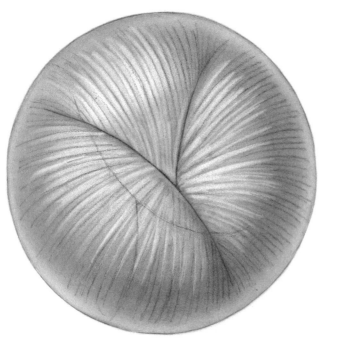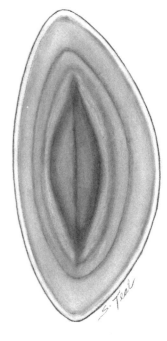

Figure 6.1. Anatomy of the lens, showing the capsule, cortex, and nucleus and the formation of Y sutures, which are the lines formed by the termination of zonular fibers.

problem arises because there is no clear, distinctive, acceptable categorization to define cataracts as seen clinically. For example, cataracts may be defined by onset, cause, or anatomy.

Cataracts Classified by the Time of Onset

Embryonal Cataracts. Cataracts can occur during gestation. Rubella cataract is the most significant and common embryonic cataract.

Congenital Cataract. Cataracts present at birth are often classified as congenital. They could be, of course, embryonal cataracts; this is a cross-over in terminology.

Juvenile Cataracts. Cataracts that occur during the first few years of life are classified as juvenile cataracts. The term is nonspecific and probably should be avoided. At times, the term infant cataract may also be used, but it is nonspecific.

Adult Onset Cataract. These are cataracts that occur in adult life. All individuals who live long enough will have some opacity of the lens which could technically be classified as a cataract. Adult cataracts represent a major cause of visual impairment in the elderly.

Cataracts Classified as to Cause

There are a number of cataracts that can be classified according to specific causes.

Galactosemia Cataract. Infants with galactosemia develop cataracts that can be prevented or reversed by appropriate therapy. Galactosemia is an inherited disorder of galactose metabolism (there is an absence of galactose-1-phosphate uridyltransferase). This enzyme is necessary to convert galactose into galactogene. Over 75% of infants with galactosemia have cataracts. The cataract is due to galactose that accumulates in the eye. The early opacities are reversible.

Steroid-induced Cataract. Steroid cataracts (see Fig. 6.7) are typical cataracts occurring in the posterior portion of the lens and are frequently referred to as posterior subcapsular cataracts. These cataracts are dose-related. They are commonly seen now in patients with renal transplants, cardiac transplants, and severe allergic conditions where steroids are required for prolonging life.

Often, in life-threatening situations, a cataract is an acceptable complication of the therapy.

Metabolic Cataracts. Cataracts associated with some metabolic imbalance can be loosely classified as metabolic. Cataracts associated with diabetes (diabetic cataracts), for example, have been referred to under this category.

Radiation Cataract. Cataracts occurring secondary to radiation, usually for cancer therapy, are radiation cataracts.

Glass Blowers' Cataract (Heat-generated). In glass blowers who are exposed to heat furnaces for many hours each working day for a number of years, cataracts can occur.

Electrical Cataract. Electrocuted patients can develop cataracts. They may be classified as electrical or as a subset of traumatic cataract.

Traumatic Cataracts. Patients with blunt trauma to the globe can develop a cataract, of highly variable appearance, after the trauma. These are referred to frequently as traumatic cataracts and less often as concussive cataracts.

Cataracts Associated with Certain Specific Diseases or Syndromes

At times, opacities are associated with certain diseases. These can be classified in a number of ways but frequently are given the tag related to the associated disease process.

Myotonia Dystrophica. Patients with myotonia dystrophica have a characteristic cataract with glistening, multicolored granules in the areas underneath the capsule and in the cortical areas of the lens.

Lowe's Syndrome. This is X-linked. Besides cataract, ocular changes include glaucoma and corneal opacities.

Others. There are also other cataracts associated with specific diseases.

Cataracts Classified by Anatomy (Fig. 6.2)

Polar. These are cataracts that are on the front portion of the lens, usually in the visual axis near the anterior capsule.

Cupuliform. These are cataracts in the subcapsular region. Cataracts most often classified in this anatomical way are cortical changes that occur with advancing age.

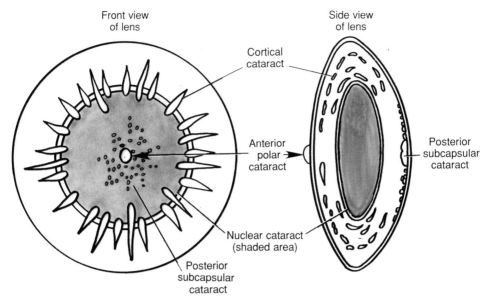

Figure 6.2.   Cataract types. This composite drawing shows the positions of cataract opacities: nuclear sclerotic cataract, cortical cataract, posterior subcapsular cataract, and anterior polar cataract.

Figure 6.3.   Using the red retinal reflex to determine lens opacities. By shining a light through the dilated pupil, the red reflex can provide retroillumination to show lens opacities. With central illumination, opacities show up as dark against a red background. In this black and white photograph, the superior portion of the lens is clear; however, the inferior portion is dark from cortical (cuneiform) cataract lens changes.

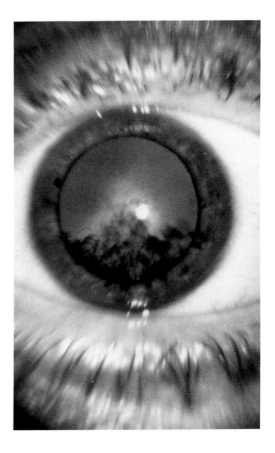

Coronary. These are opacities that are found just outside the nucleus of the lens. They are also described as supranuclear.

Cuneiform. These are opacities within the cortex of the lens. Cuneiform opacities occur with metabolic cataracts as well as age-related cataracts (Fig. 6.3).

Lamellar. A cataract change within the nucleus. Also known as a nuclear cataract or a zonular cataract. In lamellar cataract, the opacity is most dense at the outer portions of the lens nucleus and is seen as a distinct layer.

Sutural. Sutural cataracts relate to Y sutures, which are a result of the embryonic migration of lens capsule fibers. Sutural cataracts usually are seen anteriorly and posteriorly, with a distinctive upside-down or right-side-up Y appearance.

Nuclear. The entire nucleus can be involved and become opacified causing a nuclear sclerotic cataract. This condition occurs in all human beings with aging. Nuclear sclerotic cataracts (that is, densening of the nucleus) are the major reason for adult cataract removal today.

Zonular. A lamellar cataract that develops up to 12 months after birth is called *zonular*. It is usually bilateral.

Posterior Subcapsular (Fig. 6.4). Cataracts that form posteriorly in the lens or near the posterior capsule are called *posterior subcapsular*. They are usually central and may cause significant visual reduction at an early stage (Fig. 6.5).

Christmas Tree. Another name for the cataract associated with myotonic dystrophy is *Christmas tree* because of the brilliantly colored specks (iridescent dust).

Cataracts Classified According to Stage of Development

- Immature cataract opacities affect vision very little or not at all.
- Mature cataracts affect vision dramatically and usually present as whitish opacities of the pupillary area (Fig. 6.6).
- Hypermature cataract is so advanced that a breakdown of the firm lens fibers and liquifaction begin to occur. Hypermature cataract can induce inflamma-

tion in the eye by leaking toxic proteins through the intact capsule.

- Morganian cataracts are cataracts in which the nucleus moves in the liquified cortical parts of an intact lens capsule. This is an advanced hypermature cataract.
- Metabolic cataracts have causes directly related to metabolic imbalance and may be classified according to that metabolic imbalance. Examples are diabetic cataracts and galactosemic cataracts.
- Cataracts may be classified according to a toxic cause. Pilocarpine, steroids, chlorpromazine, and phospholine iodine all can produce cataracts that have variable appearances.

Clinically Important Cataracts

Age-related Cataract

With time, the human lens begins to develop opacities. These can occur both in the cortical fibers and in the nucleus.

The nuclear changes, called nuclear sclerotic cataracts, occur in all individuals. Lens fibers remain within the eye from the time of birth; lens fibers can only be concentrated centrally as new fibers are formed. With age, these fibers are compacted in the central, nuclear portion of the lens. This area develops into a hard nuclear sclerotic lens.

The first sign of nuclear sclerosis is the inability to focus at near objects, called presbyopia. Presbyopia becomes evident in middle age when people hold their reading matter and small print away from their eyes ("My arms seem too short"). Eventually, those in their 40s or early 50s need reading glasses, which are simply lenses that converge the rays to adjust for the loss of convergent power that occurs when nuclear sclerosis progresses in the lens. This is a normal and predictable process in all humans.

As nuclear sclerosis continues to progress, visual acuity can be affected. Visual acuity decreases slowly over a period of years. As the nuclear sclerosis progresses, however, visual loss may be acclerated.

Diabetes. Diabetics are known to have more rapidly advancing nuclear sclerosis, and

Figure 6.4. **A**, Posterior subcapsular cataract. A cataract may form near the capsule of the lens. These posterior subcapsular cataracts may be due to drugs, most commonly steroids, or ocular inflammation or may be idiopathic. **B**, Zonular cataract. A cataract involving the nucleus and appearing early in life. **C**, Cuneiform (or cortical) cataract. Certain opacities in the cortex of the lens are described as cuneiform.

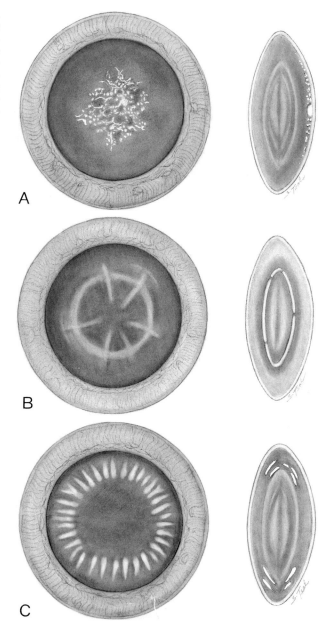

the visual loss from nuclear sclerosis can be earlier in diabetics.

Color Vision. Nuclear sclerosis not only produces loss of vision, but also alters color vision. There is a yellowish discoloration from the brownish hue of nuclear sclerosis. This brownish discoloration is the collection of adrenochrome pigment from the concentration of the cortical fibers in the nucleus.

This discoloration filters certain wavelengths of the spectrum, altering color components of the image projected on the retina.

Cortical Changes. Cortical changes can also occur with age and appear as whitish opacities. Cortical changes associated with age can be posterior (underneath the capsule in a cup form—cupuliform), or they can appear as spoke-like opacities (cuneiform). Cor-

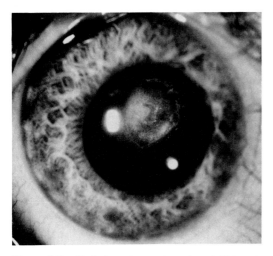

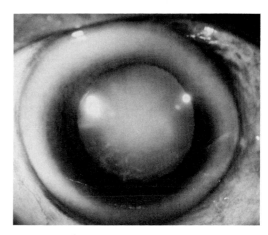

Figure 6.6. A cataract is an opacity of the lens. Here the white pupil is caused by an advanced cataract.

Figure 6.5. Posterior subcapsular cataract. This cataract is located in the back of the lens region of the posterior capsule. The position of these cataracts makes them have a dramatic and significant effect on visual acuity. Posterior subcapsular cataracts can be caused by a number of processes including steroids and inflammation but also can be part of an age-related cataract.

tical changes are frequently associated with nuclear sclerotic changes.

Social Significance. In the United States, it is estimated that more than a million cataract extractions are done a year. By far the majority of these are removals of age-related cataracts. This represents a significant economic potential for physicians and hospitals but also represents a major factor for third party payers and governmental agencies. Health care costs for cataracts alone run in the billions of dollars. This is becoming increasingly important because it is estimated that a large proportion of the population will be elderly as lifespans increase and medical advances prolong life and prevent death from previously fatal conditions.

Congenital Cataracts

Congenital cataracts, present at birth, must be treated early if vision is severely affected. Rubella cataracts will prevent the normal development of vision even if a normal visual system is present. The human eye, at birth, is not fully developed. A number of years are necessary for the development of full 20/20 vision and binocular vision that will allow depth perception (stereopsis). The presence of a cataract opacity will not allow images to be focused on the retina, impeding the total development of the visual system. For this reason, the management of congenital cataracts has been increasingly acknowledged as important.

Removal of the cataract then demands, in these newborns, visual recovery. None of the presently available alternatives is as good a replacement as the normal human lens. Spectacle corrections in infants are not possible because frames do not fit easily on the infant face. Cataract replacement by contact lenses is satisfactory in the very young child but, as children become toddlers, it is almost impossible to maintain visual correction with a contact lens because the lens is frequently lost and dislocated. Insertion is difficult for many parents, and it is unusual to find that contact lenses are a successful alternative.

Intraocular lenses are rarely placed in the eyes of young children because of the changing dimensions of the eye. The rigid intraocular lens does not allow for these changes. Also, the inflammation and healing reaction to intraocular lenses are excessive and result in unwanted scarring within the eye.

Epikeratophakia, a new procedure that is still developmental, may provide ways to develop better vision in children with congenital cataracts.

The important problem of obtaining maximal recoverable visual acuity in a child with congenital cataract continues to be a major challenge in ophthalmology.

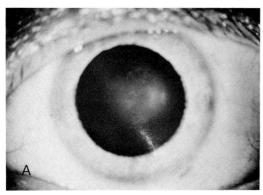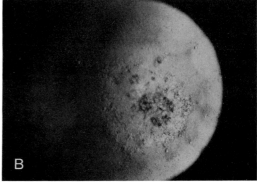

Figure 6.7. Steroid cataracts are caused by topical or systemic steroids and are dose-related. They are found in the posterior portion of the lens just under the capsule (posterior subcapsular cataracts). **A**, The cataract position. **B**, The characteristics of the change when the illumination is from behind (retroillumination).

Steroid-induced Cataract (Fig. 6.7)

Cortical steroids, either systemically or topically administered, can produce significant cataracts. These cataracts are dose-related.

In patients who require steroids, steroid cataracts are frequently accepted as a complication. This has been an increasing problem in patients with renal, cardiac, and other types of transplants. It can also be a complication with corneal transplants, where prolonged steroid administration is necessary to decrease graft rejection.

These cataracts can be anticipated and observed. Changes in vision due to steroid cataracts are not reversible, and surgery should be considered at appropriate times. This frequently means surgery in age groups (20s, 30s, and 40s) that would not previously have been thought of as potential candidates for cataract surgery. Nonophthalmologists and ophthalmologists should be aware of changing indications in these areas.

Cataract Changes That Occur with Metabolic Disturbances

Diabetes mellitus is often associated with aging cataracts having an earlier onset and more rapid progression. Also, snowflake opacities occur in the cortex in diabetics, especially in juvenile onset diabetics. Cortical changes can also progress rapidly and affect vision severely.

One mechanism causing diabetic cataracts is well known and frequent. As there is increased glucose content in the blood, there is also increased glucose content in the aqueous humor. Increased levels are also seen inside the lens, where aldose reductase converts glucose to sorbitol. Sorbitol is not metabolized and remains in the lens. A subsequent osmotic gradient develops because of this increased concentration of sorbitol within the lens itself. Water is then drawn through the lens capsule into the lens. Lens fibers swell and eventually cloud, causing loss of vision.

Lens Opacities Due to the Deposition of an Abnormal Substance

In Wilson's disease (hepatolenticular degeneration), an anterior subcapsular opacity develops in the cortex. This opacity is described as a sunflower cataract. This cataract is due to the deposition of copper and is seen as a reddish brown coloration.

Metabolic Cataract Associated with Galactosemia

Galactosemia, an inherited disorder, results from an absence of galactose-1-phosphate uridyl transferase. This enzyme converts galactose to glycogen. Without the enzyme, galactose builds up. When galactose accumulates in the blood and aqueous humor, it diffuses into the lens. Aldose reductase in the lens converts galactose to dulcitol. Dulcitol collects and is unable to diffuse out through the lens capsule. This creates an osmotic gradient.

Excess water is then taken into the lens, and cataract develops.

Rubella Cataract

A rubella cataract is usually localized to the central portion of the lens and is described as a nuclear cataract. Ocular complications due to rubella, including cataract, occur with viral infection during the *first trimester* of pregnancy. Rubella is also associated with heart defects and hearing loss. In the eye, not only cataract but glaucoma and a chorioretinitis, which appears as scattered pigmentation and scarring, are present. The lens of the eye can retain the virus for up to 3 years after birth.

HEADACHE

Migraine Headaches

Characteristics

Migraine is common and is estimated to occur in as many as 15% of the population. Women are more frequently affected than men in a 2/1 ratio, and headaches in women tend to be more severe. Eye signs, especially a diagnostic visual experience before the onset of pain (aura), often bring patients to ophthalmologists for examination.

Onset

Of adult migraine patients, 50% start having migraines before age 20. More than 10% experience them before age 10. The onset may be with menarche or puberty. Signs and symptoms are often accentuated during menopause. Migraine rarely starts after age 40 and, if migraine symptoms begin at this time, other causes should be considered (cerebrovascular disease and intracranial abnormalities).

Inheritance

Migraine may be transmitted as a dominant characteristic. Members of a migrainal patient's family will frequently have migraine symptoms.

Ophthalmic Symptoms

Areas of visual alteration (scotomas) appear as glittering lights; shimmering, silvery, jagged circles; or hemicircles (scintillations) along with blind spots (homonymous scotomas). These scintillations or scotomas may appear either separately or together. At times, the visual phenomena may not be followed by headaches. Although the shape, size, and character of the scotomas and the scintillations vary, the description by the patient is characteristic enough to establish migraine as a cause. Rarely, patients may have complete cortical blindness for short periods and recover in 10 to 15 minutes.

General Symptoms

The migraine headache, a boring, sometimes throbbing pain, is usually unilateral and is often accompanied by nausea and vomiting. Patients may have depression or nausea before the headache starts. After the headache, fatigue sets in and patients may sleep for hours after an attack.

A major feature of migraine is repeated attacks. These may be very frequent or occasional and widely spaced, but recurrence is common.

Cluster Headache

Features

- Duration—minutes to hours
- Characteristically unilateral with head or face pain
- Attacks in clusters occurring over a few days or months

Ocular Signs

A Horner's syndrome is often present and may remain after the attacks.

Onset

- Age 60 years or more
- Symptoms usually intensified by alcohol
- More frequent in men

Headache with Brain Tumor

Headaches with brain tumor tend to be over the site of the tumor. This is especially true in patients with brain tumor without papilledema.

Posterior fossa tumors are almost always accompanied by headache. Cerebellar angle tumors, however, are not associated with headache. Patients with pituitary tumors may not have headaches.

The headache due to tumor has a deep, aching, steady, and dull pain. It is not throbbing or rhythmic. The headache may be aggravated by coughing or straining. Certain positions may make it worse, especially an upright position. The headache tends to be worse in the early morning.

Headache of Hypertension

These headaches are dull and diffuse. They may be throbbing. They are often generalized but may be unilateral. The occipital region is the common location. They are usually worse in the early mornings. They may begin between midnight and 4:00 a.m. and reach a peak around sunrise. The headache is often increased by bending over, coughing, or sneezing.

Headache of Ocular Origin (Asthenopia)

Although imbalance of muscle motility or refractive errors can produce headaches, this is certainly not common. When they do occur, the headaches are typically around the eyes. They may be in the frontal area and, when they spread, they spread posteriorly from the forehead to the temples. Ocular headaches are always associated with use of the eyes. Headaches of refractive origin are cured by proper correction of refractive error. Muscle imbalance headaches are relieved by occlusion of one eye and are cured by correcting the imbalance.

Headaches of the Nasal and Paranasal Sinuses

Headaches may be associated with frontal sinusitis as well as sphenoid and ethmoid sinus disease. Frontal sinusitis causes pain around and over the frontal sinuses on the forehead, whereas sphenoid and ethmoid sinusitis causes pain behind the eyes and over the vertex of the head. If severe and of long duration, sinusitis can produce headache in the posterior part of the skull. The headache usually begins around 9:00 a.m. and becomes worse as the day progresses, ending in the evening or before retiring. Headache associated with maxillary sinusitis begins in the afternoon.

The pain may be characterized as deep, dull, and aching. There is no throbbing.

Additional Causes of Headache

- Subarachnoid hemorrhage
- Cranial (temporal) arteritis
- Trauma
- Trigeminal neuralgia

Unknown

Many patients with headache will not have ocular or other disease processes. These headaches are often posterior in the occipital region. They are frequently attributed to tension (tension headaches).

AGE-RELATED MACULAR DEGENERATION

Other Names

Age-related maculopathy, macular degeneration, senile macular degeneration

Cause

Age-related macular degeneration is the leading cause of new blindness in the United States. Its cause is not known. The primary abnormality seems to be within the retinal pigment epithelium and its biochemical relationship to the photoreceptor cells. Heredity is probably important. There has also been an implication that light-induced damage affecting the photoreceptor outer segments in the retinal pigment epithelium may accelerate the underlying dysfunction.

Normal Aging Changes

Normally, there are histologic changes in the macula that affect the outer retinal layers, the pigment epithelium, Bruch's membrane, and the choriocapillaris (Fig. 6.8). There is loss of pigment granules, formation of lipofuscin granules, and accumulation of residual bodies. Drusen (hyaline deposits) form on

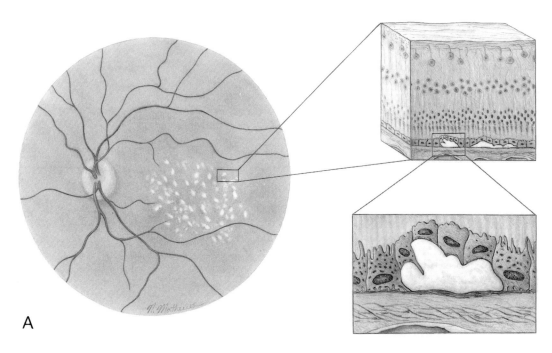

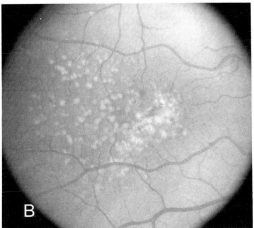

Figure 6.8. **A**, Drusen of the macula are deposits just below the retinal pigment epithelium. They show up as white to yellow-white opacities. Many times they have no clinical significance. However, they may be associated with age-related macular degeneration. Familial drusen also occur. **B**, Macular drusen are small, yellow-white, approximately round, discrete changes in the posterior pole. This photograph shows drusen in the macula.

Figure 6.9. Aging macular degeneration, a common cause of bilateral legal blindness of adult onset, is a major socioeconomic problem in the elderly population. Illustrated is the nonexudative or dry form of the condition.

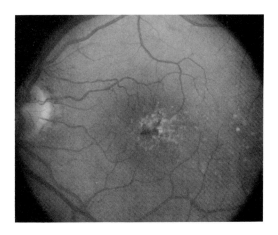

Bruch's membrane beneath the basement membrane of the pigment epithelium. Bruch's membrane may thicken and fragment. Calcification may also occur. Visual loss may be associated.

Pathologic Macular Degeneration

In pathologic macular degeneration, there are two forms: nonexudative (or the dry form) and the exudative form. In the dry form, drusen (Fig. 6.9), pigmentary changes, and atrophy are noted. Drusen may differ greatly in appearance; some are discrete and yellowish, some are calcified with sharply demarcated crystalline lesions, some are diffuse, and some are soft and associated with small serous detachments of the retinal pigment epithelium.

Various amounts of pigment clumping and atrophy accompany the drusen formation.

The exudative form is associated with macular drusen and is usually due to the development of a subretinal pigment epithelial neovascular membrane. This membrane grows from the choriocapillaris through defects in Bruch's membrane. Bleeding with neovascularization and membrane formation can be detected by fluorescein angiography. The final stage of the exudative form of macular degeneration is a disciform scar.

The exudative form (Fig. 6.10) is associated with a rapid onset of visual loss. In the dry form, however, there is a slow, gradual loss of central visual acuity. In the exudative form, the rapid visual loss may be associated with

Figure 6.10. Aging macular degeneration may show exudates from unstable vessels. This carries a poor prognosis for vision.

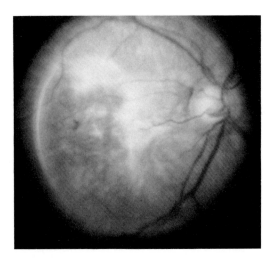

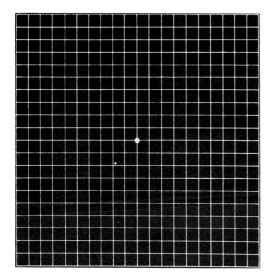

Figure 6.11. Amsler grid. The central white dot is used for fixation. One eye is tested at a time. Distortion of the lines of squares is an indication of macular disease.

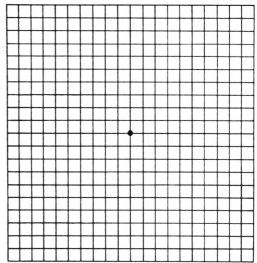

Figure 6.12. The Amsler recording chart provides a permanent record of the distortion in a patient's eye. The patient or the observer can draw the changes on the chart. The recording chart is printed in black on white for convenience of recording.

metamorphopsia. Metamorphopsia is an irregularity in central vision and can be tested with the Amsler grid (Figs. 6.11 and 6.12). Metamorphopsia indicates a need for immediate fluorescein angiography because effective laser treatment must be done early.

Both nonexudative and exudative forms are associated with drusen and aging (that is, over the age of 50). The complication of choroidal neovascularization is more likely in eyes with a confluence of hyaline drusen.

VENEREAL DISEASES AND THE EYE

Chlamydial Conjunctivitis

Other Names

Adult inclusion conjunctivitis, conjunctivitis due to *Chlamydia trachomatis,* conjunctivitis due to chlamydial oculogenitalis

Clinical Features

The incubation of chlamydial conjunctivitis is a few days to 2 weeks. It presents as bulbar conjunctival and limbal follicles, a key feature. Punctate epithelial keratitis occurs. The lesions are coarse and vary considerably in shape. Subepithelial yellow-white infiltrates occur later, especially in the superior cornea.

The conjunctiva is hyperemic, and a papillary conjunctivitis commonly evolves into a chronic follicular conjunctivitis. The inflammation is associated with preauricular lymphadenopathy.

Systemic Associations

Otitis media and pharyngitis are not uncommon with chlamydial conjunctivitis. Although rare, recurrent iridocyclitis and arthritis have been noted.

Incidence

Chlamydial conjunctivitis occurs secondary to prolonged genital infection. Ocular infection develops in 1 of every 100 to 300 patients with chlamydial urethritis.

Laboratory Testing

Giemsa stains of conjunctival scrapings reveal plasma cells, immature leukocytes, and giant cells. Typical Halberstaedter-Prowazek intracytoplasmic basophilic inclusion bodies can be seen occasionally in acute cases. (They are easily seen in neonatal chlamydial infections.) Additional tests include fluoresceinated monoclonal antibodies and enzyme-linked immunoassay.

Gonococcal Conjunctivitis

Cause

Neisseria gonorrhoeae

Clinical Features

Gonococcal conjunctivitis is acute bacterial conjunctivitis with lid edema, conjunctival chemosis, papillae that are bright red, and pseudomembranes in preauricular lymphadenopathy. The cornea shows punctate epithelial erosions (see page 26) in some cases. The erosion may be followed by subepithelial infiltrates, which can lead to corneal ulceration and perforation.

Laboratory Testing

Gram-stained smears of the conjunctival exudates show neutrophils and Gram-negative diplococci. The diplococci are frequently intracellular. Culture on chocolate agar and Thayer-Martin medium is necessary. Antibiotic sensitivity testing should be performed because resistant strains are not uncommon. Organisms should also be tested for beta-lactamase production.

Ocular Syphilitic Disease

Ocular involvement may occur with either congenital or acquired syphilis.

Primary and Secondary Syphilis

In acquired syphilis, the chancre is the characteristic lesion. It is the indurated ulcer that appears 3 weeks after exposure to the organism Treponema pallidum. Chancre usually occurs on the genitalia but has been seen rarely on the eyelid and conjunctiva. It is associated with preauricular lymphadenopathy when on the eyelid. The chancre disappears spontaneously. Weeks later, a maculopapular rash occurs, manifesting secondary syphilis. The rash characteristically involves the palms and the soles of the feet. Sometimes the eyelids are affected. The rash may leave patchy areas of depigmentation.

Syphilitic Keratitis

This is also called "interstitial keratitis." It involves nonsuppurative stromal inflammation and vascularization. Of all cases of luetic interstitial keratitis, 95% are associated with congenital syphilis and 5% are from acquired syphilis.

The keratitis, which may be associated with iritis or cataracts, occurs in patients with congenital syphilis between the ages of 5 and 20 years. Initial signs are a deep stromal infiltrate with iridocyclitis and keratic precipitates. Deep stromal neovascularization occurs, giving a characteristic "salmon patch" hue to the cornea. As a reaction subsides, corneal opacification with ridges and Descemet's membrane, endothelial cell dysfunction, and a "ground glass" haze occurs. Stromal ghost vessels may persist indefinitely. Five to 10% of cases will recur. Glaucoma occurs as a later complication in 20% of cases.

In congenital syphilis, bilateral pigmentary chorioretinopathy (salt and papper fundus), narrowed vessels, and optic atrophy may occur. In acquired syphilis, after the rash with secondary syphilis, iridocyclitis may be the sole clinical presentation. Optic neuritis and choroiditis with vitritis may occur during the late secondary stages of syphilis.

Diagnosis is made through the serologic test—the fluorescent treponemal antibody absorption (FTA-ABS) test, the microhemagglutination test for T. pallidum (MHA-TP), and the VDRL test. A false-positive FTA-ABS test is rare but may occur in patients with lupus erythematosus, hypergammaglobulinemia, pregnancy, and nonspecific spirochetal disease.

Acquired Immune Deficiency Syndrome (AIDS)

There are frequent ocular manifestations in AIDS. On occasion, these ocular problems may be the source of presenting signs and symptoms.

Koposi's Sarcoma

Koposi's sarcoma associated with AIDS may present on the lid or conjunctiva. When presented with a suspicious lesion, biopsy is recommended.

Cytomegalovirus (CMV) Retinitis (Figs. 6.13 and 6.14)

CMV retinitis shows progressive retinal destruction with fluffy white retinal infiltrates and intraretinal hemorrhages that are most

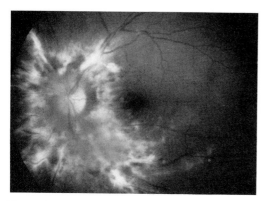

Figure 6.13. Retinitis caused by cytomegalic inclusion virus in a patient with AIDS. (Credit: Louis Lobes, M.D.)

marked along the major vessels. Histologically, full-thickness retinal necrosis with intracellular and intracytoplasmic inclusions are seen.

Additional Ocular Lesions

Cotton-wool spots and isolated retinal hemorrhages are also seen.

Infection

Numerous opportunistic infections occur in AIDS: cryptococcosis, toxoplasmosis, atypical mycobacterial infection, herpes simplex retinitis, and herpes zoster ophthalmicus. CMV retinitis is the most common infection, being seen in approximately one-third of the cases.

ULTRAVIOLET LIGHT AND SUNGLASSES

Light, of course, is composed of many different wavelengths. The visible spectrum provides energy in wavelengths that stimulate our visual system. The two ends of the spectrum, the lower end or ultraviolet (UV) radiation and the upper end, infrared radiation, are both invisible to the eye. It is the UV energy spectrum that poses the greatest problem of toxicity to the eye.

Photochemical damage to the eye, the type of damage due to UV radiation, is produced by the UV spectrum (320 to 400 nm) and the lower portion of the visual spectrum (400 to

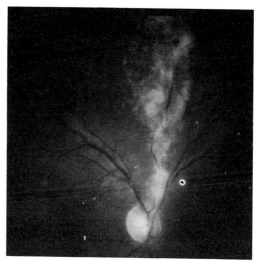

Figure 6.14. Typical CMV perivascular distribution of retinitis. (Credit: Louis Lobes, M.D.)

470 nm). The sun is the greatest source of UV radiation. UV radiation is strongest in situations where snow or water is present, where 85% of the UV radiation is reflected, as opposed to only 5% from earth or grass.

Photochemical damage occurs when nonionizing radiation is absorbed by the tissue. This radiation is below the levels that cause thermal damage. Higher levels cause heat damage. Photochemical damage is produced by photons of light, which change molecules. The new molecular structure (free radicals) causes tissue damage. Such photochemical toxicity can damage membranes, enzyme systems, and other tissue.

Lens Damage

Ultraviolet radiation has recently been implicated as causing the brown (brunescent) cataracts seen in the aging lenses of humans. It is suspected that exposure to sunlight produces this change. There is a higher prevalence of brunescent cataract in people living near the equator. Brunescent cataracts can also be produced experimentally with exposure to UV radiation. Cortical cataracts in humans have also been correlated with exposure to midrange UV light (ultraviolet B).

Certain lower wavelengths are also toxic to the retina; the most toxic are 320 to 475 nm.

Most of the ultraviolet radiation (300–400 nm) that might reach the retina is filtered before it enters the eye. UV radiation damage to the retina is lessened by the following ocular structures: 25% of the UV radiation is filtered by the cornea, 11% by the aqueous, and 64% by the lens. Less than 1% reaches the retina in the normal eye.

Removal of the normal lens increases the UV exposure of the retina. This can be significant because there are more than one million extractions of cataractous lenses in the United States each year. Each of these patients then has the potential for increased UV exposure.

In general, the following individuals are most susceptible to UV radiation phytotoxicity:

- Patients who have had their lenses removed by surgery (aphakic patients);
- Patients who are exposed to abnormal levels of UV radiation, for example, sailors or lifeguards close to the water or workers in industries using UV polymerization techniques;
- Patients treated with psoralen in UV therapy for psoriasis or vitiligo or with phototherapy for hyperbilirubinemia.

Selection of Sunglasses

There is little standardization in the production of sunglasses. The following general recommendations can help in selection: (*a*) Total transmission of the sunglass should be 10 to 20% depending on use. (*b*) Transmission of the lenses should filter the UV and blue portions of the spectrum. Wavelengths up to 470 nm should be eliminated. (*c*) Transmitted wavelengths should allow color discrimination. The degree of UV transmission by sunglasses has been shown to have no relationship to the color of the sunglass, the darkness of the tint, or the cost.

EYE DISEASE AMONG THE ELDERLY

The American population is aging, and the problem of providing health care for this elderly population will be significant over the next 2 decades. In fact, within the next 30 years people over 65 will be 17% of the population of the United States (51 million in the year 2020). Of interest to ophthalmologists is the fact that the risk of blindness is 10 times greater for those over 65 than for younger individuals.

In general, aging affects the eye with significant, if not dramatic, outcomes. A steep increase in eye disease occurs after age 40, corresponding to the onset of difficulty in near vision [presbyopia (see page 343)]. An even steeper increment in eye disease occurs at the age of 60. It is significant that more than half of all legally blind Americans are over 65.

Four major conditions affect the elderly.

Macular Degeneration

Macular degeneration is the leading cause of visual impairment for people over 65. One-third of the new cases of legal blindness in the elderly are due to macular degeneration. If vision loss of more than 20/40 is considered, 10% of those between 65 and 75 have macular degeneration, as do 20% of those over 75. Today, more than three million individuals have some age-related macular degeneration that causes visual loss. By 2020, there will be eight million cases.

Glaucoma

Glaucoma is the second most common cause of vision loss in the elderly population. The prevalence is 5% of people over 75 years of age. This is compounded by the known continuous visual field loss with age, with or without glaucoma. Of all individuals legally blind from glaucoma, 75% are over 65 years of age.

Cataract

From ancient time, cataract has been a major cause of visual loss, and it is still a considerable cause worldwide. In the United States, the introduction of advanced surgical techniques has allowed visual recovery when cataracts are surgically removed. Cataract extraction has become so common that, in the past year, an estimated one million cataract extractions were done in the United States.

More than 90% of individuals 75 to 85 years old have some cataract formulation, which causes a vision loss in approximately 30 to 45%. For unknown reasons, women have a slightly higher prevalence of cataract in all age groups.

Although the techniques are available to provide improved vision with surgery when cataracts are present, the impact of cataract surgery on the economics of health care delivery is significant. Billions of dollars of health care will need to be dedicated to cataract extractions over the coming decades.

Diabetic Retinopathy

In people over 65 years of age, diabetes is responsible for 10% of blindness. Aging has a significant effect on diabetic retinopathy. Diabetic retinopathy increases from 2% in the age group of 65 to 75 to 7% in the group over 75. The longer diabetes is present, the more common is the association with diabetic retinopathy. Severe nonproliferative diabetic retinopathy is seen in about 15% of patients 60 to 74 years old and about 11% of those over 75. Proliferative retinopathy is seen in about 4 to 5% of diabetics over the age of 60. It is estimated that 2% of those over 65 can be expected to manifest moderate to severe diabetic retinopathy.

Risk Factors

It is important to determine the risk factors that may suggest earlier evaluation and earlier treatment. Macular degeneration, for example, can be treated in a very small group of patients but must be treated within a short period early in the process. Education can emphasize symptoms to patients and physicians.

Open angle glaucoma has risk factors that are well known. Black patients and all patients with a strong family history have an increased incidence of glaucoma. Recognition of these risk factors will help in the detection and treatment of this disease. Glaucoma is a treatable disease in a majority of patients, and screening programs and educating physicians can help to identify cases and direct treatment.

The avoidance of certain factors that are known to be associated with cataract development is important. Ultraviolet rays, infrared rays, microwaves, and drug interactions (steroids) are important in cataract formation.

Knowledge of the incidence of complica-

tions and recognition of risk factors is important in the management of diabetes in the elderly.

FUNCTIONAL VISUAL LOSS

Visual system complaints may be present without any organic evidence of disease. Functional visual complaints may be due to malingering or hysteria. Malingering implies willful presentation or exaggeration of symptoms. Hysteria suggests a subconscious expression of symptoms. Hysterical neuroophthalmologic complaints occur in patients who have little insight into their condition and display a lack of concern over the incapacitating symptoms. The malingering patient usually has a secondary gain, such as a desire for compensation after an injury.

Characteristics of Functional Visual Field Loss

The most common presentation of functional visual loss is constricted visual fields or decreased visual acuity in one or both eyes. Constricted visual fields with functional loss have the following characteristics when compared to real loss. When a real (organic) field constriction occurs, the visual field will expand as the test distance is increased. In functional constriction of the visual fields, no such expansion is seen. On visual field testing with functional constriction, a *spiraling* on perimetry may be seen—that is, the gradual expansion of the field as the perimetrist moves the target circumferentially.

Detection of Monocular Functional Visual Loss

Optokinetic Nystagmus

In patients feigning severe visual loss, the presence of optokinetic nystagmus can reveal malingering. If an optokinetic strip or drum (see page 331) is viewed at a distance of 10 feet, the presence of a monocular response of optokinetic nystagmus indicates a visual acuity of better than 20/100.

Presence of Stereopsis

A standard stereopsis test, such as the fly test or the Worth four-dot test, may also help to establish malingering. To identify all of the dots on a Titmus dot test, one must have 20/30 vision in both eyes.

Use of Prisms in a Prism Shift Test

If a patient is fixating on a Snellen chart requiring 20/40 visual acuity or better and a 4-diopter base-out prism is introduced in front of the eye that is said by the patient to be bad, a compensatory shift to regain binocular fixation on the target is seen. (The prism causes the target to seem to move.) When the shift occurs, it is assumed that the eye reportedly with bad visual acuity at least sees the chart as it regains fixation.

Vertical Prism Test

If a vertical prism is placed in front of one eye while the patient is reading an eye chart with both eyes, a separation or double vision of the two lines is produced. When the patient reports seeing double letters, the patient must be seeing well out of both eyes.

Polaroid Filters

Polaroid filters may be placed in front of the eyes so that the vision of one eye can be controlled by the orientation of polarized light. Malingering may be determined by appropriate presentation or inappropriate response from the patient, who is unable to recognize whether an image is being seen by the "normal" or the "bad" eye. A pattern of allowing one or the other eye to see by changing the filter is under the control of the examiner.

OCULAR INJURIES

Traumatic Hyphema

Hyphema is the presence of blood cells in the anterior chamber of the eye (Fig. 6.15). Traumatic hyphema occurs after injury. Other types of hyphema are: (*a*) postsurgical, (*b*) associated with inflammation or tumor, and (*c*) spontaneous.

Types of Hyphema

Microscopic Hyphema. In microscopic hyphema, the blood cells are freely floating in the aqueous and must be observed with the slit lamp. The vision is usually decreased when microscopic hyphema is present.

Layered Hyphema. In layered hyphema, the blood cells settle out by gravity and form

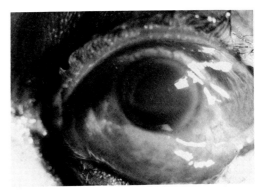

Figure 6.15. Hyphema is blood in the anterior chamber. Here the blood is layered inferiorly. This would be described as approximately a 40% hyphema, indicating that approximately 40% of the anterior chamber is filled. Hyphemas may be spontaneous, but they are most often associated with trauma.

a layer of blood, which appears as a flat line across the anterior chamber. The layering of the hyphema depends upon the position of the head. With the patient in an upright position, the hyphema will layer inferiorly. If the patient is lying down, the hyphema may layer temporally or nasally.

Layered hyphemas may be graded by the position of the top of the hyphema in the anterior chamber. For example, a hyphema may be said to fill one-quarter of the anterior chamber.

Blackball or Total Hyphema. Blood may fill the entire anterior chamber, causing a blackball hyphema. The reference is to a pool ball; this hyphema is also called "eight ball" hyphema. When the anterior chamber is filled with blood, the cornea and the anterior chamber take on a dark appearance. No iris or pupil can be seen. The effect is dark and shiny, like the eight ball in pool.

Cause

Blunt injury to the eye causes an immediate, transient, and often high rise in intraocular pressure. With this sudden increase in pressure, there is tearing of the susceptible tissue areas at the chamber angle where the iris joins the corneal scleral junction. A major arteriole system for the iris in the region may be severed with this pressure-induced tear. The result is bleeding into the anterior chamber.

Complications

Complications of hyphema are related to the severity of the initial injury. There is rough correlation of the amount of blood in the anterior chamber and the initial visual acuity with the final outcome.

Recurrent Bleeding. The major complication is recurrent bleeding. This occurs within 5 days but usually by the 3rd or 4th day after the trauma. Recurrent bleeding is associated with the need for surgical management of hyphema, glaucoma, visual loss from optic nerve damage, and corneal blood staining. Much of the therapy that is used now (aminocaproic acid) is to prevent recurrent bleeding, which seems to be related to fiber and clot dissolution within the anterior chamber.

Glaucoma. Blood cells are cleared from the anterior chamber by removal through the trabecular meshwork. The 8-μm red blood cell is squeezed through the 2- to 3-μm openings within the trabeculum. The blood cells tend to clog these openings, and there is pressure rise. Constant monitoring of the pressure after hyphema is necessary to detect this complication.

Corneal Blood Staining. Corneal blood staining is the deposition of hemoglobin breakdown products in the corneal stroma. It is related to damaged endothelium and changes in intraocular pressure. It is most often associated with increased intraocular pressure; however, it may occur in the presence of damaged endothelium with both normal and low intraocular pressures. Corneal blood staining takes months or occasionally more than a year to clear from the corneal stroma. Not infrequently, residual corneal scarring may be associated with severe corneal blood staining.

Angle Recession Glaucoma. Angle recession is the term given to the tear in the chamber angle that occurs with a hyphema. The area that is damaged has no filtration capability. Late uniocular glaucoma can occur in the traumatized eye. This glaucoma is usually related to angle tears that are greater than 180°. Patients who have had traumatic hyphema and have had gonioscopy (see page 44) indicating large angle recessions should be followed for late increases in pressure for a lifetime. Early identification of this angle change is important because the glaucoma can be difficult to manage.

Special Considerations

There is a need for hemoglobin electrophoresis in blacks. Patients with certain hemoglobinopathies, especially sickle cell traits, are susceptible to sickling within the eye, which can cause additional complications. Sickle cells are not pliable and do not easily exit from the anterior chamber because they get hung up in the trabeculum. This causes early and severe pressure rises. This can be anticipated by screening all black patients with hyphema for presence of sickle cell hemoglobinopathies.

Besides the glaucoma associated with hemoglobinopathies, there is also an increased incidence of optic nerve atrophy with hyphema in these patients. The sickling process is thought to decrease the oxygenation of the optic nerve head, making it more susceptible to damage.

Certain drugs such as Diamox increase the sickling process, causing acidosis in the aqueous. These drugs should be avoided.

Epidemiology

Hyphema tends to occur in children, who are more susceptible to ocular injuries. It also tends to occur in young adults, especially males, who are in their productive years.

In young age groups, BBs from BB guns and firecrackers are continuing major causes of trauma resulting in hyphema. In adults, sports-related injuries, especially those associated with racquetball, squash, and hockey, are major causes of hyphema, which emphasizes the need for protective eyewear in high risk sports.

Chemical Burns

Acid Burns

In general, acid burns do not cause the same degree of damage to the eye as do alkaline burns. Acid burns tend to coagulate the epithelial surface, which forms a relative barrier to further penetration by the acid. Also, the corneal stroma has a buffering capacity for solutions that are acidic.

In general, the poor prognostic indicators

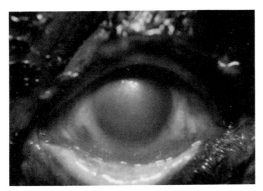

Figure 6.16. Chemical burns vary in their degree of severity according to acidity or alkalinity. Alkaline burns, especially those due to sodium hydroxide and ammonia hydroxide, are particularly devastating because the alkali penetrates the eye readily. Key features for prognosis are the appearance of the cornea and the conjunctiva. When the conjunctiva is completely burned away, the eye appears white because of lack of vessels. This, in contrast to most conditions, is a bad prognostic sign. This photograph also shows a ground glass cornea. This corneal opacification means that the cornea is totally edematous and is a poor prognostic sign.

for acid burns are complete corneal anesthesia, conjunctival and episcleral ischemia, iritis (indication of penetration of the acid), and lens opacities.

Alkaline Burns

Alkaline burns can cause severe damage to the eye (Fig. 6.16). Sodium hydroxide (lye) penetrates rapidly and causes severe intraocular damage, secondary only to that caused by ammonium hydroxide. Potassium hydroxide also penetrates readily; however, lime (calcium hydroxide) penetrates poorly because it forms calcium soaps with the epithelial membrane, which hinder further penetration (similar to acid burns). The factors that govern the severity of alkaline burns are pH, the amount of alkali, the duration of exposure, and penetration.

There may be extensive damage to the cornea and to intraocular structures including the lens, the trabecular meshwork (which can cause glaucoma), and the optic nerve (atrophy usually secondary to glaucoma). Collagenase activity destroys collagen in the cornea. The epithelium, which heals slowly, is altered, and effective corneal healing is dependant upon an intact epithelium.

The *prognostic factors* in alkali burns are:

- Degree of haze of the cornea—severe haze or "ground glass," where no iris details can be seen, has a poor prognosis (Fig. 6.16)
- Ischemia of the conjunctiva or absence of the conjunctiva also carries a poor prognosis. This appears clinically as a white eye because the vessels of the conjunctiva are destroyed.
- Total corneal anesthesia
- Ocular hypotony
- Cataract formation

Corneal Scleral Lacerations

Corneal scleral lacerations (Fig. 6.17) are caused by a variety of ocular traumas. A common cause is glass injury during a motor vehicle accident.

Corneal scleral lacerations may be associated with lid lacerations. Any lid laceration requires examination of the eye to be sure that laceration of the cornea is not present.

Lid anesthesia can be used to assist in examination for lacerations. Care should be taken so that during examination no pressure is exerted on the globe. Extrusion of intraocular contents is possible if pressure occurs.

All ocular trauma has a guarded prognosis. Corneal and corneal-scleral lacerations have a poor prognosis, especially if there is damage to intraocular contents, prolapse of vitreous or uveal tissue, or retention of an intraocular

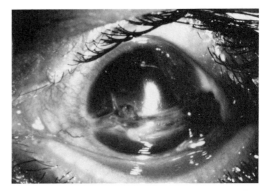

Figure 6.17. This corneal laceration shows disruption in the cornea inferiorly. Lacerations are often accompanied by anterior chamber damage, especially through the iris and lens. (Credit: George Waring, M.D.)

foreign body. Late complications include astigmatism, infection, corneal opacification due to scar tissue, and glaucoma.

Rupture of the Globe

Rupture of the globe occurs when a force applied to the globe increases the pressure within the eye until the globe explodes. This is seen with injury due to a fist, racketball, squash ball, or tennis ball and with other severe periorbital injuries.

The common sites of rupture are the *limbus,* the *equator,* and especially *under the rectus muscles,* where the sclera is thinnest. Because scleral rupture is secondary to severe injury, the prognosis is generally not good.

7

Ocular Motility

Table 7.1.
Yoke Muscles Active in Cardinal Positions of Gaze (Fig. 7.1)

Eyes up and right	right superior rectus left inferior oblique
Eyes up and left	left superior rectus right inferior oblique
Eyes right	right lateral rectus left medial rectus
Eyes left	left lateral rectus right medial rectus
Eyes down and right	right inferior rectus left superior oblique
Eyes down and left	left inferior rectus right superior oblique

Table 7.2.
Abbreviations for Extraocular Muscles

Right superior oblique	RSO
Right inferior oblique	RIO
Right superior rectus	RSR
Right inferior rectus	RIR
Right lateral rectus	RLR
Right medial rectus	RMR
Left superior oblique	LSO
Left inferior oblique	LIO
Left superior rectus	LSR
Left inferior rectus	LIR
Left lateral rectus	LLR
Left medial rectus	LMR

Table 7.3.
Muscle Functions

Muscle	Primary Function	Secondary Function	Tertiary Function
Medial rectus	Adduction		
Lateral rectus	Abduction		
Inferior rectus	Depression	Excycloduction	Adduction
Superior rectus	Elevation	Incycloduction	Adduction
Inferior oblique	Excycloduction	Elevation	Abduction
Superior oblique	Incycloduction	Depression	Abduction

Table 7.4.
Important Abbreviations

sc =	without correction
cc =	with correction
Ortho =	Orthophoria
ET =	Esotropia at distance
ET' =	Esotropia at near (⅓ m)
E (T) =	Intermittent esotropia
E =	Esophoria at distance
E' =	Esophoria at near (⅓ meter)
X =	Exophoria at distance
X' =	Exophoria at near (⅓ meter)
XT =	Exotropia at distance
XT' =	Exotropia at near (⅓ meter)
AC/A =	Accommodative convergence/ accommodation ratio
DVD =	Dissociated vertical deviation

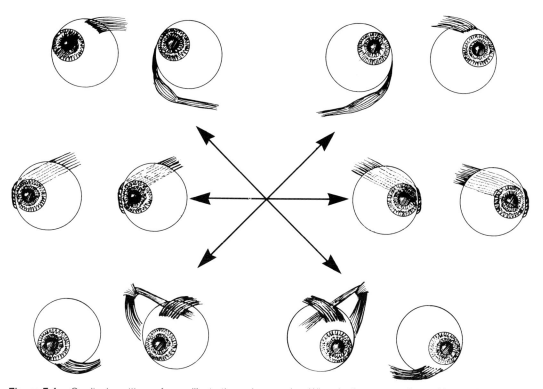

Figure 7.1. Cardinal positions of gaze illustrating yoke muscles. When both eyes are directed in certain positions of gaze, there are certain muscles that act in unison to bring those eyes into that position of gaze. These are known as yoke muscles. Illustrated are these paired muscles in the various positions of gaze.

AMBLYOPIA

Amblyopia is decreased vision without organic disease. Amblyopia is most often associated with strabismus, where reduced vision occurs from a failure to use the eye during the first few years of life, a time when stimulus to the brain from the eye is required to develop sharp visual acuity.

A newborn does not have sharp visual acuity. In fact, the visual system is only beginning to mature. It will take 4 to 5 years for 20/

20 vision and complete binocular vision to develop. If the eye cannot provide an image, the visual system will not develop properly. This has been demonstrated in animals when the eyelid is permanently closed at birth. Vision potential fails to develop, and the visual pathways show atrophy.

Amblyopia is defined as two or more lines of difference on the eye chart between the worse eye and the good eye.

There are three types of amblyopia:

- *Strabismic amblyopia* develops from crossed eyes, which do not allow adequate stimulus in proper position on the retina to develop good vision.
- *Anisometropic amblyopia* develops from unequal refractive error (greater than 2 diopters) where, with one eye focused, the retinal image on the opposite eye is not sharp enough to develop clear vision.
- *Sensory amblyopia* results from failure of the image to form on the retina due to opacities of the ocular medium, for example, cataract or corneal scars.

SUPPRESSION

Suppression is an adaptive mechanism. Suppression is when an image that stimulates a retina is not perceived. Most commonly, this occurs in strabismus patients, where abnormal alignment of the eye causes different areas of the two retinas to be stimulated, a condition that would result in double vision (diplopia). The brain chooses to ignore the image from one eye, that is, suppress the image, so that double vision does not result.

There are practical applications to suppression. People who use one eye to look through a monocular microscope, hunters who align a gun sight with one eye, and people who use a telescopic lens to view an opera singer will conveniently suppress the image not wanted in the eye that's not being used for viewing. This suppression, of course, is not complete and not pathologic.

PHORIA

A phoria is a latent tropia and is related to brain fusion of retinal images from two eyes.

A tropia is a deviation of the eyes. Both eyes are not coordinated as usual and eyes cross in (esotropia) or out (exotropia). Tropias are continually present.

A phoria is a latent tropia, that is, the deviation is present at some times and not at others. Fusion is the mechanism that keeps both eyes straight when a phoria is present. If there is loss of fusion, a deviation occurs and the phoria becomes obvious.

Fusion is the function of the visual system whereby an image is recorded on both retinas and transported to the brain where it is superimposed into one image. Each point on the retina has a corresponding point in the brain. For fusion of the two retinal images to occur, it is necessary for the exact retinal points in each eye to be aligned so that the images will be superimposed in the brain according to where they fall on the retina. When fusion is active, it has a feedback control mechanism that helps maintain ocular alignment. With a phoria, the feedback mechanism by fusion prevents the deviation. When the fusion is interrupted by covering one eye and allowing only a single image to the brain or by weakened central control due to fatigue or alcohol, a phoria occurs.

Test for Phorias

A phoria is a deviation of the eyes that occurs only at certain times (a latent tropia). Remember that in tropias the deviation is always present. However, in phorias, the abnormal deviation does not occur unless fusion is not present. To test for this, we break fusion by covering one eye. If a phoria is present, a deviation will occur.

- *Exophorias* are latent deviations outward.
- *Esophorias* are latent deviations inward.

Diagnosis

In the cover/uncover test (Fig. 7.2), each eye is covered for approximately 2 to 3 seconds. Between covering the eyes, the examiner pauses to allow both eyes to go back to the fused position. If there is movement while one of the eyes is covered, a phoria is present. Inward movement of the covered eye is an

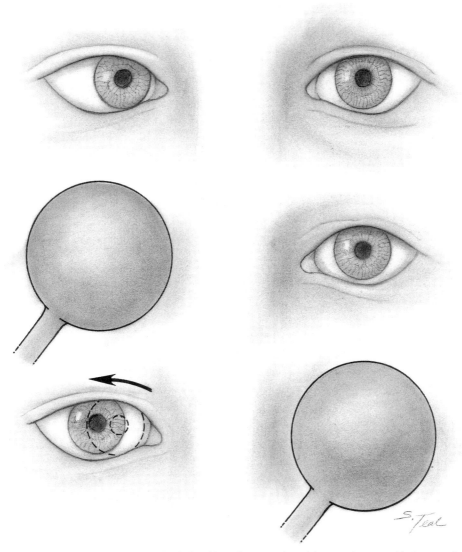

Figure 7.2. The cover/uncover test breaks fusion. Normally no motion of the eyes is seen with the cover/uncover test. However, with a latent deviation (phoria), movement of the eye that is covered is diagnostic.

esophoria; outward movement is an exophoria.

The degree of phoria may be determined by Maddox rod testing. A Maddox rod, a special lens that forms a "rod" image, produces a red-light line in front of one eye that can be compared to a dot or a white line in front of the other eye. Fusion is broken, and if a phoria is present it will be elicited. Prisms are then used to bring the two lines together. When the lines meet, the amount of prism necessary is a measure of the deviation.

Prisms can also be used, without a Maddox rod, to measure the degree of phoria. Prism power is increased until the eye movement induced by the cover/uncover test is neutralized. This quantitates the amount of phoria in prism diopters.

Importance of Phorias

Phorias may manifest when a patient becomes tired, drinks alcohol, or is under stressful situations. In some patients, the necessity of maintaining fusion to control the phoria, prevent a deviation, and avoid double vision may require an excess amount of work on the

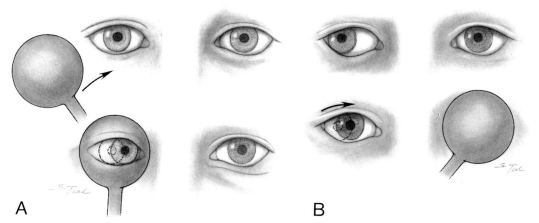

A   B

Figure 7.3. The cover/cross-cover test is used to test the presence of ocular deviation, exotropia or esotropia primarily but also hypertropias. The occlusion paddle is moved from one eye to the other and back again. The patient needs to be fixating on an object during the test. Normally no movement will occur. If there is an abnormal deviation, movement of the eye is seen with movement of the occluder.

extraocular muscle system. In these circumstances, the symptoms of brow ache or vague discomfort in and around the eyes while using the eyes may be relieved by establishing the diagnosis of a phoria and providing effective treatment. Exophoria can progress to intermittent exotropia, a permanent deviation (page 152).

ESOTROPIA

Definition

Esotropia is a constant inward crossing of the eyes (Figs. 7.3 and 7.4). The eyes cross in-

ward in other conditions also. In esophoria (page 144), the eyes cross only when one eye is occluded. Occlusion prevents the fusion of two images in the brain and, as a result, the influence of fusion on control of the alignment of the eyes is lost. When this control is broken, the eyes cross inward. This is *esophoria*. In intermittent *esotropia,* the esotropia is present at some times and not at others.

Prevalence

Esotropia is the most common type of misalignment of the eyes. Inward deviations rep-

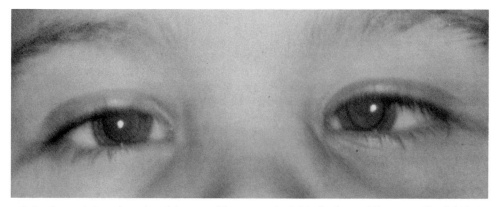

Figure 7.4. Esotropia is an inturning of the eyes. The eye on the left is fixating and the eye on the right is turned in. Note the asymmetrical positions of the light reflexes. On the left, the corneal light reflex is in the center; on the right, the light reflex is off center toward the pupillary edge. The use of light reflexes to estimate ocular deviations is known as the Krimsky test.

resent over 50% of all ocular deviations in young patients.

Causes

The two major types of esotropia are accommodative and nonaccommodative. In the nonaccommodative group, there are a number of subcategories.

Accommodative esotropia is due to a refractive error of hyperopia (farsightedness). These patients can see improvement with the use of glasses. In contrast, the nonaccommodative group requires surgery for proper alignment of the eyes. The nonaccommodative group includes inturning of the eyes that may be present from birth (congenital or infantile) and may be associated with other syndromes, may be acquired because of restrictions of one of the ocular muscles, or may be due to a neurologic deficit.

Combinations

There may be a combination of nonaccommodative and accommodative esotropia.

Nonaccommodative Esotropia

Esotropias that are present at birth (congenital) or in early infancy (infantile esotropia) are underlined. Those conditions not underlined occur later in life.

- Classic congenital esotropia
- Duane's syndrome
- Sixth nerve palsy
- Monofixation syndrome
- Möbius' syndrome
- Others
- Graves' ophthalmopathy (thyroid association)
- Medial orbital wall fracture
- Surgically caused muscle restriction
- Sixth nerve palsy
- Others

Classical Congenital Esotropia (Infantile Esotropia)

Characteristics

Congenital esotropia starts within the first 6 months of life, but the exact time is difficult to pinpoint. Family members often have a history of crossed eyes, although no distinct genetic pattern is usually found. Children with congenital esotropia are usually otherwise healthy, although this type of esotropia has been associated with cerebral palsy and hydrocephalus.

Large Deviation

Infants with congenital esotropia tend to have large degrees of inturning [greater than 30 prism diopters]. Characteristically, they develop a cross-fixation, that is, they use one eye or the other eye with equal facility but not together. The central nervous system blocks out the image of the eye not in use so that there is no double vision. Because they use both eyes with equal facility, the visual acuity tends to be good as well as equal in both eyes.

A less common alternative to cross-fixation occurs. Some esotropic infants use one eye only for all visual function. There is no cross-fixation. The eye opposite does not develop good visual acuity because of lack of use (amblyopia).

Other difficulties with alignment in the ocular system are common in congenital esotropia:

- Overaction of the inferior oblique muscles;
- Dissociated vertical deviation (page 152) (thought to be an important hallmark of esotropia);
- Nystagmus (page 112)—rotary, horizontal, or latent.

Accommodative Component

It is not uncommon to have some portion of esotropia and of congenital esotropia be associated with an accommodative component of farsightedness. Careful refraction and trial of glasses is indicated to determine the actual amount of nonaccommodative esotropia.

Accommodative Esotropia

Accommodation is the ocular mechanism for focusing the image on the retina when the object is moved from distance to near. This focus is a result of contraction of the

Figure 7.5. A,   Accommodation is the focus mechanism. It is under parasympathetic control. Ciliary body contraction loosens zonules, and the lens thickens. Accommodation results.

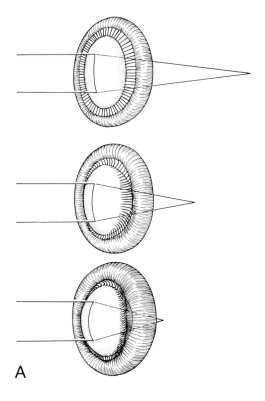

A

Figure 7.5. B,   In the emmotropic eye, an object at distance is focused on the retina. A near object without accommodation focuses behind the retina. Accommodation focuses a near object on the retina.

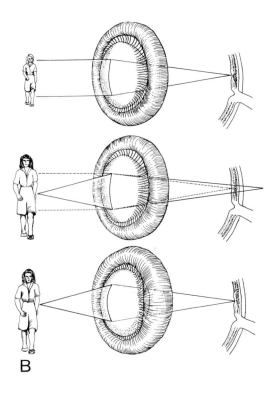

B

ciliary muscle, which changes the shape of and therefore affects the power of the lens[a] (Fig. 7.5).

The process of accommodation is naturally tied to the process of convergence. Convergence refers to the alignment of the eyes as attention is moved from distance to near. At distance, the eyes may be almost parallel in their position for observation. As the image comes closer, however, there is a need for the eyes to look progressively inward by increased contraction of both of the medial rectus muscles. This is called convergence (Fig. 7.6).

Because accommodation and convergence are normally interacting at the same time, a significant abnormality can occur when accommodation is overworked. This is commonly seen in the farsighted (hyperopic) child. In farsightedness, the refractive system is deficient, and the image is focused behind the retina. To see clearly, the child must (even at a distance) use accommodation to bring the image onto the retina. This is in contrast to the eye with no refractive error (emmetropia); in this eye, no accommodation is required at distance because the image is focused on the retina, and accommodation is used only for near focus.

The farsighted child must use accommodation at a distance and at a time when he would normally, if he were not farsighted, not need accommodation. To see up close, the farsighted child must add even more accommodation to the accommodation used at distance. This total accommodation is far in excess of what the normal person would need for keeping the image clear at near.

This excess of accommodation causes an excess of convergence. When the excess convergence occurs, the eyes cross inward (esotropia). Esotropia caused by excess accommodation as a result of hyperopia is called *accommodative esotropia.*

Accommodative esotropia usually starts

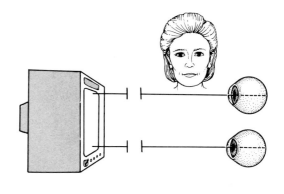

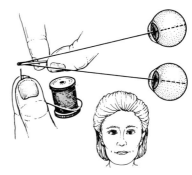

Figure 7.6. Convergence is inward turning of the eyes as an object moves from distance to near. Illustrated are eyes in relative parallel alignment for distant viewing but converging for near function, such as threading a needle. Convergence, accommodation, and pupillary constriction occur simultaneously.

between the ages of 1 and 3 years. The onset is usually abrupt. There frequently is a history of crossed eyes in the child's family.

Testing an Esotropic Child for Accommodative Esotropia

To be able to test the esotropic child, all accommodation must be relaxed to allow an accurate measure of the degree of farsightedness. To relax this accommodation, a strong parasympatholytic drug is used. The most common drugs used are atropine, homatropine, and cyclopentolate. This technique is a *cycloplegic refraction.*

Treatment

To treat accommodative esotropia, one corrects the refractive error. By doing a complete refraction and giving full correction so that accommodation is reduced, convergence

---

[a]To achieve accommodation, the circular ciliary muscle within the eye contracts. This relaxes the supporting ligaments (zonules) on the intraocular lens, and the lens is allowed to become more rounded. This adds plus power to the lens and brings the image from behind the retina onto the retina.

can be relaxed. This brings the refractive state to normal, takes away the convergence stimulus, and lets the eyes straighten.

Glasses. The degree of accommodation used by the hyperopic child must be determined by a cycloplegic refraction. Correction of the farsightedness with glasses straightens the eyes unless there is an underlying strabismic mechanism other than the accommodation esotropia. If there is excess accommodation at near even when accommodation is relaxed at a distance, bifocal lenses can be used to help further relax accommodation for near.

Drugs. Anticholinesterase drugs can be used to reduce accommodation and treat accommodative esotropia in selected cases. These drugs are rarely used today.

No Surgery. In pure accommodative esotropia, where all excess accommodation is due to refractive error, surgery is not indicated. Many cases, however, have only a partial accommodative component and often both surgery and glasses are required.

ACCOMMODATIVE CONVERGENCE/ ACCOMMODATION RATIO

Background

The AC/A ratio involves convergence and accommodation. At distance, the eyes are parallel but, as attention is directed from far to near, both eyes converge inward. This is convergence. Accommodation is the ability of each eye to focus from a distant object to a near object. Convergence and accommodation are linked by neurologic control. Under normal circumstances, the relationship between the amount of convergence and the amount of accommodation remains constant as visual tasks change from distance to near; that is, a measured amount of convergence is accompanied by a similar amount of accommodation.

Convergence is measured in prism diopters. The prism diopter (see page 345) refers to the movement of light or of an image that occurs when a prism is placed in the pathway of light. A prism diopter will divert the path of light 1 cm at a distance of 1 m.

Accommodation is measured in diopters, not prism diopters. The terminology can become confusing. This diopter for accommodation is the same diopter that is used in reference to plus and minus lenses in refraction. In this case, the diopter is the degree of power of the lens that will converge parallel rays at a distance of 1 meter. Because the accommodative mechanism involves the ciliary muscle, the zonules attached to the ciliary muscle in the lens, and the lens shape, the accommodative mechanism deals with changes in lens power.

Abnormal Accommodative Convergence/ Accommodation (AC/A) Ratio

With a normal AC/A ratio, the eyes converge when a set amount of lens focus occurs. With a high AC/A ratio, convergence at near is in excess of what would be expected with the accommodation stimulus. This usually presents clinically as straight eyes at distance and esotropia at near.

In contrast, a low AC/A ratio would be more convergence related to accommodation at distance and less convergence related to accommodation at near. This could present either as an exotropia near with normal alignment at distance or as less esotropia at near than at distance.

Two Methods of Measuring the AC/A Ratio

Measuring How Much the Convergence Changes When Accommodation Is Altered

In this method, the subject is asked to look at a target that the subject keeps in focus. The distance remains constant. Then, by the use of refractive lenses, accommodation is stimulated. For example, by placing a -2-diopter lens in front of the eye, 2 diopters of accommodation by the eye are required to keep the image in focus.

As the accommodation is changed by the use of lenses, the degree of convergence is measured in prism diopters. This technique requires skill with prisms and the cover test (Fig 7.2). The AC/A ratio is then calculated by dividing the change in lens power into the change in the prism diopters associated with the change. This is the *gradient method.*

Measuring Eye Alignment at Near and at Far

The second technique measures the alignment of the eyes at near and at far. If the patient is more esotropic at near than at distance, this is a high AC/A ratio. If the patient is less esotropic at near and more esotropic at far, this indicates a low AC/A ratio.

The normal AC/A ratio, although variable, is usually between 3.7 and 4.2.

High AC/A Ratio with Accommodation Esotropia

High AC/A ratios may occur with or without accommodative esotropia. There are certain characteristics of a high AC/A ratio that may occur with accommodative esotropia:

- *Refractive errors* may vary, but are usually *normal* for the age;
- There is little or *no distance deviation,* but the *esotropia* occurs in *near* (of moderate degree);
- The esotropia may be present only with small objects requiring a far amount of accommodation;
- The esotropia is lessened at near when +3-diopter lenses are placed in front of the eyes.

MONOFIXATION SYNDROME (MICROTROPIA)

Clinical Characteristics

Monofixation syndrome usually presents with a very small amount of esotropia (usually less than 8 prism diopters).[b] The fovea is anatomically the central area of the retina used for discrete vision. In the monofixation syndrome, in one eye there is a very small area of decreased vision directly in the center of the fovea (central scotoma). The area around this scotoma in the fovea sees normally and the eyes are able, under most circumstances, to achieve some fusion of images in the central nervous system and usually present with binocular viewing. However, decreased vision (amblyopia) is a common finding, although it is most often slight. Steropsis is usually present although, because of the loss of vision, the quality of the steropsis is altered (reduced stereo acuity).

Cause

- It may be a primary condition without identifiable cause.
- It may follow the treatment of a larger amount of esotropia either with glasses or by surgery.
- It can occur when there is a difference in the refractive error between the eyes (anisometropia).
- It may occur with a small macular lesion that causes loss of foveal vision (central scotoma).

EXODEVIATIONS

Definition

There are three exodeviations:
1. Exotropia. Exotropia is an outward deviation of the eyes that is consistent (Fig. 7.7). There is no fusion.
2. Intermittent exotropia. This is an outward deviation of the eye that is present at some times and not at others. When the deviation is not present, the fusion mechanism controls alignment of the eyes.
3. Exophoria. Exophoria is an outward deviation of the eyes that occurs only when the fusion mechanism is broken by covering one eye (cover/uncover test, Fig 7.2). When the fusion mechanism is intact and both eyes are functioning, the eyes are in proper alignment.

Exophoria

The degree of exodeviation in exophoria with one eye covered is usually small. The patient may have symptoms of ocular fatigue (asthenopia), especially with long periods of detailed visual work and reading.

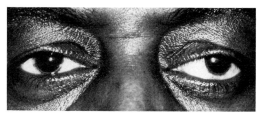

Figure 7.7. Exotropia is an outward deviation of the eyes. Here the patient's right eye is fixated straight ahead and the left eye is deviated laterally. (Credit: George Waring, M.D.)

---

[b]This syndrome may also present with exotropia or even no crossing of the eyes.

Intermittent Exotropia

Onset

This condition usually begins in childhood, from infancy to about age 4 years. Some patients with intermittent exotropia will decompensate into constant exotropia.

Clinical Characteristics

- Bright light causing eye closure. Exposure to sunlight as when walking from a dark room into bright sunlight can cause a reflex closure of one eye.
- Suppression. When the deviation is present, temporal hemiretinal suppression may occur. The deviation causes the image to fall in a retinal area that does not correspond with an appropriate similarly stimulated area in the opposite eye. Suppression assures that, during the time of deviation, the misplaced image will not be perceived. This develops with deviations in children less than 10 years of age. When the eyes are straight with fusion present, retinal correspondence functions normally.
- The exodeviation may be aggravated by certain factors: distant viewing, distraction, illness.
- Amblyopia (vision loss without evidence of organic disease) is rare in individuals with exodeviation.
- A high accommodative convergence to accommodation ratio (AC/A) (page 150) is usually present.
- Oblique muscle dysfunction may be present, and vertical deviations may occur.
- Deviation may progress, with distance fixation being involved first. Later, near fixation is involved. This is variable.

Exotropia

Characteristics

- Found mostly in adults after uniocular visual impairment or from a decompensated intermittent exotropia.
- Double vision is unusual.
- If the exotropia is large, oblique muscle

overaction is common. [A large X pattern may be present (page 258)].
- Congenital exotropias do occur.

Exotropia may occur with third nerve lesions. Third nerve palsies are rare in children, but are common in adults. They are caused by a variety of processes: diabetes, aneurysm, trauma, neoplasm. Third nerve palsies are accompanied by ptosis of the lid, pupillary abnormalities, and abnormal horizontal-vertical movements of the eye.

Classification of the Exodeviation

The basic exodeviation is constant at near and far. However, there is variability and two subclassifications are used.

1. Divergence Excess

This consists of exodeviation that is greater at distance than at near fixation.

Diagnosis. A true divergence excess remains greater at distance than at near when tested on remeasurement with a +3.00 lens in front of the eyes or if deviation remains constant after a period of uniocular occlusion. A simulated divergence excess refers to a change in the degree of deviation when a +3.00 spherical lens is used in front of each eye or when one eye has been occluded for 30 to 45 minutes.

Mechanisms of Tests. Uniocular occlusion removes binocular fusion impulses and the +3.00 lenses decrease the effect of accommodation on the fusional system.

2. Convergence Insufficiency

This is diagnosed when the exodeviations are greater at near than at distance.

DISSOCIATED VERTICAL DEVIATION (DVD)

Diagnosis

While the patient is gazing forward, either eye may drift upward into an elevated position. This may occur when one eye is occluded or may occur when the subject becomes inattentive to gaze.

The key point in diagnosis is that the eye that drifts upward then comes back to the original position and the fellow eye, which is the fixating eye, shows no movement whatsoever. (This differentiates the condition from hypertropia where, if the elevated eye comes down to a horizontal position, the opposite eye will show movement and be depressed.)

Characteristics

- The eye that drifts almost always drifts in the upward position.
- This eye may also turn outward and rotate outward on elevation.
- The condition usually is bilateral, but is not always symmetrical. On occasion, it may be unilateral only.
- It may also be associated with nystagmus (page 112) and congenital esotropia (page 147).

Cause

Unknown

Differential Diagnosis

Rule out the following when making this diagnosis:

- Overaction of the inferior oblique;
- Presence of a hypertropia.

VERTICAL DEVIATIONS
Definition

Vertical deviation is one eye higher or lower than the other. The terminology is based on which eye is looking at an object. If one eye is fixated on an object and the other eye is higher, the condition is called *hypertropia*. If, however, one eye is fixated and the other eye is lower, this is called *hypotropia.*[c]

---

[c]Hyperphorias and hypophorias also exist. Hyperphoria or hypophoria is when one eye is higher or lower than the other, but only one or the other eye is occluded. This occlusion prevents fusion of images, and the control fusion contributes to maintaining ocular alignment. For further information regarding phorias, see page 144.

In evaluation of vertical deviations, there are two general categories, commitant and incommitant. If the difference in the alignment between the two eyes is the same in all positions of gaze (cardinal positions), then the deviation is described as *commitant.* Most vertical deviations do not start out in this way; however, after time, they come closer and closer to being more equal in all fields of gaze, especially when a muscle paralysis is the cause. If the vertical deviation is more marked in one field of gaze than in others, it is described as *incommitant.*

Causes of Vertical Deviation

There are two major causes of vertical deviation: (*a*) decrease or lack of a nerve stimulus to muscle and (*b*) friction of muscle movement due to scar tissue or some mechanical restriction.

Differential Diagnosis of Vertical Deviation

- Dissociated vertical deviation (page 152)
- Inferior oblique muscle overaction
- Superior oblique muscle overaction
- Paralysis of the superior oblique muscle
- Brown's syndrome (page 263)
- Double elevator palsy
- Inferior oblique muscle palsy
- Fractures of the orbital floor with soft tissue and muscle entrapment
- Restriction due to Grave's ophthalmopathy

THREE-STEP TEST
Use

This is the test used in patients with vertical muscle imbalance, primarily to help localize superior oblique palsy.

Background

This test isolates the involved superior oblique muscle causing a vertical imbalance

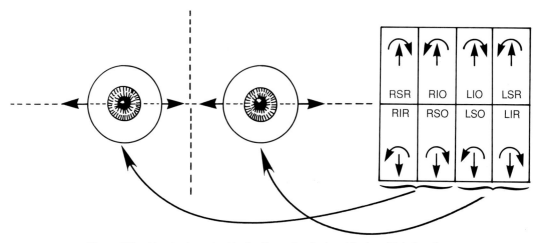

Figure 7.8. Muscles important in the three-step test and their multiple functions.

between the two eyes. Twelve extraocular muscles work together to keep the eyes aligned and in position, six muscles on each eye. Depending on the position of the eye, some muscles have multiple functions. They may not only pull the eye in or out or up or down, but may also have a rotating function.

Rotation of the eye, called cycloversion, can be induced by tilting the head to the right. The eyes will rotate to keep the ocular (and the retinal) position upright. To be specific, head tilt to the right rotates the left eye outward and the right eye inward. Keep in mind that these inward and outward rotations of the eye are done by muscles that also function to lift or depress the eye.

When the eye looks in, the oblique muscles do most of the elevating and depressing. When the eye looks out, the vertical rectus muscles do most of the elevating and depressing. The superior muscles (SR, SO) rotate the eye in (intort) and the inferior muscles (IR, IO) rotate the eye out (extort) (Fig. 7.8).

When a patient is unable to maintain the alignment of the eyes vertically, we can narrow down the number of possible muscles involved from 12 to 8. The lateral and medial recti have functions only in horizontal gaze and would not be involved in the up or down movement of the eye. Therefore, we have the two vertical rectus and the two oblique muscles, in each eye, for a total of eight.

The three-step test, which is based on iso-

lation of one of the eight possible muscles, is as follows:

1. Find out which eye is higher than the other.
2. Find out whether the difference between the two eyes is greater in left gaze or in right gaze.
3. Tilt the head to the left and then to the right and see in which position the vertical imbalance between the two eyes is greater.

These three steps isolate the multiple functions of each of the muscles and help determine the muscle that is weak. We can follow this process through by example. Remember:

- Elevate the right eye—RSR, RIO;
- Elevate the left eye—LSR, LIO;
- Depress the right eye—RIR, RSO;
- Depress the left eye—LIR, LSO.

The above muscle functions are important in steps 1 and 2.

- Right eye rotate in—RSR, RSO;
- Right eye rotate out—RIO, RIR;
- Left eye rotate in—LSR, LSO;
- Left eye rotate out—LIO, LIR.

The above muscle functions are used in step 3.

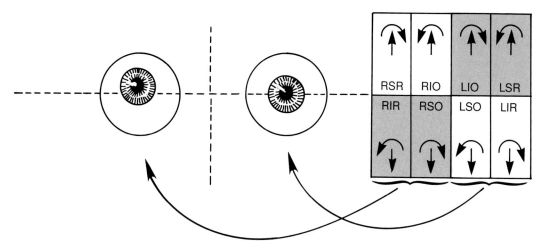

Figure 7.9. Three-step test, step 1. The right eye is higher than the left in primary gaze (frontal gaze). The muscles that might be involved are *shaded*. For right eye, RIR, RSO, or for left eye, LIO, LSR.

A Sample Patient Evaluated with the Three-Step Test

A patient describes double vision, with objects above and below each other. Eight muscles are involved in vertical movements (right superior oblique, right inferior rectus, right inferior oblique, right superior rectus, left inferior oblique, left inferior rectus, left superior oblique, left superior rectus). The three-step test will determine which of the muscles is not functioning.

Step 1

We determine, using the alternate cover test (Fig 7.3), that in looking straight ahead the right eye is higher than the left eye (Fig. 7.9). This means one of two things: either those muscles that pull the right eye down are deficient or those muscles that elevate the left eye are deficient. Those muscles that pull the right eye down are the right inferior rectus and the right superior oblique and those that lift the left eye are the left inferior oblique and the left superior rectus. On the diagram (Fig. 7.9), the muscles involved in the vertical deviation isolated by step 1 are shaded. We now have four possible muscles.

Step 2

Is the deviation worse in left gaze or right gaze (Fig. 7.10)? In our example, the difference in vertical alignment is worse in left gaze. By referring to Figure 7.10, we can identify the muscles involved in keeping the eyes aligned in left gaze: the right inferior oblique and the right superior oblique for the right eye and the left superior rectus and the left inferior rectus for the left eye. The boxes indicating these muscles are shaded.

Step 3 (Fig. 7.11)

Is the vertical difference worse with the head tilted to the left or to the right? In our sample patient the difference is worse when the head tilts to the right (Fig. 7.11). With head tilting, the rotators of the eye come into play; therefore, muscles that assist in rotation of the eye in the right-tilted head position are deficient. With the head tilted to the right, the right eye must rotate in and the left eye must rotate out to maintain alignment. In Figure 7.11, those muscles that are active in rotation of the eye in a right-tilted head position are shaded. These are the muscles that will rotate the right eye inward and the left eye outward: right superior rectus, right superior oblique, left inferior rectus, and left inferior oblique.

The various functions in different head positions and in different fields of gaze are isolated. We can now combine our information from each step to find out which muscle has been involved in all three steps of the test. Combine the shaded boxes of our previous diagrams and find that only one muscle is

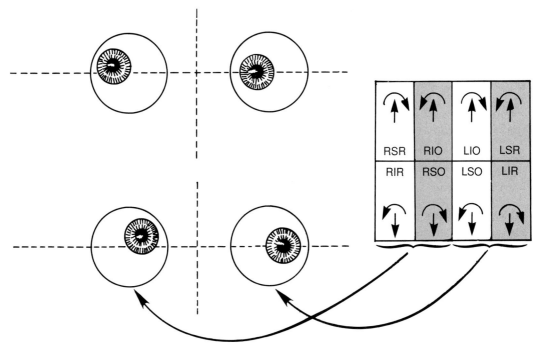

Figure 7.10. Three-step test, step 2. On looking to the right and then the left, the deviation is greater in left gaze. Those muscles that might be involved are *shaded.* For the right eye, RIO, RSO, and for the left eye, LSR, LIR.

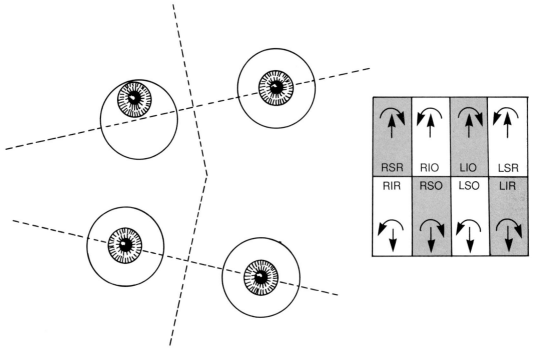

Figure 7.11. Three-step test, step 3. When the head is tilted to the right and then to the left, the deviation is worse when the head is tilted to the right. Muscles that might be involved are *shaded.* For the right eye, RSR, RSO, and for the left eye, LIO, LIR.

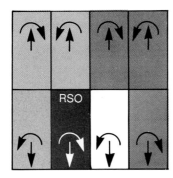

Figure 7.12. Three-step test, combining results. By summarizing the three parts of the three-step test, we can see that the only muscle that is identified in all three stages of localization is the right superior oblique *(darkest shading)*. The three-step test isolates the right superior oblique as the muscle affected.

shaded 3 times in this three-step test (Fig. 7.12). In our example, this is the right superior oblique. By using the three-step test, we have discovered that the right superior oblique is the paretic muscle.

DUANE'S RETRACTION SYNDROME

Cause

Electrophysiologic studies have shown that Duane's syndrome results from a paradoxical innervation of the lateral rectus muscle. In essence, the nerve stimulus decreases when it should be increasing (when the eye is turning outward) and increases when it should be decreasing (when the eye is turning inward). This paradoxical firing causes the medial rectus and the lateral rectus to contract simultaneously. This is a co-contraction and causes the globe to be pulled back into the orbit. As time progresses, the involved muscles become fibrotic. Fibrosis is secondary to the primary process of paradoxical innervation.

Clinical Features

- The involved eye is unable to move out or laterally (absence of abduction).
- There is restriction to the involved eye turning inward (restricted adduction).
- The globe retracts into the orbit a few millimeters when there is an attempt by the involved eye to look inward (adduction).
- The space between the lids narrows due to the retraction of the globe on attempted looking inward to the involved eye.

Important Aspects of Duane's Syndrome

- Left eye more frequently involved than right eye, can be bilateral, and may involve right eye only.
- Bilateral in 15 to 20% of cases.
- Vertical upshooting (or downshooting) of the involved eye may be present and is a helpful diagnostic sign.
- Retraction of the globe with inturning of the involved eye.
- More frequent in females than in males.
- Of all patients with strabismus, 1% have Duane's retraction syndrome.
- Patients turn the head to the involved side to compensate for the lateral gaze position that the eye must assume.
- As time develops, an esotropia becomes prominent.

Clinical Types

Clinically there are three types of Duane's syndrome:

- Type 1: Limitation of outward movements (abduction) of the involved eye.
- Type 2: Limitation of inward turning of the involved eye (adduction).
- Type 3: Limitation of both inturning and outturning of the involved eye (abduction and adduction).

Syndromes That Have Increased Frequency of Association with Duane's Retraction Syndrome

- Klippel-Feil anomalies of the spine;
- Wildervanck's syndrome (a combination of Klippel-Feil anomalies, sensorineural deafness, and Duane's syndrome).

8

Medical Ophthalmology

OCULAR ALBINISM

Albinism is congenital hypopigmentation. Ocular albinism may or may not occur with other general forms.

Characteristics

Ocular albinism is generally divided into two types: (*a*) congenitally subnormal visual acuity with nystagmus and (*b*) normal to moderately reduced visual acuity with no nystagmus. Both are characterized by decrease of pigment in ocular structures.

Both types of ocular albinism have similar clinical features: (*a*) iris transillumination (light from the interior of the eye normally blocked by iris pigment now shines through, giving the iris a red hue), (*b*) hypopigmented eye grounds, and (*c*) light sensitivity (photophobia).

Albinism and Syndromes

Tyrosinase enzyme activity is important in the biosynthesis of melanin and has been used to differentiate albinism. In general, tyrosinase-positive and tyrosinase-negative individuals can be determined clinically: tyrosinase-negative subjects have no pigmentation of the skin, hair, or eyes; tyrosinase-positive persons have partial pigmentation. For the clinician, the tyrosinase test is limited in its application to patient care.

Ocular albinism is associated with a number of syndromes. There are two important syndromes that are life-threatening. The Chédiak-Higashi syndrome is associated with a susceptibility to infections in young children. The Hermansky-Pudlak syndrome is associated with bleeding abnormalities. Patients experience easy bruising and bleeding due to a platelet abnormality.

COTTON-WOOL SPOTS

Definition

Cotton-wool spots (Fig. 8.1) are focal areas of superficial retinal whitening that have fluffy margins and are generally small (occupying less than one-quarter of the diameter of the optic disc).

Importance

Even a single isolated cotton-wool spot may be an indication of systemic disease. Any patient who presents with cotton-wool spots as an isolated or as one of multiple findings and who does not have a reasonable established diagnosis should be investigated for an occult systemic disease.

158

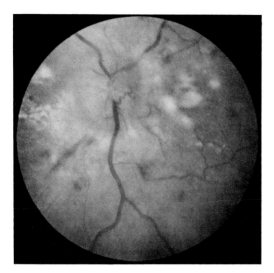

Figure 8.1. Cotton-wool spots. Cotton-wool spots, here illustrated around the disc as fluffy white patches, are areas of edema secondary to retinal ischemia. Cotton-wool spots can be seen in hypertension, diabetes, and vessel occlusions due to emboli, as well as a number of other conditions.

Cause

Cotton-wool spots are due to local ischemia from obstruction of a retinal arteriole. Cotton-wool spots can be reproduced experimentally by injecting minute glass spheres into the vascular system of primates to cause the occlusion.

Causes of cotton-wool spots are listed in Table 8.1. In the differential diagnosis of cotton-wool spots, the following diseases are most common.

Diabetes Mellitus

Of cotton-wool spots, diabetes is the most common cause. Of a single cotton-wool spot without other physical signs or symptoms and without a history of diabetes or other systemic illness, diabetes remains the single most important cause. For these patients, a 3-hour glucose tolerance test should be considered.

Systemic Hypertension

Systemic hypertension is a common cause of cotton-wool spots. The cotton-wool spot may or may not be associated with arterial narrowing. The presence of cotton-wool spots is associated with high diastolic pressures. The presumed mechanism is prefibrinoid ne-

crosis with occlusion of the precapillary arterioles.

Collagen Vascular Disease

The following collagen vascular diseases should be considered when cotton-wool spots are seen: dermatomyositis, systemic lupus erythematosus, and polyarteritis nodosa. Antinuclear antibody titers should be drawn to rule out this possibility.

Cardiac Valvular Disease

Mitral regurgitation and mitral valve prolapse (Barlow syndrome) should be considered in the differential diagnosis. Echocardiography can be used to help in diagnosis.

Carotid Obstruction

Arteriography should be done to rule out stenosis of the internal carotid artery when in-

Table 8.1.
Causes Associated with Cotton-Wool Spots

Common Causes
Diabetes mellitus
Systemic hypertension
Collagen vascular disease
   Systemic lupus erythematosus
   Dermatomyositis
   Polyarteritis nodosa
   Scleroderma
   Giant cell arteritis
Cardiac valvular disease
   Mitral valve prolapse
   Rheumatic heart disease
   Endocarditis
AIDS
Leukemia
Trauma (Purtscher's retinopathy)

Less Common Causes
Radiation retinopathy
Central retinal artery obstruction
Retinal venous obstruction
Metastatic carcinoma
Severe anemia
Acute blood loss
Aortic arch syndrome
Intravenous drug abuse
High altitude retinopathy
Onchocerciasis
Acute pancreatitis
Dysproteinemias
Papilledema
Papillitis
Rocky Mountain spotted fever
Leptospirosis

---

dicated. Cotton-wool spots can be seen on the same side as carotid stenosis.

Leukemia

A seemingly healthy person can present with cotton-wool spots with myelomonocytic leukemia. A complete blood count will help establish this diagnosis.

AIDS

Cotton-wool spots can be seen in the fundi of patients with acquired immune deficiency syndrome (AIDS). These are frequently associated with signs and symptoms compatible with cytomegalovirus, an opportunistic infection associated with AIDS.

Trauma (Purtscher's Retinopathy)

Cotton-wool spots can be seen in patients who have sustained severe body trauma, especially to the chest and long bones. These cotton-wool spots (see color Fig. C.31) may be uniocular or binocular. They are thought to be due to emboli released into the blood stream as a result of the trauma.

Radiation Retinopathy

Patients who have received radiation in and around the eye (e.g., radiation for sarcoma of the orbit or for sarcoma or carcinoma of the choroid) may have cotton-wool spots that dominate the fundus picture.

Intravenous Drug Abuse

In young people, especially those with a history of drug abuse, cotton-wool spots could be caused by emboli due to intravenous injection.

Metastatic Carcinoma

Metastatic carcinoma has been known to present with the isolated finding of cotton-wool spots. The exact mechanism is unknown.

Giant Cell Arteritis

Cotton-wool spots have been seen with giant cell arteritis where the optic disc is normal in appearance and the remainder of the posterior pole is normal. The opposite eye has a history of sudden vision loss and has evidence of acute anterior ischemic optic neuropathy. The sedimentation rate is increased.

Laboratory Tests

The occurrence of cotton-wool spots without a reasonable clinical explanation should stimulate the physician to consider the following tests: 3-hour glucose tolerance test, blood pressure, complete blood count, antinuclear antibody titers, erythrocyte sedimentation rate, and questioning for history of trauma or drug abuse. The HTLV-3 titer is indicated if AIDS is suspected as a diagnosis.

HYPERTENSIVE RETINOPATHY

Essential hypertension is an increase in systemic blood pressure. As 22 million Americans have hypertension, the changes seen on ophthalmoscopy are all the more important. Hypertension differs from hypertensive disease. Hypertension is blood pressure elevation only. Hypertensive disease suggests involvement of the kidneys, brain, heart, and eyes. Hypertensive disease occurs in approximately 5% of the population.

Retinal Changes in Hypertension (Fig. 8.2)

Generalized Narrowing

Significant elevation of blood pressure for an appreciable period results in attenuation or narrowing of the arterioles. This narrowing of the caliber of the vessel has a definite relation to the increase in the diastolic pressure.

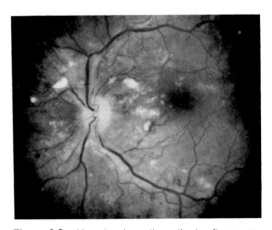

Figure 8.2. Hypertensive retinopathy is often superimposed on the more chronic changes of arteriolar sclerosis. (Credit: Paul Sternberg, M.D.) (See color Fig. C.31.)

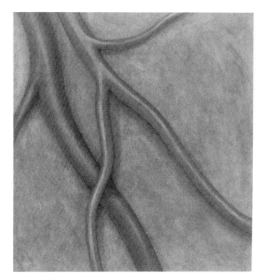 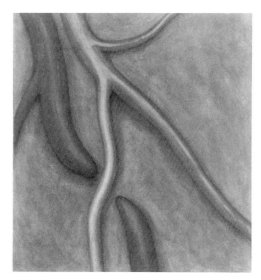

Figure 8.3. Gunn's sign. Gunn's sign is a change in the vein at the site of an arteriole crossing. It is seen especially in hypertension, where arteriolar sclerosis makes the arteriole walls thicker and the artery less pliable. The crossing of the artery causes a tapered appearance of the vein as it crosses underneath.

The size of the abnormal vessel may be compared to that of those without hypertension. More commonly, the ratio of the artery to the vein is established. Normally, the ratio is 2:3; that is, the artery is two-thirds the size of the vein. With arteriolar narrowing the ratio may decrease to 1:3.

Sclerosis of the Arterioles. Arteriolosclerosis (i.e., diffuse hyperplastic sclerosis) occurs when the diastolic pressure remains elevated. It is a compensatory reaction. The wall of the arteriole becomes thickened. There is hyperplasia of the muscle in the media, and the intima becomes thickened by fibers in elastic tissue. Hyaline degeneration eventually occurs, and narrowing of the central lumen of the vessel results.

Sclerosis causes a change in the light reflex. Early, there is an increase in the light reflex from the vessel. The reflex decreases with progression of the sclerosis. It is sometimes described as a "copper wire." With continued sclerosis, the vessel becomes whitish and is likened to a silver wire. In the end stage of sclerosis, there is no visible blood in the column and the vessels appear as fibrous, white cords.

Focal Constriction. Focal constriction is a localized, symmetrical narrowing of the arterioles. The arteriole abruptly narrows and abruptly increases in size. The segments characteristically vary in length, number, and location. Focal constriction is seen most frequently with elevated diastolic pressure of greater than 110 mm Hg. The severity of the constriction is also related to the acuteness of the development of hypertension.

Crossing Changes. Various crossing changes of the artery and vein occur. Compression of the vein by the arteriole (Gunn's sign) (Fig. 8.3) and a change in the course of the vein under the artery (Salus' sign) are seen in hypertensive arteriole disease. The vein may also bank, which is an increase in vein size due to dilation or swelling of the vein peripheral to the crossing.

Crossing changes occur over a period of many years. High diastolic pressures hasten their development.

Not all crossing changes result from hypertension. Some crossing changes can be seen in aged individuals without hypertension.

Hemorrhages

Hemorrhage is the change most commonly associated with hypertension. Most hemorrhages are in the nerve fiber layer and form "flame-shaped" hemorrhages. Deeper hemorrhages, or blot hemorrhages, are not as frequent as nerve fiber layer hemorrhages. Hemorrhages alone are not of great significance; however, they are significant when accompanied by retinal residues.

Cotton-Wool Spots

Focal ischemia causes cotton-wool spots (or soft exudates) (Fig. 8.1). These appear suddenly and clearly within a few weeks. Aneurysms may be seen around the cotton-wool spots.

Pathologically, these are ischemic areas. (Histologically, cytoid bodies, which result from degenerative changes in the axon, occur within the cotton-wool spots.) These cotton-wool spots are usually located in the posterior pole near the optic disc. They may be few or many.

Edema Residues

Residues appear as yellowish white deposits and vary in size from small dots to areas as large as the optic disc. They accumulate in the posterior pole. Around the macula they may form a "macular star." These residues have a low fat content and appear gray or silver. They can be differentiated by this characteristic from the residues in diabetes, which are waxy in appearance. Histologically, the residues are lipid-containing macrophages in the deeper layers of the retina.

Arteriole Straightening

At crossing changes, arteriole narrowing and straightening occurs so that the branches come off at right angles. The significance of this is not fully understood.

Vessel Sheathing

Increase in the optical density of the vessel wall reflects increased light because of vessel sheathing. Parallel sheathing to the vessel represents lateral thickening. Sheathing in hypertension is associated with arteriovenous crossing changes.

Papilledema

In severe forms of hypertension (the malignant phase), papilledema is an essential finding. Papilledema is most often actual swelling of the disc due to ischemia caused by arteriolar occlusion and leakage of individual vessels. The disc first becomes blurred on the nasal side. Edema then progresses to include

Table 8.2.
Keith-Wagner-Barker Classification: A Classification of Ophthalmoscopic Retinal Findings Correlating with the Hypertensive Disease State

Group 1
Slight narrowing of the arterioles
Mild elevation of blood pressure
No impairment of cardiac, cerebral, or renal function
Group 2
More definite narrowing of retinal arterioles, focal constriction, sclerosis
Blood pressure levels sustained and higher
Satisfactory cardiac, cerebral, and renal functions
Group 3
Group 2 findings plus retinopathy, including cotton-wool spots with or without hemorrhages
Blood pressure higher and sustained
Mild impairment of cardiac, cerebral, and renal function possibly present
Group 4
Findings in group 3 plus neuroretinal edema and papilledema
Severe focal constriction and chronic arteriolosclerosis
Blood pressure persistently elevated
Impairment of cardiac, cerebral, and renal function

the entire nerve head. Retinal edema accompanies the disc edema. Papilledema can also be caused by increased intracranial pressure due to hypertensive encephalopathy.

Prognosis

The development of papilledema, hemorrhages, and exudates all have prognostic significance. In patients who have retinopathy without papilledema, the mean life expectancy is less than 3 years. In hypertensive retinopathy with papilledema, the mean life expectancy is less than 1 year.

A number of classifications are used for hypertensive retinopathy. The Keith-Wagner classification (Table 8.2) classifies retinal changes by correlating with the generalized vascular changes of hypertension. The Scheie classification (Table 8.3) separates arteriolosclerotic changes and hypertensive changes in the belief that they have different significances and should be graded separately.

GRAVES' OPHTHALMOPATHY

Other Names

- Graves' disease
- Infiltrative ophthalmopathy

Table 8.3.
Scheie Classification of Hypertension

	Hypertension
Grade 1	Slight generalized attenuation of retinal arterioles
Grade 2	Obvious arteriolar narrowing with focal areas of attenuation
Grade 3	Grade 2 plus retinal exudates, cotton-wool spots, and hemorrhages
Grade 4	Grade 3 plus optic nerve edema
	Arteriolosclerosis
Grade 1	Broadening of arteriolar light reflex; minimal A/V crossing changes
Grade 2	Obvious broadening of arteriolar light reflex and A/V crossing changes
Grade 3	Copper-wire arterioles and more marked A/V crossing changes
Grade 4	Silver-wire arterioles and severe A/V crossing changes

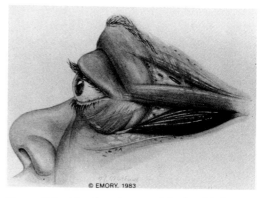

Figure 8.4. Muscle enlargement in thyroid disease. The extraocular muscles are enlarged to 7 or 8 times normal size in Graves' ophthalmopathy, which is frequently associated with thyroid abnormalities. Illustrated is swelling of the inferior rectus muscle. The inferior rectus and the medial rectus are the muscles most often involved, although all four muscles may be involved. Diagnosis by computed tomographic scanning is helpful (see page 276).

- Congestive ophthalmopathy
- Thyroid eye disease
- Eye changes in Graves' disease
- Malignant exophthalmus
- Endocrine exophthalmus
- Dysthyroid ophthalmopathy

Graves' Disease—a Triad of Clinical Manifestations

Graves' disease is associated with hyperthyroidism (90%) with diffuse goiter, ophthalmopathy (50%), and dermopathy (15%). The hyperthyroidism may be due to multiple causes.

The ophthalmopathy that is often associated with thyroid abnormalities may be present without thyroid abnormalities. Of those patients who present with ophthalmopathy, one-third will develop some thyroid signs within a 5-year period.

Cause

The exact cause is unknown. However, there is every indication that this is an immune phenomenon affecting the ocular muscles (Fig. 8.4). Immune complexes (thyroid globulin) and antithyroid globulin are thought to reach the orbit by the superior cervical lymph channels. These channels drain both the thyroid and the orbit. These immune complexes are thought to bind to extraocular muscles while stimulating the characteristic inflammation. The muscles are infiltrated with lymphocytes, plasma cells, mass cells, and deposits of hyaluronic acid. Circulating antibodies to ocular muscles can be detected in a high percentage of patients.

Characteristics

- *Women* affected 8 times more frequently than men
- *Onset* between 20 and 40 years of age
- *Variable association* with hyperthyroidism, or euthyroidism

Clinical Signs

Lid Retraction

Retraction of the upper and/or lower lid may occur unilaterally or bilaterally. This may be accompanied by scleral show (Fig 12.4) and produces the common association of thyroid stare.

Lid Lag

On downgaze, the thyroid patient has a lag in the falling of the lid with the globe as it moves downward (Fig. 8.5).

Proptosis

Unilateral or bilateral proptosis of the globe may occur in thyroid disease. Thyroid dysfunction is the most common cause of either unilateral or bilateral proptosis in the adult.

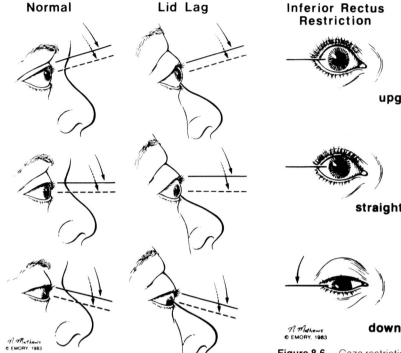

Normal   **Lid Lag**

Figure 8.5. Thyroid lid lag. On the *left*, downward motion of the normal lid and eye are simultaneous. On the *right*, in affected thyroid patients, the lid lags behind the downward motion of the globe.

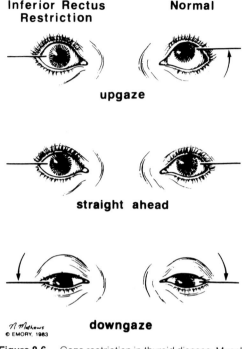

Inferior Rectus Restriction   **Normal**

upgaze

straight ahead

downgaze

Figure 8.6. Gaze restriction in thyroid disease. Muscle involvement in Graves' ophthalmopathy, most often associated with thyroid disease, is initially an inflammatory response. This frequently restricts eye movements in certain fields of gaze. Illustrated is restriction of the right eye on looking upward due to fibrotic changes in the inferior rectus muscle.

Eyelid Edema

Swelling of the eyelids due to edema may be an early sign of Graves' ophthalmopathy.

Conjunctival Injection over the Rectus Muscles

A characteristic sign, especially visible over the lateral rectus muscles, can occur in thyroid disease involving the ocular muscles.

Ocular Motility (Gaze) Restriction (Fig. 8.6)

Ocular motility may be restricted. Most characteristic is inhibited upgaze due to involvement of the inferior rectus muscle. Although all muscles may be involved, the inferior rectus is most commonly involved, and the medial rectus is second most commonly involved.

To determine muscle involvement, the forced traction test is used. In the forced traction test, anesthesia is placed on the conjunctiva and the muscle tendon is grasped with a forcep. Motion is directed in the field of gaze in which the muscle would be relaxed. Inhibition of motion indicates fibrosis of the muscle. For example, if the interior rectus is fibrotic from thyroid disease, the forced traction test will show inhibition to movement in upward gaze. Involvement of the medial rectus may simulate an abducens nerve palsy.

Complications

Optic Neuropathy

Vision may deteriorate because of compression of the optic nerve by swollen muscles. When multiple muscles are involved, especially in the posterior orbit, swelling of the posterior ocular muscles may compress the optic nerve. Careful monitoring of visual acuity and visual fields is necessary. Only a small percentage of patients will develop optic neuropathy; however, the complication can be serious. It is more common to see optic neuropathy with only mild or no proptosis, making the suspicion of this complication all the more important. Computed tomographic scanning can help determine whether thyroid disease is the cause of optic neuropathy by showing enlargement of the muscles.

Corneal Complications

Corneal drying may occur because of inappropriate blink and inadequate distribution of tears across the cornea. This is a frequent occurrence due to lid retraction and proptosis, which widens the palpebral fissures. Usually, mild corneal and conjunctival staining produce symptoms that are treated with artificial lubricants. However, in a small number of cases (usually less than 5%), corneal complications from drying may be severe. Rarely, perforation may cause severe visual loss.

Restriction of Ocular Motility

Double vision (diplopia) may occur as extraocular muscles are involved. After the acute cellular infiltrative phases of Graves' ophthalmopathy, fibrosis occurs, restricting ocular motion. This may result in ocular motility problems and severe visual symptoms.

Diagnosis of Thyroid Disease

Hyperthyroidism

Clinically, a number of signs should be sought by the ophthalmologist when Graves' ophthalmopathy and involvement of the thyroid are suspected. The general evaluation should include observation for:

- Presence of tachycardia at rest;
- Tremor;
- Weight loss with increased appetite;
- Thyroid gland enlargement.

Hypothyroidism

Grave's ophthalmopathy may also be associated with hyperthyroidism. Clinical indications include:

- Signs of depressed metabolism including lethargy;
- Weight gain with a decreased appetite;
- Weight gain bradycardia.

Euthyroid Graves' Disease—Clinical Evaluation

Two-thirds of these patients have an autonomously functioning pituitary thyroid axis. In testing for euthyroid Graves' disease, one must exclude the possibility of active thyroid changes. First, test T_4 and T_3 resin uptake, which estimates T_4. Second, if the first test is normal do a serum T_3. Third, if the other tests are normal, use a thyrotropin-releasing hormone (TRH) test. This shows normal release of thyroid-stimulating hormone (TSH). If this test is normal, then euthyroid Graves' disease is a probability.

Dermopathy in Thyroid Disease

The dermopathy is characterized by localized myxedema (pretibial myxedema), a peau d'orange appearance to the skin, and plaque-like or nodular changes, usually on the anterior legs or on the feet.

LEUKEMIAS

Ocular structures are involved as part of the systemic disease process in approximately half of the cases of leukemia. Ocular changes are more frequent with acute leukemia such as myelogenous, monocytic, or acute lymphocytic leukemia.

Clinical Features

Iris

Involvement of the iris is characterized by general thickening. Small nodules are often seen in the pupillary margin. Tumor cells may collect in the anterior chamber, simulating a hypopyon. Infiltration of the chamber angle can occur, and glaucoma can result.

Retina

Retinal involvement in leukemia includes tortuous veins, infarcts in the nerve fiber layer, perivascular sheathing, hemorrhages, and Roth's spots (page 352). Preretinal and vitreous hemorrhages can also be seen. Yellow infiltrates may be seen in the retina.

Optic Nerve

Leukemic infiltration of the optic nerve head causes disc swelling. The color is pink to gray. This is most often seen unilaterally, an important differential point from papilledema, which is bilateral.

Retinal Pigment Epithelium

The retinal pigment epithelium usually remains intact in leukemic infiltrations.

GIANT CELL ARTERITIS (TEMPORAL ARTERITIS)

Associated Systemic Process

Polymyalgia rheumatica

Definition

Giant cell arteritis is an active inflammatory process of the arteries of the body associated with a disease process. It generally begins with a low grade fever, anorexia, malaise, and weight loss. It affects *elderly* patients. Frequently, there is frontotemporal or occipital head pain with scalp tenderness. Approximately one-third of the patients will have bilateral blindness if untreated.

Characteristics

Giant cell arteritis is a disease of elderly patients. The average age of patients is in the 70s, with a range of approximately 60 to 85.

There are definite examples of familial giant cell arteritis. The incidence of giant cell arteritis or polymyalgia rheumatica is about 10 times higher in family members of patients with giant cell arteritis than in the general population.

The disease is more common in women.

Presentation

Polymyalgia rheumatica may be the presenting symptom complex in approximately 10% of patients with giant cell arteritis. This includes cerebrovascular disease, fever, myalgia, and anorexia. One-third to one-half of all patients with giant cell arteritis will have some of these associated symptoms. Fatigue, muscle aching and stiffness, weight loss, and fever (especially before the onset of illness) are common features.

Headaches

Almost all patients with giant cell arteritis have headache pain, especially severe in the temporal region. The temporal artery may be felt as firm and tortuous and very tender to touch. The patient may complain of inability to brush hair because of scalp tenderness at the temple and may have difficulty putting glasses on over the ears.

Jaw Muscle Pain

One-quarter to one-half of all patients will have pain while eating. This can be pain while chewing or pain within the tongue itself.

Visual Symptoms

Visual manifestations may not be the first presenting symptoms. Loss of vision is relatively uncommon as the initial complaint. Double vision (diplopia) is a more common visual symptom.

Visual Loss

Visual loss in giant cell arteritis frequently is transient in the beginning stages. In the first few days or hours before the attack of more premanent visual disturbance, the patient may experience gray patches or blurred vision. Many patients will have a prior diagnosis of amaurosis fugax.

When sustained loss of vision occurs, it is often abrupt. One eye is usually affected. The second eye is affected 1 to 10 days afterward (If the second eye is not involved within 6 to 8 weeks, the chances of the second eye becoming blind are not great.)

Visual loss is high in untreated patients. Of untreated patients, 65% will develop bilateral involvement. Of those, 27% will be totally blind. Steroids greatly improve the visual outcome.

Ocular Muscle Involvement

Double vision (diplopia) is a very common transient and permanent symptom of giant cell arteritis. Of the ocular motor nerves, the abducens (VI) and the ocular motor nerve (III) are responsible for the diplopia in about equal incidence. When the third nerve is involved, it is involved with pupil sparing, similar to diabetes or hypertensive third nerve palsies.

Ophthalmoscopic Findings

Fundus findings are related to focal ischemia (cotton-wool spots). Giant cell arteritis is a consideration in the differential diagnosis of cotton-wool spots (page 279).

Usually the optic nerves are involved 3 to 12 weeks after systemic signs occur. Both optic nerves may be involved simultaneously or one after the other. If they are involved at separate times, the interval of involvement may be anywhere from a few days to a number of years.

The disc appears pale, and there may be swelling of the optic nerve. Small nerve fiber layer hemorrhages may be seen around the disk (peripapillary hemorrhage). The retinal arteries may appear constricted. Cupping of the optic disc with optic atrophy may occur late.

Papilledema is commonly seen and may be associated with nerve fiber layer hemorrhages in the peripapillary area. Cotton-wool spots are frequent. Retinal veins may be present.

Involvement of the optic nerve with decreased vision may be retrobulbar. When retrobulbar ischemic optic neuritis is present, the disc may be normal.

Visual Fields

Visual fields may be variable. Classically, the upper or lower half of the central portion of the visual field is involved (altitudinal hemianopsia). Also characteristic are sector-shaped central defects. Central scotomas breaking into the periphery are also seen.

Pupillary Signs

A Marcus-Gunn pupil (afferent pupillary defect) may be present. There may also be a dilated pupil secondary to paralysis of the pupillary sphincter if there is severe general ischemia to the eye. A tonic pupil may be present because of involvement of the ciliary ganglion.

Ocular Manifestations of Giant Cell Arteritis in Order of Frequency

- Ischemic optic neuritis (swollen, pale optic disc)
- Diplopia in 10 to 30% (amaurosis fugax)
- Optic atrophy
- Ischemic retinopathy
- Occlusion of central retinal artery
- Ischemic retrobulbar neuritis

Laboratory Findings

Anemia

Normochromic microcytic anemia may be present in two-third or more of the cases.

Sedimentation Rate[a]

Abnormal sedimentation rates are a most important laboratory tool. Only about 2% of patients with giant cell arteritis have a normal sedimentation rate. All others will be abnormal. Elevated sedimentation rates are diagnostic and can help in monitoring the results of therapy.

White Blood Count

The white blood count is often elevated, especially in association with fever.

Abnormal Serum Proteins

A marked increase in the alpha-2-globulin fraction is seen. There is also an increase in alpha-2-glycoprotein.

Diagnosis with Temporal Artery Biopsy

Biopsy of the temporal artery can provide a positive diagnosis of temporal arteritis. However, false-negative biopsies (when the patient has the disease, but the temporal biopsy does not show it) are common. They may occur in as many as 25 to 60% of temporal artery biopsies. There are ways to improve the effectiveness of a temporal artery biopsy.

- Biopsy involved arteries or sections of arteries that are tender or hardened.
- Orient the biopsy specimen so that cross-sections are cut.
- Know the pathology of both acute arteritis and healed arteritis so, when healed arteritis is present, the diagnosis is not missed.

Pathologic Features of Active Arteritis

Marked thickening and edema of the intima, chronic inflammation and necrosis, disruption of the internal elastic lamina, and inflammation with lymphocytes, macrophages, and giant cells in the intima, media, and adventitia of the vessel wall are present.

---

[a]Method of determining normal sedimentation rate for age: men—divide age by two; women—add 10 years to age and divide by two.

Features of Healed Arteritis

Diffuse marked intimal thickening, fibrosis in the intima and media, fragmentation of the internal elastic membrane, and scarring in the adventitia are present.

Skip Areas in Artery Biopsy

Although skip areas can be found in temporal artery biopsies, they are infrequent. By careful selection of the temporal artery biopsy site and by doing bilateral temporal artery biopsies, the false-negative rate is greatly decreased.

Need for a Temporal Artery Biopsy

A positive temporal artery biopsy is helpful in managing steroid therapy. Even more important, a normal temporal artery biopsy has clinical significance. Evidence suggests that patients who do not have positive biopsies may not need steroids.

Important Facts to Remember about Temporal Arteritis

- There are two major ways, other than sedimentation rate (which is not specific for temporal arteritis), to determine the diagnosis of temporal arteritis. Most important is a response to steroids. Second is a temporal artery biopsy that is positive.
- It is a disease of older individuals, with the average age in the late 60s to early 70s.
- It is unusual in black patients.
- If a biopsy is performed, it should be done within a few weeks after the start of steroid therapy. Active arteritis changes may be absent in 7 to 8 weeks.
- A temporal artery biopsy is strongly indicated in patients who have contraindications to steroid therapy—peptic ulcer disease, osteoporosis, or diabetes mellitus.
- The sensitivity of temporal artery biopsy can be increased by the recognition of both active arteritis and healed arteritis.

PHAKOMATOSES

General

The phakomatoses are a group of diseases that are congenital, and all have a dominant hereditary pattern. They have widely varying symptoms both in the eye and systemically and are important for the ophthalmologist to understand because of the varied presentations.

Two categories are vascular anomalies of mesodermal origin: von Hippel-Lindau disease and Sturge-Weber syndrome. Two are neuroectodermal dysplasias: tuberous sclerosis and neurofibromatosis.

A variant of the angiomatosis is called the Wyburn-Mason syndrome and is discussed elsewhere (page 383).

Hamartomas

All of the phakomatoses are disseminated hamartomas. They involve not only ocular structures but also the central nervous system. Hamartomas are tumors composed of cells that would normally be present in the involved tissue. (Tumors of congenital origin that are composed of cells normally not present in the area are called choristomas.)

Neurofibromatosis

Other Names

Recklinghausen's disease, von Recklinghausen's disease

Inheritance

Dominant

Onset

The condition is congenital, but signs and symptoms do not appear until late childhood or early adulthood.

Skin Characteristics

Dermal pigmentation is striking. Called *café au lait spots* (Fig. 8.7), they may be as

Figure 8.7. This is a café au lait spot. This high magnification of skin pigmentation characteristic of neurofibromatosis was taken from the arm.

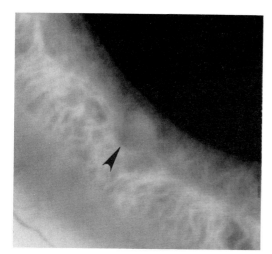

Figure 8.8. The iris can be an important structure for the diagnosis of neurofibromatosis in patients who have other signs of the disease. The iris nodules tend to be round, tan to brown, and single or multiple. Illustrated is a small nodule near the pupillary margin.

small as 1 mm or many centimeters in size. They are light or dark brown. They are found in 10% of the general population but are significant when they exceed 1.5 cm in diameter because lesions of this size are almost always associated with neurofibromatosis.

Axillary freckling and pigmentation are pathognomonic of neurofibromatosis.

Subcutaneous tumors arising from Schwann cells of the peripheral nerves (plexiform neuromas) stand out under the skin. These tend to be long and feel like worms under the skin. Solitary neurofibromas of the skin that are pedunculated (fibroma molluscum) may be scattered throughout the body and are not infrequently found on the eyelids.

Ophthalmologic Findings

Iris. Neurofibromas of the iris are small, round, tan, elevated lesions that usually must be observed with the magnification provided by the slitlamp (Fig. 8.8). When multiple, they may result in iris color changes and are important in the differential diagnosis of heterochromia (Fig 16.35).

Retina. Retinal tumors are the same as those described in tuberous sclerosis (page 170).

Glaucoma. Glaucoma in adults has been associated with neurofibromatosis.

Proptosis. Proptosis, forward displacement of the globe, may result from orbital involvement by the tumors of neurofibromatosis.

Optic Nerve. Glioma of the optic nerve is found in 10% of patients. (Retinal gliomas are rare.)

Central Nervous System Changes

Neurofibromatosis may involve the meninges, cerebrum, sympathetic nerves, and cranial nerves. The acoustic nerve is particularly susceptible.

Sturge-Weber Syndrome (Encephalotrigeminal Angiomatosis)

Nonocular Characteristics

Cutaneous hemangiomas are seen in the distribution of the branches of the trigeminal nerve, most often the first branch, occasionally the first and second branches, and rarely all three branches. The nasal mucosa, buccal mucosal, and conjunctiva may also be involved. Vascular hyperplasia of the cheeks and lips are present in 40% of patients.

The characteristic feature is the port-wine stain, a flat venous hemangioma. It is usually unilateral.

Hemangioma can occur in the meninges and the choroid. (The choroidal lesion is a hemangioma.) Because of the meningeal involvement, neurologic signs are common. Epilepsy, hemiplegia, and mental retardation occur.

Glaucoma

Glaucoma from unknown causes is associated with Sturge-Weber disease and is an important differential diagnosis in the evaluation of unilateral glaucoma.

Ophthalmologic Findings

Yellow lesions that are circular and elevated are seen. By depression of the sclera externally, lesions seen by ophthalmoscopy may disappear or decrease in size. Vascular anomalies of the eye occur, including telangiectasia of both the conjunctiva and the episclera. Telangiectasia involvement of the iris may result in heterochromia.

Tuberous Sclerosis (Bourneville's Disease)

Characteristically, the triad of tuberous sclerosis is mental deficiency, epilepsy, and adenoma sebaceum. The most important ophthalmoscopic findings are astrocytic hamartomas and giant drusen of the optic nerve head.

Lesion

Retinal lesions are astrocytic hamartomas. They appear as gray-white tumors with nodules (mulberry-like). The hamartomas are about 1 disc diameter in size. Characteristically, they are located in the posterior pole near the optic nerve, but they may be found elsewhere. There is no relationship to the surrounding vasculature, and there is no retinal reaction around the tumors. Portions of the hamartomas may break off and mestatasize within the eye.

Lesions similar to astrocytic hamartomas in the retina are also found in the cerebrum, basal ganglion, brain stem, and cerebellum. *Epilepsy* and *mental deficiency* are common.

Giant Drusen

Giant drusen of the optic nerve head, which appear as translucent or yellow-white hyaline bodies within the nerve head tissue, can be seen in tuberous sclerosis.

Characteristics

There is no racial preference. The sexes are affected equally.

Cutaneous Lesions

Adenoma sebaceum are small lesions from 1 to 8 or 9 mm in size. They are reddish brown papules. They are distributed in a butterfly fashion over the nose, cheek, and nasolabial folds. They are thought to be angiofibromas.

The most common skin lesion is the shagreen patch, which is usually located on the back. This lesion has a pigskin or orange peel appearance.

"Ash leaf" lesions are congenital white macules on the trunks and limbs. They are seen in the majority (86%) of patients. They may range from 1 to 100 mm in size. They can be linear or oval, with one end rounded and the other end pointed, giving rise to the description of ash leaf. They are better seen with Wood's lamp. They are an important early diagnostic sign of tuberous sclerosis.

Other cutaneous manifestations of importance are nevi, fibromas, and *café au lait spots.* Koenen's tumors (small fibromas localized to the sides of the nails or sublingual), white pedunculated tumors on the palpebral conjunctiva, and reddish to yellow tumor-like thickenings on the bulbar conjunctiva have been seen.

Tuberous sclerosis has been associated with many other conditions including rhabdomyosarcoma of the heart, additional tumors of the thyroid and kidney, and spina bifida.

Onset

Signs and symptoms usually start before age 6.

Von Hippel-Lindau Disease (Angiomatosis of the Retina and Cerebellum)

Terminology

Von Hippel's disease involves retinal angiomatosis and is named after the person who first described it. Lindau's disease are the ocular findings described with angiomatous cyst of the cerebellum and angiomatosis retinae. Von Hippel-Lindau disease refers to the typical ophthalmologic findings and is associated with hypernephroma, kidney cyst, pancreas cyst, ovarian cyst, and anomalies of the skull.

Characteristics of von Hippel-Lindau Disease

Of the cases, 20% are familial. Heredity is dominant. Penetrance is incomplete. The onset of symptoms is usually in the 30s.

Retinal Findings

Round, elevated, red tumors of the retina are 2 to 3 disc diameters in size. Running to and from these tumors are large vessels. The lesions are *bilateral* in half of the patients. Lesions are most commonly found in the *periphery,* although they may occur anywhere in the retina.

Course

The course of these tumors is highly variable. Tumor enlargement, hemorrhages and exudates, and retinal detachment may develop. Late complications include glaucoma and phthisis bulbi.

Patients who have cyst of the cerebellum have about a one in five chance of having retinal angiomas. Lesions in the central nervous system consist of large endothelium-lined sinusoidal hemangiomas. They are usually in the cerebellum but may involve the medulla and spinal cord.

9

Ocular Inflammation

Uveitis	Ankylosing Spondylitis	Endophthalmitis
Sarcoidosis	Relapsing Polychondritis	Endogenous Endophthalmitis
Toxoplasmosis	Subacute Sclerosing	Exogenous Endophthalmitis
Presumed Ocular	Panencephalitis	Clinical Evaluation of a Patient
Histoplasmosis Syndrome	Masquerade Syndrome	with Endophthalmitis
Behçet's Disease	(Iridocyclitis)	Causes of Endophthalmitis
Juvenile Rheumatoid Arthritis	Reticulum Cell Sarcoma and	Endophthalmitis Due to Drug
Pars Planitis	Uveitis	Abuse

UVEITIS

Definition

Uveitis is inflammation of the uvea. The uvea consists of the iris, the ciliary body, and the choroid. Uveitis is an inflammatory response that occurs because of many ocular insults and is a general term.

Terminology

Uveitis is the most common term applied to ocular inflammation. Many other terms may be used for more specifically identified inflammation sites.

Subclassification

- *Iritis* is inflammation of the iris. This is usually localized in the anterior segment. Trauma is a frequent cause.
- *Cyclitis* is inflammation of the ciliary body. This term is not in common use.
- *Iridocyclitis* is inflammation of the iris and the ciliary body. Sarcoidosis frequently causes iridocyclitis.
- *Choroiditis* is inflammation of the choroid.
- *Chorioretinitis* is inflammation of choroid and retina. The retinal inflamma-

tion predominates. Histoplasmosis is an example.
- *Retinochoroiditis* is inflammation of the retina and choroid. The choroidal inflammation predominates. Toxoplasmosis is an example.
- Posterior uveitis is inflammation limited to the back part of the eye.
- Anterior uveitis is inflammation limited to the front of eye.

Inflammation of the Anterior Segment

Other Equivalent Terms. Uveitis; anterior uveitis; iritis; iridocyclitis

Features. The symptoms of anterior segment inflammation are variable according to cause and severity. In most patients, there is some decrease in vision. Light sensitivity and tearing may occur. Pain is variable and rarely severe. Redness may occur. Especially from increase in size of the deep scleral vessels.

Establishing the Diagnosis. When the eye is red from vascular injection, 2.5% Neo-Synephrine can be used to help differentiate between conjunctivitis (superficial inflammation of the surface lining of eye) and uveitis (deep internal inflammation). Conjunctival vessels will blanch when 2.5% Neo-Synephrine is applied. The deeper scleral vessels

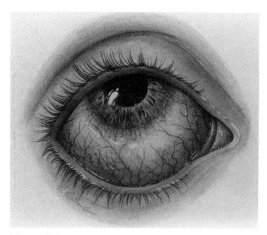

Figure 9.1. Ciliary flush is an increase of the size of the vessels around the limbus. These vessels are within the superficial sclera underneath the conjunctiva. The ciliary flush is important because it indicates the presence of intraocular inflammation. To differentiate it from simple conjunctival hyperemia, Neo-Synephrine drops can be used. Neo-Synephrine will usually blanch the conjunctival vessels; however, the ciliary vessels, because they are deeper, remain visible.

that are enlarged and inflamed by uveitis will not be affected.

The deep scleral vascularization is usually in the perilimbal area. This is known as ciliary flush (Fig. 9.1).

1. Ciliary Flush. Intraocular inflammation dilates the vessels at the scleral limbus. Clinically, this appears as a reddish flush running in a band just behind the limbus. This flush is under the conjunctiva, where vessels may also be enlarged and inflamed. To differentiate between conjunctival hyperemia and ciliary flush, a drop of 2.5% Neo-Synephrine on the eye will constrict and blanch conjunctival vessels but leave scleral vessels unchanged. The presence of ciliary flush indicates the presence of intraocular inflammation.

2. Flare. Flare is an indication of released protein in the anterior chamber, which occurs with ocular inflammation. Using the slitlamp (see page 360), a narrow slit beam or a small, circular beam is directed through the anterior chamber. When protein is present, the beam, as it passes through the aqueous fluid, takes on a grayish appearance. The slitlamp beam is similar to a beam of light from a movie projector in a dark movie theatre. In the theatre, the reflection of the beam is due to particles

in the air. In essence, anterior chamber flare is due to reflection from protein particles in the aqueous (see color Fig. C.5).

You can imagine a flare (or practice slitlamp techniques) by thinking of adding a few drops of milk to a small, clear container of water. As the milk diffuses and mixes with the water, the water illuminates in the path of the slit beam.

Flare is graded on a scale of 0 to 4+. In early stages of learning to use the slitlamp, the examiner may find determination of flare to be difficult. Every eye should be routinely checked for flare when using the slitlamp.

3. Cells. Cells due to inflammation, white cells of various types, float in the anterior chamber. While shining a small slitlamp beam through the aqueous, these cells will be visible as small, illuminated specks. Continued experience with the slitlamp is necessary to become efficient in recognizing cells. These are graded on a scale of 0 to +4. Blood cells can also be seen in aqueous with the slitlamp but are rarely associated with uveitis and are seen most often after trauma or surgery.

4. Keratitic Precipitates (KPs). Cellular conglomerates appear on the back of the cornea as round globules and may be small or large. These may be tan-colored to darkly pigmented, white, or even translucent. These are usually associated with granulomatous inflammation, sarcoid, for example.

5. Synechiae. Synechiae are adhesions either between the iris and the lens or between the iris and the cornea. Adhesions to the lens capsule are known as posterior synechiae. Adhesions to the cornea (in the chamber angle) are known as peripheral anterior synechiae.

6. Cataract. Prolonged inflammation may result in cataract. Cataract formation in the posterior portion of lens (posterior subcapsular cataract) is the most common type, although other opacities in other parts can be seen.

7. Glaucoma. Because the inflammation may obstruct the outflow of aqueous through the chamber angle structures, glaucoma may result (known as inflammatory glaucoma).

8. Hypopyon. Inflammatory cells can layer in the inferior of the eye, causing a white to yellow appearance to the inferior part of the cornea (Fig. 9.2).

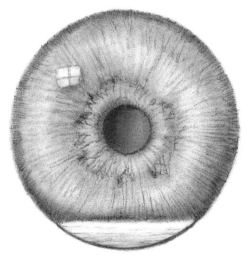

Figure 9.2. Hypopyon is a layering of white cells in the anterior chamber. Because of gravity, the cells layer inferiorly. The white cells indicate inflammation, and hypopyon is frequently associated with inflammation from infection (see Fig. 1.11).

Inflammation of the Posterior Segment

Other Terms. Choroiditis, chorioretinitis, posterior uveitis, vitritis, pars planitis, retinochoroiditis

Presentation. Vision loss is usually the presenting symptom. Because of the inflammatory debris that may occur in the vitreous, floaters may be perceived moving in the field of vision and may also be a common presenting symptom. These floaters are described as darkish to gray to black objects hanging or skirting through the visual field.

Establishing the Diagnosis.

1. Cells in the Vitreous. Cells and sheets of cells can be seen in the vitreous. These are best observed with the Hruby lens or Volk lens or with the use of the gonioprism lens (Fig 3.8).

2. Retinitis. Edema of the retinal layers may appear as whitish clouding of the retina. The boarders of areas of inflammation tend to be indistinct. The most common cause of retinitis is toxoplasmosis. As the lesions in toxoplasmosis heal, the borders of the retinal lesions become more distinct.

3. Choroiditis. Inflammation of the choroid appears as patches of white or gray and sometimes yellow areas of inflammation with

distinct edges. The retina is normal. When healed, these choroidal areas form white scars with pigmented borders.

4. Macular Edema. Edema in the foveal (macular) region seriously decreases vision. This edema is most often associated with pars planitis (inflammation in the periphery, or anteriorly near the ciliary body, of the retina). It is not frequently seen with anterior segment inflammation and is rarely seen with specific posterior segment disease.

5. Neuritis. Neuritis may also be called papillitis if the optic disc is inflamed. When the optic nerve becomes inflamed, the term neuritis is used.

6. Vasculitis. Vasculitis is cuffing of the retinal vessels, with small puffs of white around the vessels. Either the arteries or the veins may be involved. For example, in toxoplasmosis, arteries (periarteritis) are involved, whereas, in sarcoidosis, veins (periphlebitis) are involved.

7. Retinal Pigment Epithelial Changes. Retinal pigment epithelium may be involved in certain inflammations and can cause specific characteristic changes in conditions such as sympathetic ophthalmia, Vogt-Koyanagi-Harada syndrome, and certain viral conditions.

8. Neovascularization. Neovascularization of the retina, subretina, and optic nerve may result from chronic inflammation in the posterior portions of the eye.

Tests for the Workup of Uveitis

- Complete blood count
- Urinalyses
- Chest x-ray
- Erythrocyte sedimentation rate
- Rheumatoid factor
- Antinuclear antibody
- FTA-ABS
- VDRL
- X-ray of the sacroiliac joint
- HLA-B27 (ankylosing spondylitis)
- HLA-B5
- *Toxoplasma* and *Toxocara* antibody titers
- Angiotensin converting enzyme

- Gallium scan
- Serum electrophoresis
- Serum immune complex levels
- PPD skin test for tuberculosis
- Skin test for mumps
- Skin test for *Candida*

Classification of Uveitis

- Ankylosing spondylitis
- Herpesvirus
- Juvenile rheumatoid arthritis
- Reiter's disease
- Rheumatoid arthritis
- Sarcoidosis
- Toxoplasmosis

- Behçet's disease
- Bilateral acute retinal necrosis
- Birdshot choroidopathy
- Collagen vascular diseases
- Cytomegalic virus inclusion disease
- Drug abuse
- Fuchs' heterochromic iridocyclitis
- Mycobacteria
- Ocular toxocariasis
- Pars planitis (acute multifocal placoid pigment epitheliopathy)
- Presumed ocular histoplasmosis
- Relapsing polychondritis
- Reticulum cell sarcoma
- Serpiginous choroidopathy
- Subacute sclerosing panencephalitis
- Syphilis
- Uveal effusion
- Vogt-Koyanagi-Harada syndrome

Ocular Sarcoidosis (Ophthalmic Sarcoidosis)

Ocular Involvement

Approximately one-quarter of all patients with active sarcoidosis will have involvement of the eye or of tissue around the eye. Of those patients with ocular involvement, approximately one-half will not have ocular symptoms.

Ocular Manifestation

The ocular manifestations of sarcoidosis are related to the granulomatous inflammation. Anterior uveitis, the most common manifestation, tends to be chronic, with dense keratic precipitates (see Fig C.6). Iris nodules are seen and are called Busacca or Koeppe nodules, depending on position. On occasion, light keratic precipitates have been observed without serious sequelae.

Granulomatous changes may be seen in the choroid and retina. Complications of the anterior granulomatous reaction may result in cataracts, glaucoma, band keratopathy, and severe loss of vision.

Millet seed nodules can be seen on the eyelids. Conjunctival nodules and cysts occur on the conjunctiva and can be significant as a site for diagnostic biopsy. Scleritis and episcleritis are not common in sarcoid. Lacrimal gland involvement occurs in about 6% of patients with sarcoidosis and presents as swelling of the gland. Gallium scans of the lacrimal gland in presumptive sarcoidosis can help to establish a diagnosis, as can direct biopsy.

Rarely, the orbits can be involved with protrusion of the eye (proptosis).

Differences in the Pediatric Age Group

Pediatric ocular sarcoidosis divides itself into two different subsets that are related to age. Children under 5 years of age usually have uveitis, joint involvement, and skin rash. Pulmonary disease is present in about one-third of these patients.

In children 8 to 15 years old, all have lung involvement. There is also involvement of the eye, skin, liver, and spleen in 30 to 40% of these cases. However, joint involvement is rare.

Chorioretinal granulomas can be seen in either of the pediatric age groups. Biopsy of the conjunctiva can be important to diagnosis in both age groups. Lacrimal gland involvement in children under 15 years of age has not been reported.

Differential Diagnosis of Sarcoid Granulomatous Disease

- Fungal
- Microbacterial

- Spirochetal
- Parasitic
- Neoplastic conditions
  —Lymphomas
  —Hodgkin's disease
- Immunologic disease
  —Allergy
  —Systemic lupus erythematosus
  —Giant cell arteritis
  —Wegener's granulomatosis
- Reaction to chemicals
  —Starch
  —Silica
  —Zirconium
  —Beryllium

General Diagnostic Approach

There is no single diagnostic criterion for sarcoidosis. The diagnosis must be logically arrived at after a series of progressive steps.

Clinical Findings. If the clinical signs are compatible with the suspected diagnosis of sarcoid, laboratory and radiographic tests should be ordered.

Laboratory Tests.

Angiotensin Converting Enzyme. Angiotensin converting enzyme is not a specific test for sarcoidosis, and the serum concentration of the enzyme can be increased in a number of other conditions. Although it is helpful when serum levels are high to suggest sarcoidosis, it is not positive in all patients. The angiotensin converting enzyme levels are elevated in only half of patients with inactive sarcoidosis, and in patients with active sarcoidosis the enzyme is increased only 60 to 90% of the time.

Lysozyme. Although lysozyme, an enzyme produced by sarcoid granuloma, may be increased in the serum, this is a nonspecific test.

Calcium. Increased absorption of calcium in the intestine and a subsequent increase of calcium in the urine are due to increased sensitivity to vitamin D or increased activity of 1,25-dihydroxy-vitamin D in sarcoid. Hypercalcemia is seen in 2 to 10% of patients with sarcoidosis. However, increased calcium levels in the urine are found twice as often as increased serum calcium. A 24-hour urinary calcium determination may help establish the diagnosis.

Kveim Test. This test requires the injection of a suspension of human sarcoid tissue, from either lymph nodes or spleen, and observation of the reaction. There are many disadvantages to this test: it takes 4 to 6 weeks for a reaction to occur, the test requires a biopsy and a histologic interpretation of the test site, and it is difficult to obtain proper sarcoid human tissue properly prepared for the test.

HLA Typing. Because of widespread differences in patients with sarcoid among different populations when compared by inherited histocompatibiltiy antigens (HLA), HLA typing has not been used as a diagnostic tool.

Radiologic and Physiologic Tests.

X-rays.

Chest X-ray. There are five stages of x-ray findings in patients with suspected or diagnosed disease: stage 0—normal chest x-ray; stage 1—hilar adenopathy; stage 2—hilar adenopathy associated with parenchymal involvement; stage 3—parenchymal involvement without adenopathy; stage 4—fibrosis. Hilar adenopathy is bilateral and is associated in 50% of the cases with paratrachial adenopathy.

Bone X-rays. Bone involvement can be seen in sarcoidosis: "funneling" with trabecular remodeling, lytic punched out cyst, or destructive lesion.

Gallium Scans. Gallium citrate scans are used to detect inflammatory disease. These scans are more sensitive than routine chest films for determining the pulmonary involvement of sarcoid.

Gallium scans are also used to determine the status of the lacrimal gland. More than 80% of patients with active sarcoidosis show increased lacrimal gland uptake. The scan suggests a direct biopsy of the lacrimal gland when increased uptake is present.

Pulmonary Function Test. Pulmonary function test can be an early diagnostic clue and may be abnormal before x-ray findings. The earliest abnormal pulmonary physiology is a decrease in the diffusing capacity. A decrease of static lung volume is also common in these patients.

Biopsy. If the clinical signs as well as laboratory and radiologic techniques are suggestive, biopsy can be useful in establishing a diagnosis. Disirable biopsy sites are those where suspicious lesions, either on the skin or on the conjunctiva, can be found. Such sites yield a high positive result.

Blind conjunctival biopsy, although advocated as a possible diagnostic tool by most physicians, gives disappointing results. If there is no suspicious conjunctival lesion, other biopsy sites are recommended (lacrimal gland, salivary glands). Transbronchial biopsy may be indicated if other diagnostic tests have not been conclusive and a diagnosis must be established.

Toxoplasmosis

Definition

Ocular toxoplasmosis is caused by *Toxoplasma gondii.* This organism is a common cause of inflammation in the posterior portion of the eye (posterior uveitis).

Nature of the Infection

The initial infection with *Toxoplasma gondii* is usually subclinical. This primary infection affects lung, heart, and brain (pneumonia, myocarditis, or encephalitis). After the initial infection, the organism remains encapsulated in large cysts. *Toxoplasma gondii* causes antibodies; in fact, the organism is extremely common and 50% of the adult population have positive antibodies to this organism.

Congenital Infection

Toxoplasmosis can be transmitted to the unborn child during acute infection in the mother. Congenital passage of the disease to the fetus occurs only during the acute infection. Acute infection occurs only once. Therefore, those who are antibody-positive or who have had one child with congenital toxoplasmosis will not give birth to a child with congenital toxoplasmosis.

Association with Immunosuppression

Once the body accommodates to the organism, the immune response usually controls the parasite and there is no dissemination or proliferation. However, when the immune system is compromised (as in immunosuppression from disease or from drug therapy), those previously infected with *Toxoplasmosis gondii* are at considerable risk of developing serious ocular complications of the disease.

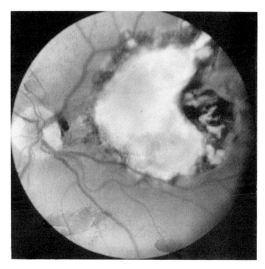

Figure 9.3. Toxoplasmosis scar. This large, inactive toxoplasmosis scar shows a white, atrophic, scarred retina with a surrounding halo of pigment that makes the diagnosis highly likely. Such scars can be from congenital or acquired toxoplasmosis. (See color Fig. C.30.) (Credit: Paul Sternberg, M.D.)

Pathology

Toxoplasmosis gondii organisms have been found only in the retina. Organisms cause retinitis associated with cells in the vitreous. The posterior vitreous face may detach, and cellular precipitates on the posterior face of the vitreous may cause a decrease in vision.

Establishing the Diagnosis

Antibody Titers. A positive antibody test to *Toxoplasmosis gondii* is only suggestive of a possible diagnosis of an invasion in the retina causing a posterior uveitis. As 50% of the population have a positive antibody test, the presence of antibody titers is not pathognomonic. Changing antibody titers also are not helpful because ocular lesions alone do not affect, in most circumstances, the systemic titers.

Clinical Appearance (Fig. 9.3). This is a focal lesion involving the retina and causing necrosis. It is usually a circumscribed, white or slightly yellowish white lesion that has indistinct or fluffy borders. Lesions vary in size from a few millimeters to 5 or 6 disc diameters. The overall appearance of the lesion is constant in color and consistency. *Exudative cells in the overlying vitreous are common* and represent a key diagnostic feature when the differential diagnosis of presumed ocular histoplasmosis syndrome (POHS) is considered. Satellite scars, small scars close to or in the area of the active lesion, are highly suggestive of an active toxoplasmic retinitis. Inactive satellite scars are frequently seen in congenital toxoplasmosis.

The diagnosis is established by a combination of clinical appearance and antibody testing. A positive antibody titer, even a 1:1 dilution, is significant.

Additional Laboratory Tests for Toxoplasmic Disease.

- Indirect fluorescent antibody test.
- Indirect hemagglutination
- Enzyme-linked immunosorbent assay (ELISA)
- Fluoroimmunoassay (FIAX)

These tests are used to reassess a negative antibody titer in a patient who has a lesion consistent with toxoplasmosis.

Presumed Ocular Histoplasmosis Syndrome (POHS)

Other Names

Histoplasmic choroiditis, presumed ocular histoplasmosis (POH), histoplasmosis

Clinical Ophthalmologic Features

Three ophthalmic findings establish the presumed ocular histoplasmosis syndrome: (*a*) perifoveal subretinal neovascular membrane, (*b*) typical choroidal scar in the same or the opposite eye, and (*c*) typical scars surrounding the optic nerves. Only 85% of patients will have typical optic nerve scarring. The diagnosis is established if a central membrane and a peripheral choroidal scar are present. The causative agent has not been isolated, and diagnosis remains "presumed."

Long-standing Disease Process. The condition is acquired in early life, and ocular changes progress with exacerbations and remissions. The patient is usually unaware of the disease process until the fovea is involved with neovascular membrane.

Basic Lesion. The basic peripheral lesion is round, subretinal, and approximately 200 to 500 μm in size. It is nonpigmented in the early stages, and the edges are distinct. The retina over the lesion is normal and flat, and there are never any cells in the vitreous.

These lesions are asymptomatic. The lesion undergoes evolution wtih time, changes appearance, and develops pigmentation. Characteristic atrophic spots with central pigmentation, called *histo spots,* develop. Histo spots may be single or numerous; they may be scattered or grouped in tracks throughout the midperiphery of the fundus. In endemic areas, the incidence of histo spots in the population is between 2 and 3%. (The risk of subretinal neovascular membrane developing from a peripheral choroidal spot is 1/100 or less, much less than the risk of foveal spots.)

A second change seen in lesions that are close to the fovea is a small serous detachment of the retina over the lesion. The patient may notice a relative paracentral scotoma (see page 357). The symptoms, however, are usually minimal.

In lesions near the fovea, the third type of evolution is the appearance of a subretinal neovascular membrane from the choroidal scar. There is a yellow nodule, which is subretinal and has a gray border with an overlying serous retinal detachment with hemorrhages and sometimes exudates.

It is not known why peripheral choroidal lesions rarely develop subretinal neovascular membranes. Subretinal neovascular membranes develop with macular choroidal lesions. We also do not know why choroidal lesions develop throughout the life of the patient.

Peripapillary Scars. As mentioned, 85% of patients with presumed ocular histoplasmosis syndrome will have scarring around the optic disc. The scarring consists of a partial or complete rim of atrophic choroid and pigment epithelium. The atrophic area around the disc has a line of pigmentation at the inner margin of the scar. This is in sharp contrast to the choroidal atrophy seen in normal eyes and in myopic eyes, which has pigmentation at the outer border of the scar. This scarring in presumed ocular histoplasmosis syndrome also has a somewhat nodular configuration.

Subretinal neovascular membranes can grow from the peripapillary scars but have a better prognosis than foveal subretinal neovascular membranes. In patients without scars near the fovea but with scarring around the disc, the chance of developing membranes is only 3 to 4%.

Natural History

The subretinal neovascular membrane, because it is the most important aspect of the evolution of the disease, is the degree of evolution of the disease process most often considered. After the onset of a subretinal neovascular membrane, a central or paracentral disciform scar will eventually occur. This process takes at least 2 years.

Visual loss is dependent upon two factors: (*a*) the closeness of the subretinal membrane to the center of the fovea (membranes with an edge closer than ¼ disc diameter to the center of the fovea have the worst prognosis) and (*b*) the size of the neovascular membrane (the larger the membrane, the poorer the prognosis).

Involvement of the fellow eye also relates to prognosis. A patient who has a choroidal scar in the opposite eye has a greater than 20% chance of developing a neovascular membrane in that eye within 5 years.

Systemic Involvement

Most patients with presumed histoplasmic choroiditis (or presumed ocular histoplasmosis) have (*a*) a positive skin reaction to the intracutaneous injection of 1:1000 histoplasmin and (*b*) chest x-ray evidence of healed pulmonary histoplasmosis. However, it is important to emphasize that the fungal organism has never been cultured or demonstrated in histologic section of a typical retinal lesion. HLA-B7 is found in association with presumed histoplasmosis syndrome.

Behçet's Disease

Definition

Behçet's disease primarily involves the eye, mouth, genitals, and skin. Joints, the gastrointestinal tract, and the central nervous system may also be affected.

Manifestations

More than 75% of patients have eye signs. Ophthalmologists may be the first physicians to see the patient because 30% of patients will seek medical care because of eye signs. This does not mean that eye signs are the first signs to appear, but they are the signs that bring a patient to a doctor. Oral aphthous ulcerations are the earliest manifestations, by history, in 80% of patients.

Behçet's disease most often affects males and has a higher incidence among the Japanese. Clinically, the ocular sequelae seem to be worse in the Japanese than in other races.

Onset

Behçet's disease starts most often during the third decade of life.

Ocular Signs

When the eye is involved, vision is lost 3 to 4 years after the onset. Complications can be severe, and about 25% of patients will be disabled by blindness.

An anterior uveitis is often the presenting ocular sign. Hypopyon is commonly associated with Behçet's disease, but hypopyon may be transient and may be only a late manifestation.

Anterior segment uveitis frequently obscures the necrotizing retinal vascular lesion that is present in 50% of patients. Cataract formation caused by the inflammation is common. Optic nerve atrophy from secondary glaucoma due to effects of inflammation is an additional threat to vision.

Oral Mucosal Ulcerations

Mucous membrane ulcerations of the mouth have a predilection for the lips, cheeks, and tongue. The palate, tonsils, and pharynx, which are more frequently involved in the lesions of Reiter's syndrome or Stevens-Johnson syndrome, are rarely involved in Behçet's disease.

The lesions of Behçet's disease have a discrete border and heal without scarring in 7 to 10 days. In contrast, the lesions of Stevens-Johnson syndrome tend to have irregular borders, and those of Reiter's syndrome tend to be heaped.

Skin Manifestations

Skin lesions heal early and may not be present when other signs are seen. Even without active lesions, examination of the skin may show pigmentation, which is frequently a mark of a resolved lesion.

Lesions usually occur on the lower extremities. They may be seen also on the buttocks, arms, neck, and face. The lesions are erythematous, are slightly elevated, and have subcutaneous induration. They are tender.

Some lesions will have the bluish color of erythema nodosum and will also be tender. These lesions occur with a fever.

Genital Lesions

Genital lesions are found on the scrotum and on the vulva. The lesions in males tend to be more painful than those in females.

Other Changes

When joints are affected, the knee is the most characteristic. Bouts of arthritis are usually seen with fever and erythema nodosa lesions.

Gastrointestinal symptoms are present in 50% of patients. Patients suffer from malabsorption and indigestion. Ileocecal ulcers often perforate. The gastrointestinal changes can be diagnosed radiologically.

Central nervous system involvement occurs in 25% of patients in a variety of presentations such as meningoencephalitis or benign intracranial hypertension. Cranial nerve palsies, peripheral neuropathies, paralysis, and brain stem signs can occur.

Psychological changes occur in 50% of patients. They may have memory impairment, dementia, or character disorders.

Mechanism

The underlying problem is an occlusive vasculitis. Evidence points to an immune phenomenon as the basis for the vasculitis. Circulating immune complexes have been found, and cell immunity has been demonstrated to antigens extracted from oral mucosa.

Genetic studies show a three- to four-fold increase of HLA-B5 in patients with Behçet's disease. HLA-B27 and HLA-B12 have been associated with arthritic and mucocutaneous forms of the disease.

Classification of the Disease—Complete/Incomplete

In the *complete form* of the disease, all four of these manifestations must be present:

- Recurrent aphthous lesions of the mouth;
- Skin lesions;
- Eye lesions;
- Genital ulcerations.

The *incomplete form* of the disease is (*a*) when three of the four major signs of the complete form are present or (*b*) when there are eye signs of recurrent anterior inflammation and/or retinal vasculitis associated with one other major sign of the complete form.

Juvenile Rheumatoid Arthritis

Other Names

Still's disease, polyarticulate juvenile rheumatoid arthritis, monoarticular rheumatoid arthritis, pauciarticular rheumatoid arthritis

Onset

Onset is usually from 2 to 4 years of age. It is more common in young girls.

Ocular Signs

Iridocyclitis and associated cataracts and glaucoma are frequent. The inflammation and the cataract can occur in a white eye, which makes diagnosis difficult and may delay diagnosis.

Juvenile rheumatoid arthritis presents in distinct types: Still's disease, polyarticular juvenile rheumatoid arthritis, and pauciarticular rheumatoid arthritis.

Course

Ocular inflammation is rare when the systemic disease is most severe. Therefore, ocular signs are most often seen with the pauciarticular variety of juvenile rheumatoid arthritis. Approximately 25% of these patients will have ocular signs.

The ocular inflammation is nongranulomatous. At times, fine keratitic precipitates are present. Inflammation of the posterior segment is unusual. However, vitreous floaters may be common. Choroiditis has been reported. Patients are usually seronegative for rheumatoid factor but positive for antinuclear antibody.

Pars Planitis

Other Names

Peripheral uveitis, chronic cyclitis

Incidence

This is a common inflammatory disease of young adults in their 20s and 30s. Another peak incidence is during the teenage years.

Characteristics

This ocular inflammation can be seen in a completely white eye (shares this feature with juvenile rheumatoid arthritis and reticulum cell sarcoma). The disease is usually bilateral; however, one eye may be more involved then the other.

Symptoms. There are floaters and decreased vision (if the macula is affected with cystoid edema). Characteristically, there is no pain, photophobia, or external signs of inflammation, such as ciliary flush. Synechiae are very rare.

Findings. There is an exudation over the pars plana, which forms a "snow bank." "Snowballs" may also be seen in the vitreous over the pars plana area. In some cases, a few fine, white, keratitic precipitates (see Fig C.6) may be noted on the endothelium of the cornea. The anterior chamber reaction is usually very minor.

The snowball opacities are preretinal and concentrated inferiorly. On occasion, there may be a peripheral vasculitis that involves veins and not arterioles. Common with the condition is cystoid macular edema, which affects vision.

Ankylosing Spondylitis (Marie-Strümpell Disease)

This occurs most frequently in young men in their 20s and 30s. HLA-B27 antigen is positive in over 90% of patients. The sedimentation rate is often elevated. Sacroiliac x-ray films show ankylosis of the spine. Tests for rheumatoid factor are negative.

Ocular Signs

Ocular changes may be unilateral or bilateral, although when bilateral they almost never occur in both eyes at the same time. This is primarily an iridocyclitis. Approxi-mately one-half of patients who show x-ray evidence of ankylosing spondylitis are asymptomatic.

Relapsing Polychondritis (Chronic Atrophic Polychondritis)

This is an uncommon disorder characterized by inflammation of the cartilage throughout the body. It presents as an arthritic disorder. It occurs in both sexes and begins between 20 and 60 years of age. The cause is unknown.

Nonocular Presentations

Inflammation of the ears (pinnae) is the most common feature. One or both ears become red or swollen and are painful. Repeated attacks cause resorption of the ear cartilage and floppy, drooping ears.

Arthralgia and arthritis are often seen. Nasal cartilage can also be resorbed after inflammation, resulting in a saddle nose deformity.

Association with Systemic Diseases

Relapsing polychondritis may be associated with rheumatoid arthritis, systemic or discoid lupus erythematosus, ankylosing spondylitis, ulcerative colitis, or sarcoidosis.

Ocular Signs

Episcleritis is the most common ocular sign. Conjunctivitis and keratitis also appear. Scleritis involves primarily the anterior portion of the eye. Many patients have kerato-conjunctivitis sicca (see page 28).

Involvement of the retina and optic nerve is less common in anterior ocular complications. Chorioretinopathy, both active and inactive, has been associated with this disorder. Optic neuritis has also been reported.

Subacute Sclerosing Panencephalitis (SSPE)

SSPE occurs mainly in children and young adults. It occurs months or years after an apparent recovery from rubeola infection. It is suspected to be a slow measles virus infection.

Ocular Changes

Focal retinitis with edema occurs. Hemorrhages and folds in the retina correspond to areas of acute retinal necrosis that have left pigmented scars.

Nonophthalmologic Signs

SSPE may be accompanied by concomitant lethargy, muscle weakness, seizure activity, and personality disorders. The disease is frequently fatal.

Masquerade Syndrome (Iridocyclitis)

Iridocyclitis (anterior uveitis) presenting in older patients should be considered to have possible metastatic tumor to the anterior segment. Primary tumor of the lung is the most common cause of this *masquerade syndrome.* Patients present without other signs of tumor and frequently present before diagnosis of the primary tumor. There are no detectable lesions on the iris or in the angle or ciliary body. The major symptom is flare caused by increased capillary permeability.

Masquerade syndrome in the eye can respond to topical steroids. A high index of suspicion should be maintained in elderly patients presenting with a first episode of iridocyclitis.

Reticulum Cell Sarcoma and Uveitis

In an older patient who presents with an inflammation of the vitreous (vitritis) or uvea (uveitis), the possibility of a reticulum cell sarcoma must be entertained. The vitritis or uveitis can be unilateral or bilateral. This reticulum cell sarcoma diagnosis should especially be considered when the older patient has no history of uveitis.

The workup often includes a CT scan, a spinal tap, and a diagnostic vitrectomy. Diagnosis is important because these patients respond to vitrectomy and radiation therapy.

Differential Diagnosis of Granulomatous Uveitis

- Sarcoidosis
- Tuberculosis
- Secondary syphilis
- Cryptococcus
- Toxoplasmosis

Rare causes:
  Brucellosis

Coccidioidomycosis
Leprosy and histoplasmosis

In older patients presenting with an initial iridocyclitis, include in the differential diagnosis:

- Leukemia
- Lymphoma
- Melanotic melanoma
- Leiomyoma
- Metastatic carcinoma

ENDOPHTHALMITIS

There are two forms: (*a*) endogenous endophthalmitis (intraocular inflammation due to blood-borne organisms) and (*b*) exogenous endophthalmitis (intraocular inflammation due to external sources, usually after surgical procedures or injuries to the eye).

Endogenous Endophthalmitis

Characteristics

Organisms reach the eye by the blood, usually in patients who are seriously ill or have severely compromised immune systems. The inflammation starts in the posterior segment of the eye, causing blurred vision.

Prognosis

Endogenous endophthalmitis frequently results in severe loss of vision and may result in loss of the eye.

Susceptible Patients

Certain classes of patients may develop endogenous endophthalmitis:

- Patients with neoplastic disease such as lymphoma or leukemia;
- Patients on corticosteroid or antimetabolite therapy;
- Patients with hyperalimentation;
- Chronic intravenous drug abusers.

Most Common Organisms

Fungal organisms are most common: *Candida, Aspergillus,* and also infrequently *Cryptococcus* and *Coccidiomycosis.*

Exogenous Endophthalmitis

The onset of postoperative bacterial endophthalmitis usually occurs within 24 to 48 hours after the entry of the bacteria, which is usually at the time of surgery. Operations that most commonly precede endophthalmitis are cataract extraction, glaucoma surgery, and repair of injuries.

Incidence

After glaucoma filtration surgery, the incidence of endophthalmitis is as high as 2%. After cataract extraction, the incidence is less than 0.1%.

Organisms

Staphylococcal organisms, *S. epidermidis* and *S. aureus,* are the most common causes of bacterial endophthalmitis. In addition, Gram-negative microorganisms such as *Pseudomonas, Aerobacter,* and *Proteus* should always be considered. *Pneumococcus* is an uncommon cause.

Source of Infection

The most common source of exogenous endophthalmitis is the patient's skin and lid margins. Other common sources, especially where multiple cases are seen, are the respiratory tracts of operating personnel.

Prophylaxis

- Many surgeons use topical antibiotics before operation.
- At the time of operation, subconjunctival antibiotics may be injected at the end of the procedure.

Patients Especially Susceptible

Immunologically compromised hosts, patients with leukopenia, patients with diabetes, patients with prolonged operations, and patients with foreign substances from trauma in the eye are at risk.

Signs and Symptoms

The eye is painful. There is loss of vision. Characteristically, the lids become erythematous and swollen with edema. The conjunctiva becomes edemedous and hyperemic. As the process progresses, the cornea decompensates and becomes opaque with edema. The anterior chamber fills with white cells, and the vitreous becomes hazy.

Differential Diagnosis

Bacterial endophthalmitis usually starts within 24 to 48 hours. Fungal endophthalmitis takes 3 to 4 or more weeks to develop after the operation. Sterile iridocyclitis is usually delayed until 5 to 10 days after the operation. *Aerobacter proprione* can present as a low grade infection for months or years.

Clinical Evaluation of a Patient with Endophthalmitis

As soon as the diagnosis is suspected, immediate laboratory samples are considered: aqueous samples by aqueous tap; vitreous samples by vitreous aspiration. The vitreous tap is important as it may be positive when the aqueous tap is negative on culture. At the time of vitreous tap, the vitreous can be injected with appropriate concentrations of antibiotics.

Causes of Endophthalmitis

There are three major divisions of endophthalmitis:

- Post-cataract extraction;
- Filtering bleb;
- Posttraumatic.

The most common organisms isolated are:

- Post-cataract extraction—*Staphylococcus epidermidis* and *Staphylococcus aureus;*
- Filtering bleb—*Streptococcus* and *Haemophilus influenzae;*
- Trauma—*Bacillus* species.

Endophthalmitis Due to Drug Abuse

Patients who use intravenous drugs may develop metastatic endophthalmitis from particulate matter injected into the veins. Substances used to dilute drugs—talc, cornstarch, and other particulates—have been implicated. The condition may present as a single focus or as multiple foci of inflammation.

10

Tumors

Rhabdomyosarcoma	Retinoblastoma
Glioma	Metastatic Tumors to the Eye
Fibrous Histiocytoma	Malignant Melanomas of the Iris
Lymphomas	Choroidal Hemangiomas
Sebaceous Carcinoma	Choroidal Nevi
Uveal Melanomas	Melanocytoma of the Optic Nerve

Both intraocular and intraorbital tumors are dealt with by ophthalmologists. This chapter outlines the major signs and symptoms of tumors commonly associated with ophthalmologic practice. Intraocular tumors, such as melanoma and retinoblastoma, are the most important tumors in adults and children, respectively. Orbital tumors of both adults and children, such as gliomas, are also covered.

RHABDOMYOSARCOMA

Rhabdomyosarcomas occur throughout the body but are found in the orbit more frequently than any other site. Rhabdomyosarcoma is the most common primary malignant orbital neoplasm of children.

Clinical Signs

This tumor characteristically produces a rapidly progressing unilateral proptosis (Figs. 10.1 and 10.2). Usually, presentation is proptosis of sudden onset in a child 7 to 8 years of age. Lid swelling accompanies the proptosis. Chemosis around the orbit may be marked.

Origin

This is a highly malignant neoplasm of the embryonic mesoderm. The tumor is differen-

tiated into different types: (*a*) embryonal, which have elongated cells called strap cells or racquet cells and cross-striations or Z bands on cells (Z bands are created by actomycin filaments); (*b*) alveolar; and (*c*) differentiated. The alveolar type has the worst prognosis. Approximately 7% of all rhabdomyosarcoma throughout the body are in the orbit.

The median age of onset of rhabdomyosarcoma is 6 years. Of patients in this age group, 85% have embryonal tumor histology.

GLIOMA

Glioma of the optic nerve is a benign astrocytic tumor that occurs in childhood. Although it is almost never detected at birth, it is probably present and can be considered a congenital tumor. Pathologic examination classifies it as a hamartoma, and it is associated with von Recklinghausen's disease in 30 to 50% of patients.

It is a slow-growing tumor. Glioma is usually discovered during the first decade of life, at 4 to 5 years of age. The two most common signs are *decreased vision* and forward displacement of the eye *(proptosis)*. Additional signs are optic atrophy, papilledema, strabismus, nystagmus, and vein obstruction. One-third of all patients will have café au lait spots.

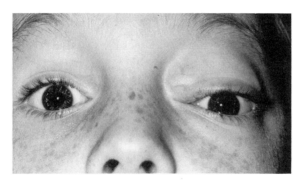

Figure 10.1. Rhabdomyosarcoma of the orbit. Rapid progressive forward displacement of the eye (proptosis) in a child demands that rhabdomyosarcoma be ruled out. Proptosis, which may be a straightforward displacement of the globe as illustrated, can also be down and out. The character of the proptosis will depend upon the position of the tumor within the orbit. (Credit: Ted Wojno, M.D.)

X-ray

One of the characteristic signs is enlargement of the optic canal on x-ray examination. When glioma is suspected, special radiographic views of the canal should be requested.

Intracranial involvement may result in a fatal outcome. Intracranial involvement with glioma is characterized by visual loss, optic atrophy, and signs of increased intracranial pressure. Intraorbital gliomas are characterized by visual loss, papilledema, and proptosis. The unilateral proptosis in intraorbital glioma rarely exceeds 3 mm.

The proptosis of a glioma, because it is in the muscle cone, protrudes the eye forward, is nonpulsatile, and cannot be reduced. The tumor is nonpalpable because of its location.

In children, where it is difficult to measure visual acuity, gliomas may be indicated by the presence of strabismus, an afferent pupillary defect, optic disk edema, or optic atrophy.

There is a rare malignant optic glioma that occurs in adults, primarily men. Characteristically, it progresses rapidly. This is a malignant astrocytoma, which should be differentiated from the hamartoma of childhood.

FIBROUS HISTIOCYTOMA

This is the most common mesenchymal orbital tumor of adults. The orbit is the site of predilection of this tumor, but it is also seen in the lacrimal sac and in the conjunctiva. It is frequently misdiagnosed.

Signs and Symptoms

Congestion of the eye is seen. Motility disturbances occur. There is a decrease in the uncorrected visual acuity. Histiocytoma occurs in patients in their 40s, with the median age being 43. There is equal sex distribution. Progression is slow, usually over a period of years. The superior orbit is a site of predilection. Pathologic findings are spindle-shaped fibroblast-like cells and histiocytes.

Course

The courses vary. Most tumors are benign, but 25% become locally aggressive. Ten percent become frankly malignant.

LYMPHOMAS

B cell lymphomas may affect the eye and the orbit, the conjunctiva, the lacrimal gland, and the muscle cone. Orbital lymphoma is a

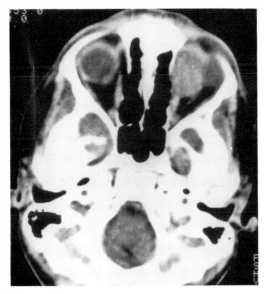

Figure 10.2. Rhabdomyosarcoma shown by computed tomographic (CT) scan of the orbit. (Same patient as in Fig. 10.1) (Credit: Ted Wojno, M.D.)

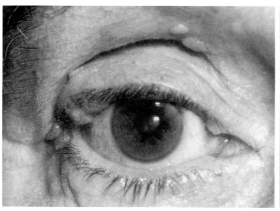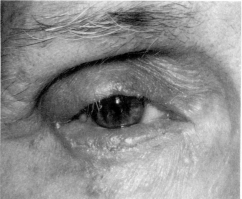

Figure 10.3. Meibomian gland carcinoma is slow-growing and may present as inflammation of the eyelid. Both of these examples of meibomian gland carcinoma show lid thickening, which at times may be diffuse and extensive. Misdiagnosis as chalazion (see page 209) is not uncommon. In chronic recurrent chalazia, the possibility of the presence of meibomian gland carcinoma should be considered. (Credit: Ted Wojno, M.D.)

common cause of unilateral forward displacement of the eye (proptosis) in an elderly patient.

Malignant lymphomas may also present as posterior uveitis. Diagnosis may require vitreous biopsy for confirmation.

T cell lymphomas, such as Hodgkin's disease, do not involve the eye or the orbit.

SEBACEOUS CARCINOMA

Sebaceous carcinoma is not synonymous with meibomian gland carcinoma (Fig. 10.3). Although sebaceous carcinoma can arise from meibomian glands, it also comes from other sources. Sources of sebaceous carcinoma are meibomian glands, Zeis' glands, caruncle, and eyebrow.

Clinical Characteristics

The most common position for sebaceous carcinoma is the upper lid. In contrast, basal cell carcinoma is usually found in the lower lid.

This diagnosis may be delayed because the condition can simulate a chronic unilateral blepharitis and conjunctivitis. Because most bacterial blepharitis is bilateral, the occurrence of a chronic unilateral conjunctivitis should make one suspect sebaceous carcinoma. The clinical signs are extremely variable:

- A nodular mass appears as a chalazion. (A chalazion is not infrequently associated with sebaceous carcinoma because they have similar positions of origin.)
- If the tumor arises from Zeis' glands, it is usually on the lower lid at the base of the lashes.
- The lid may be ropey and thickened, with loose lashes.
- Chronic unilateral blepharitis is simulated.

Frequent Misdiagnosis

In one study, 7% of the cases had the correct clinical diagnosis made at the time of biopsy. In a review of initial pathology readings, only 50% were correct.

Metastasis

Sebaceous carcinomas do metastasize, and lymph nodes should be palpated.

Demography

- Female predominance—2/1
- Upper lid to lower lid—2/1
- High mortality rate

Treatment

The treatment is surgical incision. Sebaceous cell carcinomas do not respond well to radiation.

Chronic Unilateral Blepharitis and Conjunctivitis

In chronic unilateral blepharitis and conjunctivitis in an older individual, the lid margin is thickened and lashes may be lost or loose. Possible sebaceous carcinoma should be considered. In contrast, bacterial conjunctivitis, rosacea, and staphylococcal blepharitis are usually bilateral.

UVEAL MELANOMAS

Melanomas of the uveal tract arise from melanocytes of neurocrest origin.

Cell Types

Melanomas are classically divided into three cell types: spindle A, spindle B, and epithelioid. Differentiation of the cell type is important for determining prognosis and malignant potential. The epithelioid melanoma is the most rapid-growing tumor, is most frequently associated with metastasis, and has the worst prognosis. The histologic classification has been changed recently from the classic descriptions.

Callender's Classification

Callender's classification divides uveal melanomas into six cell types: spindle A, spindle B, fascicular, mixed, necrotic, and epithelioid. The mixed cell tumor type is composed of both spindle cells and epithelioid cells.

McLean's Classification

McLean's classification has more recently divided spindle A melanomas into three groups: spindle cell nevi, spindle cell melanomas, and mixed cell melanomas. Each classification is related to prognosis because there is no mortality in the spindle cell nevi type;

however, there is almost a 50% mortality in the mixed cell melanoma group.

Onset

Most melanomas are diagnosed after the age of 50.

Bilaterality

Malignant melanomas that are bilateral are extremely rare. Choroidal nevi, by contrast, are frequently bilateral.

Race Predilection

Melanomas are rare in blacks and are unusual in orientals. Melanomas are predominantly found in whites.

Factors Predisposing to Melanomas

Ocular Melanocytosis (Melanosis Oculi)

This condition is usually unilateral but may be bilateral occasionally. Slate-gray to brown areas of pigmentation are seen in the episcleral regions. The conjunctiva moves freely over these areas. In the involved eye, the iris may have diffuse hyperpigmentation or may show a dense sector of pigmentation. Choroid may also show diffuse or sector distribution of pigmentation.

The malignant melanomas that arise in these patients usually are found in the choroid and/or the ciliary body. Melanomas do not arise from the episcleral pigmentation. This pigmentation may also be associated with optic disc hyperpigmented tumors, known as melanocytomas.

Oculodermal Melanocytosis (Nevus of Ota) (see page 328)

In this condition, the ocular pigmentations seen in ocular melanocytosis are combined with hyperpigmentation of the periocular skin. This condition is more common in orientals and blacks; however, the melanomas that occur in these patients are seen in whites only.

Malignant melanomas are also known to occur in this condition in other areas such as skin, meninges, and brain. This is almost always on the side of the hyperpigmentation.

Neurofibromatosis

Patients with neurofibromatosis have an increased incidence of uveal nevi and melanomas. They also have an increased incidence of other cancers.

The majority of melanomas in patients with neurofibromatosis occur in the iris, although posterior uveal melanomas are known to occur.

Factors Affecting Prognosis

The following factors have been reported to affect prognosis:

- Cell type;
- Tumor size;
- Age of patient at the time of enucleation;
- Location of tumor;
- Extrascleral extension;
- Amount of pigmentation;
- Integrity of Brook's membrane;
- Height of tumor.

Metastasis

Because there are no lymphatics in the orbit, metastasis of malignant melanomas is by blood. Metastasis from iris melanomas is extremely rare. However, metastasis from ciliary body and choroidal melanomas is common. It is estimated that 20 to 50% of patients with choroidal melanomas die of metastatic disease. The most common *sites of metastasis* of ocular melanomas are the liver and the lung (in that order).

Understanding of the nature of ocular melanomas is rapidly developing. The controversial aspects of treatment, including enucleation and radiation, are being investigated. The association of melanomas with the dysplastic nevus syndrome (B-K mole syndrome), an inherited condition, is an interesting clinical association.

Differential Diagnosis of Melanoma and Hemorrhage

General Considerations

The differential diagnosis between ocular hemorrhage and melanoma is important. Although less likely today with modern diagnostic techniques, in years past, many eyes were removed because of the fear of melanoma when the diagnosis was actually hematoma. Observation is still the primary evaluation technique. Here are differential features that can assist in making the diagnosis clinically.

In melanomas:

- There are feeder vessels from the choroid;
- Retinal pigment epithelium over the melanoma shows a patchy atrophy;
- There are often characteristic clusters of orange pigment on the intact pigment epithelium;
- With fluorescein angiography, there is a progressive increase in fluorescence (hyperfluorescence).

In hematomas:

- There are no observable vessels;
- There is a smooth pigment epithelium without patchy atrophy;
- There is no characteristic orange pigment on the pigment epithelium, which is uniform;
- Fluorescein angiography shows that the hemorrhage remains hypofluorescent.

MRI in Differentiating between Intraocular Melanomas and Hemorrhage

With T1-weighted early images and T2-weighted late images, a melanin-containing tumor shows up bright on the early images and dark on the late images. A melanotic tumor shows bright throughout the series.

If hemorrhage is present, the magnetic resonance imaging (MRI) pattern will vary according to the time that the hemorrhage has been present. Acute hemorrhages give bright images throughout the MRI sequence. Old, inactive hemorrhages show bright early images and late dark images.

RETINOBLASTOMA

This tumor is the most common intraocular malignancy of childhood (Fig. 10.4). It is

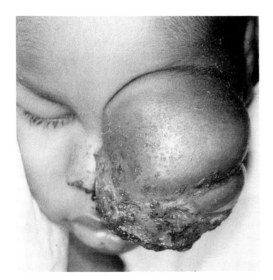

Figure 10.4. Far-advanced retinoblastoma in a child. Retinoblastoma is the most common intraocular malignancy in children. It rarely progresses to this advanced stage. It is a genetically determined tumor.

second only to the uveal melanomas as the most common primary intraocular malignancy in humans.

There is no predisposition for race, sex, or right or left eye. The tumor is bilateral in 25 to 30% of cases.

The tumor is diagnosed at an average age of 18 months. Bilateral cases are usually recognized earlier, at an age of about 12 months. Unilateral cases are recognized later, at an age of about 23 months.

Hereditary

About 5% of patients who develop retinoblastomas have a family history of the disease. The hereditary form is known to be autosomal dominant, with incomplete penetrance estimated at 60 to 95%.

In 95% of the cases, the tumor is thought to be spontaneous (sporadic). In 5%, a specific constitutional chromosomal abnormality has been shown, a deletion of the long arm of chromosome 13.

Clinical Features

The most common presenting sign is a white pupil (leukocoria). The second most common sign is crossed eyes (strabismus).

Early lesions are seen as flat, transparent or slightly white masses in the sensory retina. As

the lesion grows, the tumors are less transparent and may become solid white. As a tumor becomes larger, it grows into the vitreous cavity. There are no retinal vessels visualized over the hazy white mass. Seeding may occur into the vitreous cavity. Inflammation may be stimulated.

Tumors that grow into the subretinal space (exophytic) show retinal vessels apparently on the surface of the tumor. Tumors that grow into the vitreous are known as endophytic. As a tumor grows, cells may be deposited in the anterior chamber and a hypopyon (Fig. 9.2) may result.

Approximately one-half of the children with retinoblastoma have rubeosis iridis (vessels on the iris) at the time of diagnosis. Spontaneous bleeding from the vessels may cause hyphema (blood in the anterior chamber).

Important diagnostic points are helpful in distinguishing retinoblastoma from other causes of white pupil, such as persistent hyperplastic primary vitreous (PHPV) and rubella oculopathy. In retinoblastoma, the eye is of normal size, as opposed to PHPV where the eye is often smaller. The lens is also clear in retinoblastoma, the development of cataract (lens opacity) being extremely rare. PHPV is almost always associated with lens cataract.

Advanced retinoblastoma may involve the optic nerve. The tumor extends through the lamina cribrosa into the retrolaminar portion of the nerve. Orbital extension also occurs. The tumor invades the choroid and then gains access to the orbit through the scleral emissaria. Distant metastasis occurs, as does direct extension into the intracranial spaces by way of the optic nerve subarachnoid space.

Spontaneous Regression

Retinoblastoma undergoes spontaneous regression in certain individuals. Regressed retinoblastoma appears as a shrunken, calcified mass, often with sclerotic feeder vessels and scattered pigmentation.

Histology

Histologically, retinoblastomas show interesting and characteristic changes. *Fleurettes* are composed of groups of tumor cells that contain pear-shaped processes representing differentiation along lines of outer segments of photoreceptors. *Homer-Wright rosettes* consist of radially arranged cells around a central triangle of neurofibers. (Homer-Wright rosettes also are found in neuroblastomas and medulloblastomas.)

Flexner-Wintersteiner rosettes are also seen. These consist of columnar cells arranged around a clear central lumen.

Diagnosis

Orbital x-ray films may show intraocular calcification of the tumor. (Other conditions that can cause intraocular calcification are retinal astrocytoma, advanced Coats' disease, angiomatosis retinae, and nematode endophthalmitis.)

Ultrasound

Ultrasound is valuable for showing some typical features of retinoblastoma. Characteristic of B scan is attenuation or absence of soft tissue echoes in the orbit directly behind the areas of calcification within the tumor.

CT Scan

CT scanning may detect and delineate retinoblastoma.

Aqueous Enzymes

The aqueous to plasma ratio of lactate dehydrogenase is elevated in patients with retinoblastoma but not in patients with other conditions simulating retinoblastoma. Another enzyme, phosphoglucose isomerase, has also been shown to have an elevated ratio.

Cytology

Aqueous or vitreous humor cytology may be definitive. The malignant cells can be identified in cases of retinoblastoma.

METASTATIC TUMORS TO THE EYE

Characteristics

Metastatic tumors to the eye most often involve the uvea, although rarely the retina can be involved. The most frequent tumor type for metastasis is *carcinomas*. Metastatic sarcomas are extremely rare. Metastatic melanomas to the choroid have been reported but are extremely rare.

Origin

The most common source of metastatic cancer is *breast*. *Lung* is the second most common. These two cancers make up the majority of metastatic disease to the eye. Less common are gastrointestinal, kidney, and pancreas cancers.

Onset

Metastatic disease to the eye is most often seen in patients 40 to 70 years old.

Ocular Involvement

More than 90% of metastatic disease involves the choroid. Most often the posterior segment and frequently the macula are involved. Macular involvement usually causes decreased vision, which may be the presenting sign. The iris is involved in less than 5%. Even more unusual is involvement of the ciliary body.

Of metastatic ocular tumors, 19% are bilateral at the time of presentation. Approximately one in five have multiple foci. The appearance of multiple foci is an important diagnostic feature in these lesions.

Clinical Characteristics

Iris

Iris metastatic tumors tend to be friable and loosely cohesive. They are characterized by rapid growth. Glaucoma is a frequent association with these tumors.

Choroid

The choroidal tumors appear as a creamy yellow, plaquoid, irregular or multinodular tumor. Sometimes these tumors may be raised and dome-shaped. A serous retinal detachment is associated with 75% of these tumors.

The retinal pigment epithelium over the tumor is frequently altered. Also, a golden brown pigmentation consisting of clumped macrophages with lipofuscin and pigment can help establish the diagnosis.

MALIGNANT MELANOMAS OF THE IRIS

Incidence

About 3 to 10% of all malignant melanomas of the uvea occur on the iris. There is a predisposition in whites; these tumors are rarely seen in blacks. Males and females are affected equally. The left and right eyes are also affected equally. There is a tendency for the tumors to be located in the inferior portion of the iris. Superior iris melanomas are so unusual as to make the diagnosis suspect.

Clinical Appearance

Localized

Localized iris melanomas are usually well demarcated with variable pigmentation. They tend to be an irregular, elevated mass. The tumor replaces the iris stroma. Satellite lesions, which are similar but smaller lesions, are occasionally present near the larger tumor.

Diffuse

Diffuse iris melanomas are more difficult to diagnosis. There is an insidious darkening of the involved iris. A glaucoma, usually painless, is often present in the involved eye.

The iris is thickened, with loss of the usual iris crypts. Gonioscopy should be done to rule out involvement of the angle. When the angle is involved, there is an irregular nodularity in the inferior angle.

The configuration of the tumor has been described as multiple nodules or "tapioca." Such tumors are usually without extensive pigmentation.

Iris melanomas seem to relate to a spectrum of closely related conditions: diffuse iris melanoma, tapioca melanoma, neurofibromatosis, iris nevus syndrome, Chandler's syndrome, and essential iris atrophy.

The pigmentation of iris melanomas is extremely varied. In differential diagnosis, especially when the tumor does not contain extensive pigment, iris melanoma can be confused with other conditions such as sarcoidosis and the associated granulomatous iridocyclitis, metastatic tumors, and leiomyomas.

In iris melanomas, there are frequently vessels. Often these are prominent feeder vessels that arise from the greater circle of the iris. Fluorescein angiography may be helpful in detecting these vessels. The presence of vessels differentiates an iris mass from an iris nevus.

Differential Diagnosis of Iris Melanomas

- Localized melanoma
- Iris nevus
  (Nevi do not grow; melanomas do)
- Leiomyoma
- Tumors metastatic to the iris (no predilection for inferior quadrant, most often breast or lung)
- Iris cyst
- Foreign body
- Essential iris atrophy
- Hemangioma of the iris

Differential Diagnosis of Diffuse Melanomas

- Congenital
- Heterochromia
- Iris nevus syndrome
- Siderosis
- Hemosiderosis
- Pigmentary glaucoma

CHOROIDAL HEMANGIOMAS

Types

There are two types of choroidal hemangiomas, circumscribed and diffuse. The circumscribed hemangiomas show as a red-or-ange mass always in the posterior pole. The location is rather typical. One-half of circumscribed hemangiomas are seen in the macular area totally or partially within the temporal arcades. The other hemangiomas are on the nasal side or above the optic disc.

Circumscribed hemangiomas are 3 to 12 mm in diameter and can be 1 to 6 mm in height. In both hemangiomas, changes are seen in the retinal pigment epithelium. These appear as dark black clumps. Hemangiomas may be associated with serous retinal detachment.

Diffuse hemangiomas appear as red-orange thickening of the posterior choroid. They are often associated with the Sturge-Weber syndrome (see page 169). With diffuse hemangiomas, there may be external changes: dilated episcleral vessels or telangiectatic conjunctival vessels.

Diffuse hemangiomas may be associated with serous detachment of the retina. Glaucomas may also be associated.

Diagnosis of Hemangiomas

Fluorescein Angiography

The patterns of fluorescein angiography are variable and not diagnostic.

Ultrasound

A-scan ultrasonography is frequently useful in determining differences between hemangioma and melanoma. The acoustic hollowness and choroidal excavation seen with choroidal melanoma on B-scan are rarely seen with choroidal hemangioma. A-scan in hemangioma shows an initial high spike at the surface of the lesion followed by relatively high internal reflectivity within the tumor. Also, mushroom-shaped configurations seen with choroidal melanomas do not occur with hemangiomas.

CHOROIDAL NEVI

Incidence

This is a common intraocular tumor that occurs in 1 to 2% of the general population. (An incidence of 6.5% of autopsied eyes has been reported.) Lesions are very rare in infants and children. Nevi become more prominent at puberty.

Position

Of all choroidal nevi, 90% occur posterior to the equator. In fact, more than half are easily visible within the range of the direct ophthalmoscopic view of the posterior pole.

Clinical Features

In general, choroidal nevi appear as flat or minimally elevated slate gray lesions (Fig. 10.5). The edges are not sharply demarcated but do appear distinct. The pigmentation may vary, some being without pigment (amelanotic), pigmented, or partially pigmented. The majority are between 1.5 and 5.0 mm in size, but they may vary from 0.5 to 10 mm. The nevus is usually flat but may obtain a thickness of 2 mm or more.

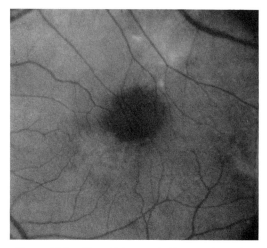

Figure 10.5. Choroidal nevus in the macular region.

Drusen are often associated with larger nevi. These are distinct yellow drusen that occur on the surface of the tumor at the level of the retinal pigment epithelium. Orange pigment is also seen over large choroidal nevi. Orange pigment flecks are commonly seen without clinical significance; however, large, defined geographic areas of orange pigment are associated at times with malignant transformation.

Differential Diagnosis of Nevi

- Small malignant melanomas of the choroid
- Hyperplasia of the retinal pigment epithelium
- Congenital hypertrophy of the retinal pigment epithelium
- Hamartomas and subretinal hemorrhage

Diagnosing Choroidal Nevi

1. The indirect ophthalmoscope is usually sufficient to make the diagnosis.

2. Visual field defects can be associated with nevi. A visual field defect does not imply a malignant lesion.

3. There is no special appearance of choroidal nevus on fluorescein angiography. Heavily pigmented nevi tend to have hypofluoresc-

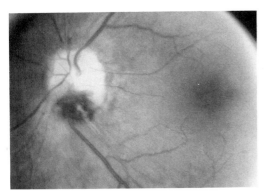

Figure 10.6. Melanocytomas are pigmented tumors seen at the disc margin in blacks. For the most part, they are considered to be benign.

ence. Less pigmented nevi tend to have hyperfluorescence.

Relation to Choroidal Melanomas

The differential diagnosis between choroidal nevi and melanomas may not be easy clinically. There is evidence that malignant melanomas do arise from preexisting benign nevi. In general, pigment and lesions higher than 2 mm and greater than 5 mm in diameter are highly suggestive of malignant melanoma. Although benign nevi are known to increase in size, photographic documentation of increased size is generally a reliable indication of malignant change.

MELANOCYTOMA OF THE OPTIC NERVE

Melanocytoma of the optic nerve is usually not diagnosed until later life but is probably present at birth. It is almost always *unilateral*. There is a slight predominance of women over men. There is a heavy predominance of melanocytomas in *blacks*. The melanocytomas that occur in whites tend to be in individuals of Italian or Hispanic descent.

Most patients are asymptomatic unless the tumor is large. An afferent pupillary defect is involved in 30% of cases. This can be true even with normal visual acuity.

Usually there is an elevated jet-black mass that is located at the edge of the optic nerve (Fig. 10.6). Although the color can vary, the large majority will have some black pigmentation. These tumors can be seen to grow in a small number of cases over a period of years. Rapid growth is uncharacteristic.

Malignant transformation, although unusual, is known to occur. The lesion should be followed with serial photographs. Enlargement should make the observer suspicious of low-grade malignant change.

11

Lacrimal System

This section discusses the lacrimal system, which is responsible for the production, distribution, and drainage of tears.

Tears are a fluid with layers of water, mucus, and oil. Each component has a different anatomical and physiologic origin. Distribution of the tears requires an intact lid system to allow the blink to spread the tear film. Tears are drained through the lacrimal system. The drainage process requires significant action of the muscles of the eyelids.

Because of its importance in external disease diagnosis, the tear film is discussed primarily in the external disease section (page 28). The lacrimal gland is discussed separately under conditions that involve the lacrimal gland, such as sarcoid or Sjögren's syndrome. In this chapter, the lacrimal drainage system is discussed, and significant diseases that affect the system are presented.

ANATOMY OF THE LACRIMAL SYSTEM (Fig. 11.1)

Lacrimal Gland

The lacrimal gland is an exocrine gland. It is located in the superior lateral quadrant of the orbit. The position is important because orbital masses may also present in the superior orbital quadrant. The lacrimal gland is divided anatomically by the levator aponeurosis into two lobes. The two lobes are referred to as orbital and palpebral.

Ducts from the lacrimal gland empty secretions into the superior cul de sac 5 mm above the lateral tarsal border. Ducts from the orbital portion of the lacrimal gland run through the palpebral lobe.

Innervation

The fifth cranial nerve acts as the reflex afferent pathway, and the seventh cranial nerve acts as the efferent pathway.

Accessory Lacrimal Glands

Krause's and Wolfring's glands are also exocrine glands. They are located in the superior fornix of the conjunctiva above the superior border of the tarsus. These glands have no nerve supply.

Lacrimal Drainage System

Punctum

The punctum is the hole in the lid margin through which the tears are drained. There is a superior punctum and an inferior punctum on the upper and lower lids, respectively. These are located at the inner margin of the lid. To function well, the punctum should be inverted slightly and against the globe.

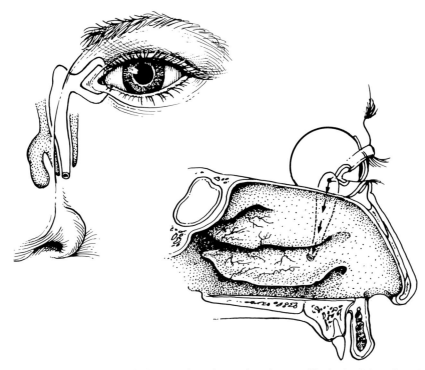

Figure 11.1.   The lacrimal system as it drains tears from the eye into the nose. The lacrimal ducts form the common canaliculus, which empties into the lacrimal sac. The lacrimal sac drains into the nasal lacrimal duct, which empties into the nose.

Ampulla

The ampulla lies between the punctum and the next portion of the drainage system, the canaliculus. The ampulla is 2 mm in length. It is a larger channel than either the punctum or the canaliculus. It is vertical to the lid margin.

Canaliculus

There is a canaliculus in both the upper and the lower lid. Each is 8 to 10 mm long. In 9 of 10 patients, the upper and lower canaliculi combine to form the common canaliculus. It is the common canaliculus that enters the lateral wall of the tear sac. It is here that *Rosenmüller's valve* prevents the reflux of tears from the sac back into the canaliculi.

Lacrimal Sac

The lacrimal sac lies within the lacrimal sac fossa and within the structure of the medial canthal tendon. The dome of the sac reaches above the tendon. The nasal lacrimal sac is 10 mm long.

Nasal Lacrimal Duct

The nasal lacrimal duct runs from the lacrimal sac into the nose. In the nose, the lacrimal duct opens through an ostium that is partially covered by a mucosal fold beneath and lateral to the inferior turbinate. This mucosal fold is called the *valve of Hasner.*

PHYSIOLOGY OF THE LACRIMAL SYSTEM

The active removal of tears (evaporation also occurs) depends upon a pump mechanism maintained by eyelid closure while blinking. The orbicularis muscles actually compress the ampullae and shorten the horizontal canaliculus. This moves the punctum medially with lid closure. This action is more superficial. Deeper action occurs as the orbicularis muscle, which is firmly attached to the lacrimal sac fascia, contracts, causing an expansion of the sac and creating a negative pressure or suction that pulls the tears from the canaliculus.

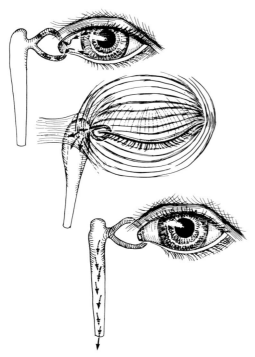

Figure 11.2. The lacrimal pump is an active mechanism that occurs with the blink (orbicularus muscle). The blink causes suction in the lacrimal sac and lacrimal ducts to move tears from the lacrimal lake into the nose.

Blinking controls this pump mechanism. On eye opening, the tear sac collapses, forcing tears into the duct and the nose. The punctum moves laterally and fluid enters into the ampullae and canaliculus. On eye closing, the sac is expanded, drawing the tear fluid into the sac, the punctum moves medially, the ampullae are compressed, and the horizontal canaliculi are shortened (Fig. 11.2).

DEVELOPMENTAL ANOMALIES

- Obstruction of the nasal lacrimal duct. Embryologically, the duct is the last portion of the lacrimal system to canalize (about the time of birth). It may be occluded at the time of birth (valve of Hasner).
- Complete stenosis of the punctum
- Absence of the punctum
- Duplication of the punctum

OUTFLOW DISORDERS
Punctal Disorders

- Agenesis and dysgenesis
- Stenosis causes nonfunctioning of a punctum. Usually only one punctum is necessary for drainage from the eye.
- Eversion of the punctum

Canalicular Disorders

- Obstruction (trauma, medications causing toxicity, viral infections, autoimmune disorders)
- Canaliculitis due to bacterial, viral, chlamydial, or fungal organisms
- Trauma
- Neoplasms

Lacrimal Sac Abnormalities
Dacryocystitis

See page 197.

Dacroliths

These are shredded epithelial cells and lipid with or without calcium. Cast formations may also occur within the lacrimal sac. *Actinomyces israelli* or topical medications such as epinephrine may produce stones of this type.

Lacrimal Sac Tumors

These are rare. They usually present as a mass above the medial canthal tendon and are associated with epiphora and chronic inflammation of the lacrimal system.

Trauma to the Lacrimal Sac

Nasal Lacrimal Duct Obstructions
Congenital Obstructions

Obstructions are common. They are due to membranous block of the valve of Hasner. They occur in 2 to 4% of full-term newborn infants within the first 2 weeks. One-third are bilateral. Most resolve spontaneously 4 to 6 weeks after birth.

Acquired Obstructions

Chronic sinus disease, injury to the nasal orbital area, and dacryocystitis may all produce an acquired obstruction of the nasal lacrimal ducts. The most common cause is involutional (age-related) stenosis. Women are twice as frequently affected as men. Additional causes of acquired obstruction are granulomatous diseases such as sarcoidosis and Wegener's granulomatosis.

SPECIFIC DISEASE PROCESSES

Canaliculitis

Definition

Canaliculitis is inflammation of the canalicular portion of the tear drainage system.

Characteristics

This occurs primarily in adults and is much more common in women. The lower canaliculitis is involved twice as often as the upper. It frequently presents as a chronic unilateral conjunctivitis. Follicles may be present around the inner canthus. The chief symptom may be persistent weeping on the involved side.

Signs are dilation of the punctum, injection of the lid margin, and mucopurulent material or concretions on expression of the canaliculitis material.

Diagnosis is by expressing the material from the canaliculitis. Conjunctival scrapings may also show organisms.

Causes

- Bacterial—*Actinomyces, Streptococcus,* and others
- Fungal, especially *Candida* and *Aspergillus*
- Viral (herpes simplex virus)
- *Chlamydia*

Dacryoadenitis

Definition

Dacryoadenitis is inflammation of the lacrimal gland. This is an uncommon condition that is usually unilateral and is more common in children.

Cause

The most frequent cause is mumps. Other causes include viruses other than mumps—measles, influenza, mononucleosis, and others. Bacterial causes include gonorrhea, *Staphylococcus, Streptococcus,* tuberculosis, and syphilis. Fungal and parasitic causes are rare.

Chronic inflammation of the lacrimal gland is most frequently caused by sarcoidosis. This is most common in blacks. Rare causes are tuberculosis and syphilis.

Signs and Symptoms of Dacryoadenitis

- Pain—specific
- Swelling of the lid
- Redness—specific
- Conjunctival ingestion
- Ptosis and inflammation of the palpebral lobe of the lacrimal gland, affecting lid function
- Inflammation of the orbital portion of the gland causing orbital symptoms

Dacryocystitis

Definition

Inflammation of the lacrimal drainage system

Cause

This is caused by a congenital or an acquired nasal lacrimal duct obstruction. In newborns, it is due to a nonfunctioning nasal lacrimal duct. In adults, it presents with nasal congestion with edema of the nasal mucosa and nasal polyps, which lead to obstruction (Fig. 11.3). It may also be due to drugs, tumors, and injuries.

Organisms most commonly seen are:

- *Streptococcus*
- *Staphylococcus*
- *Haemophilus influenzae*
- *Pseudomonas aeruginosa*
- *Proteus mirabilis*
- *Candida albicans*
- *Aspergillus*

Figure 11.3. Dacryocystitis, infection, and inflammation of the lacrimal system are illustrated, with swelling over the lacrimal area (to the *right* of the cotton-tipped applicator). Purulent discharge is present. (Credit: George Waring, M.D.)

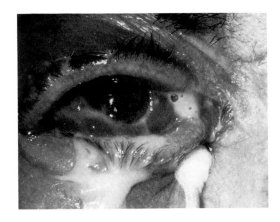

EXCESSIVE TEARING IN ADULTS (EPIPHORA)

Definition

Epiphora is excessive tearing.

Differential Diagnosis

- Absence of lacrimal system
- Stenosis
- Canaliculitis
- Neoplasm—frequently basal cell carcinoma
- Radiation exposure
- Drugs
- Postsurgery or posttrauma
- Stevens-Johnson syndrome
- Pemphigoid
- Dacryocystitis—dacrolyths
- Tumor of the lacrimal sac
- Nasal sinus surgery
- Involutional changes
- Tumor of the sac
- Maxillofacial fractures

Important Clinical Point

With masses in the nasal lacrimal region: if the mass is above the medial canthal tendon, it is most often tumor; if it is below, it is most often dacryocystitis.

Evaluation of Epiphora in Adults

- Fluorescein dye disappearance test. Fluorescein is placed in both conjunctival fornices, and the disappearance is noted over 5 minutes. An abnormal test is an inequality of fluorescein removal from both sides.
- Probing of the lacrimal system
- Scintigraphy (radioactive tracer)
- Dacrocystography and macrodacrocystography (also subtraction macrodacrocystography)
- Computed tomographic scan for tumors
- Clinical examination for stones from a canaliculitis

COMMONLY CONFUSED DEFINITIONS

Blepharoptosis

Blepharoptosis is another name for ptosis or drooping of the eyelid (see page 202).

Blepharochalasis

Blepharochalasis is specifically related to relaxation of the skin and the tendons of the eyelids and loss of elasticity after chronic or recurrent edematous swellings of the eyelids. The cause is unknown, but it does show a familial trait. The disease is of young people; one-half of the patients have the onset between the ages of 11 and 20.

Blepharophimosis

Blepharophimosis is a decrease in the dimensions of the lids, which are otherwise normally differentiated. It is associated with ptosis, telecanthus, and epicanthal inversus.

Dermatochalasis

Dermatochalasis is excessive skin on the eyelids. This may hang down in redundant folds, characteristically in the upper lids, and produce visual field decrease.

ADDITIONAL TOPICS FOR STUDY

- Schirmer test (see page 30)
- Jones test (see page 309)
- Tear film (see page 28)

12

Eyelids

This section deals with common eyelid lesions that are first diagnosed in or most often associated with the eyelids. No attempt has been made to be all inclusive. Conditions that secondarily affect the eyelids, such as neurofibromatosis or sarcoidosis, are not included in this section.

EYELID ANATOMY

Muscles of the Eyelid

Orbicular Muscle

The orbicular muscle, a protractor, is innervated by the seventh cranial nerve. It closes the eyelids on contraction. Portions of the muscle also surround the lacrimal drainage system (canaliculi) and provide action to drain tears. Portions of the obicularus muscle are found in the pretarsal, the preseptal, and orbital areas.

Levator Muscle

The levator muscle, a retractor of the upper eyelid, originates in the back of the orbit at the apex and moves forward into the lid muscle. The muscle portion of the levator is 40 mm long, and the aponeurosis is 14 to 20 mm long. The levator aponeurosis inserts on the superior tarsus. Laterally, the levator aponeurosis forms a septa that courses through the lacrimal gland. The levator muscle is innervated by the third cranial nerve.

Müller's Muscle

The superior tarsal muscle of Müller arises on the underside of the levator aponeurosis about 12 mm above the superior tarsal border. This muscle is important because of its sympathetic innervation. The muscle can provide 2 mm of lift of the upper eyelid and, when there is sympathetic interruption, such as Horner's syndrome (see page 93), the lid will droop (ptosis).

Superior Eyelid Crease

The superior eyelid crease curves near the superior border of the tarsus. The crease is created by the attachments of the levator aponeurosis to the pretarsal orbicularis bundles. The crease may be lacking in orientals, but is an important landmark in the caucasian lid and serves as a basis for diagnosis when displaced, as well as a surgical landmark.

Orbital Septum

The orbital septum is a thin sheet of fibrous tissue. It arises from the periosteum overlying the superior and inferior orbital rims. In the upper eyelid, it fuses with the levator aponeurosis approximately 3 mm above the tarsal border.

The orbital septum is the barrier between the orbit and the eyelid. It acts to limit the spread of infection and hemorrhage. Orbital fat is found behind the orbital septum, and in elderly patients this orbital fat can herniate into the eyelids as the septum becomes thin.

Tarsus

There is a tarsus in both the upper and the lower lid. The tarsus is a fibrous tissue plate. It acts as a skeletal base for the eyelids. The upper tarsus measures 8 to 12 mm vertically in the center. The lower tarsus is 4 mm or less. The tarsus is approximately 1 mm thick. Both the upper and lower lid tarsi taper as they course medially and laterally.

Conjunctiva

The conjunctiva lines the inner portion of the upper and lower lids. Conjunctiva contains mucin-secreting goblet cells and the accessory lacrimal glands of Krause and Wolfring. The accessory lacrimal glands are found mainly in the upper eyelid tissue between the superior tarsal border and the fornix (see Fig. 2.1).

Canthal Tendons

For each eye, there is a medial and a lateral canthal ligament. These support the upper and lower eyelids. The medial canthal ligament originates from the anterior and posterior lacrimal crest. The lateral canthal ligament attaches to the lateral orbital tubercle just inside the orbital rim. Lack of integrity of either of the canthal ligaments causes functional lid problems.

Eyelid Margin (Fig. 12.1)

The eyelid margin contains the junction of the conjunctiva and the skin—the mucocutaneous junction. The eyelid margin also contains the gray line, an avascular zone just anterior to the mucocutaneous junction. The gray line divides the eyelid into anterior and

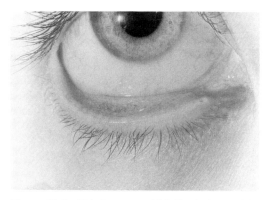

Figure 12.1. This is a normal lid. The lashes and lid margin are illustrated. On the lid margin, meibomian gland orifices can be seen. On the right side of the lid, the inferior lacrimal punctum can be seen. Normal global and palpebral conjunctiva are also demonstrated.

posterior portions. It is an important landmark for surgery.

The posterior border of the eyelid margin is sharply defined and fits snugly against the globe. Along this posterior border rides the tear film meniscus. As the lid closes, it acts as a distributor for the tear film over the cornea.

On the eyelid margins, the openings of the meibomian glands are seen. There are 25 in the upper lid and 20 in the lower lid. The meibomian glands are sebaceous-like glands imbedded in the tarsus of each lid.

Eyelashes originate from the anterior portion of the eyelid. There are about 100 lashes in the upper lid and 50 in the lower lid.

Blood Supply

The eyelid is supplied by two major sources:

- The ophthalmic artery and its branches (the ophthalmic artery arises from the internal carotid artery);
- The external carotid artery by way of arteries of the face.

There is extensive collateral circulation between these two systems.

Venous drainage occurs both pretarsal and posttarsal. Pretarsal tissues drain into the angular vein immediately and into the superior temporal vein laterally. Orbital veins drain the posttarsal tissue.

Lymphatic Drainage

Lymphatic drainage is important because some infections characteristically involve lymph nodes related to the eyelids. Lymphatic fluid from the medial portion of the eyelids drains into the *submandibular* nodes under the jaw. Lymph channels draining from the lateral portions of the eyelids go first into the preauricular nodes in front of the ear and then to the deeper cervical nodes. Characteristically, epidemic keratoconjunctivitis, a virus-induced infection, and bacterial infections that result in Parinaud's syndrome will cause lymph node enlargement in the *preauricular* regions.

Nerves

The eyelids are innervated by the third cranial nerve, the seventh cranial nerve, and the sympathetic system.

PTOSIS

Measurement of Levator Function

Levator function is measured with a millimeter rule held in front of the eye. The excursion of the upper eyelid margin from downgaze to upgaze is measured. Good levator function is considered to be a total of 8 mm or more from extreme downgaze to extreme upgaze. Five to 8 mm is moderate function, and less than 4 mm is considered poor function.

To make the test effective in long-standing ptosis, the examiner holds the frontalis muscle on the forehead above the eye to prevent its use in elevating the ptotic eyelid. Patients with long-standing ptosis will use the frontalis for this motion.

Evaluating Lid Crease Position

Lid crease is the indentation in the skin of the upper eyelid in the primary position. In patients with unilateral ptosis, the position of the lid crease in the abnormal upper lid differs from that in the normal lid. The superior lid crease above the lash margin is measured with a millimeter rule held vertically at the center of the lid. The distance will be increased when the lid is ptotic.

Definition

Ptosis (Fig. 12.2) (also called blepharoptosis) is a drooping of the upper lid. The upper

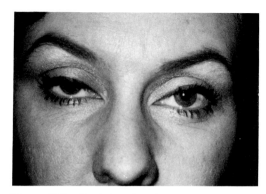

Figure 12.2. Ptosis is a drooping of the eyelid. In this patient, the right eyelid droops so that the pupil is almost entirely covered. Normally, the upper lid covers approximately 2 mm of the iris coloration of the eye when the eyes are directed in primary gaze. (Credit: Ted Wojno, M.D.)

eyelid is in an abnormally low position when the eye is looking straight ahead.

The normal upper eyelid rests at a point approximately 2 mm below the upper limbus of the globe when the eye is looking straight ahead. The lower lid normally rests 1 mm above the lower limbus. The palpebral fissure (the opening between the upper lid and the lower lid) for men is between 7 and 10 mm and for women is 8 to 12 mm. These measurements should be confirmed when evaluating lid function.

Classification

Congenital

Congenital ptosis is present at birth and is divided into three distinct categories.

Myogenic Ptosis. Myogenic ptosis refers to defects in development or function of the levator muscle.

Neurogenic Ptosis. Neurogenic ptosis results from improper innervation during embryonic development.

Aponeurotic Ptosis. Aponeurotic ptosis is caused by a defect in the levator aponeurosis that prevents proper elevation of the lid.

Acquired Ptosis

Definition. An acquired ptosis is any ptosis that develops after birth.

Aponeurotic Ptosis.

Age-related (Also Called Involutional Ptosis). Clinically, age-related ptosis can be diagnosed when the outline of the cornea can actually be seen through the skin of the upper lid. Age-related ptosis is due to a defect in the levator aponeurosis. With absence or a defect of the aponeurosis, the upper lid is thinned and the corneal shape can be seen under the skin with the lid closed.

Trauma.

Intraocular Surgery. Ptosis is not uncommon after cataract surgery.

Myogenic Acquired Ptosis.

- Chronic progressive external ophthal-moplegia
- Myasthenia gravis (defect in myo-neural junction)

Neurogenic Acquired Ptosis.

- Ocular motor (third nerve) palsy
- Horner's syndrome (sympathetic system disrupted)

Mechanical Acquired Ptosis.

- Tumor
- Scar formation (cicatricial)
- Trauma

Pseudoptosis.

Dermatochalasis. Excessive skin on the upper lid, dermatochalasis, can cause a droop of the eyelid.

Small globe. A small globe due to injury or inflammation that results in an abnormal shape (phthisis bulbi) can simulate a ptosis. Because of the lack of support of a full globe, the lid appears to be lower on the side with the shrunken globe.

ECTROPION

Definition

Ectropion is a turning out of the eyelid so that the eyelid margin does not approximate to the globe (Fig. 12.3). Ectropion usually involves the lower lid. The tear film distribution function of the lid may be disrupted, resulting in drying of the eye, inflammation, and visual loss from corneal opacification.

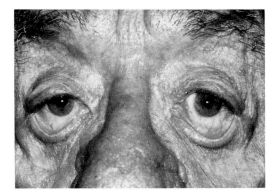

Figure 12.3. Ectropion is an outward turning of the lid. It usually involves the lower lid and can lead to corneal exposure. This patient shows severe bi-lateral lower lid ectropion. (Credit: Ted Wojno, M.D.)

Causes

There are many causes of ectropion.

Congenital

Congenital ectropion may be an isolated finding but is frequently associated with other congenital eyelid abnormalities. It involves the *upper lids.*

Atonic

Involutional. Involutional ectropion is secondary to relaxation of the tissue of the lids. It is common in the elderly. This loss of eyelid tone results in eversion of the lid margin. Complications then develop from the sagging lid including conjunctiva hypertrophy and chronic inflammation secondary to improper wetting of the globe and conjunctiva. Involutional ectropion is most frequently seen in the *lower lid.*

Paralytic Ectropion. This follows temporary or permanent seventh nerve palsy or paralysis. Because of lack of lower lid closure, chronic irritation occurs secondary to evaporation of the tear film.

Scarring (Cicatricial) Ectropion

This may occur on the upper or lower eyelid secondary to either thermal or chemical burns, mechanical trauma, lid surgery, or chronic inflammation such as discoid lupus erythematosus.

Inflammatory Ectropion

This is usually secondary to acute or chronic inflammation. An allergic condition or a localized or diffuse dermatitis is the most common cause.

Mechanical Ectropion

This is caused by eyelid tumors or, more commonly, by fluid accumulation in the lid, herniation of fat, or poorly fitting glasses that evert the lid.

Checklist for the Diagnosis of Lower Lid Involutional Ectropion

1. Lid Loose?

Check to see that there is no greater displacement possible than 6 to 10 mm on mechanical distortion of the lower lid with thumb and forefinger. To *determine lid laxity,* the lower lid can be distorted by the thumb and forefinger of the examiner. Simply pinch the lower lid. Normally there is no greater movement than 6 to 10 mm on this mechanical distortion. After distortion, the lid should bounce back immediately. If there is more than 6 to 10 mm of excursion or if the lid does not return briskly to its original position, laxity is present.

2. Lid Snappy?

With mechanical distortion of the lower lid outward away from the globe, does it snap back or is it loose?

3. Punctal Position?

Is the punctum in its normal position at the inner lid against the globe and slightly inverted? Is the medial canthal tendon tight so the punctum does not move more than 3 to 4 mm on attempts at lateral displacement? Greater movement indicates abnormality.

4. Loss of Lid Retractors?

This can be seen with a deep inferior fornix and sometimes a white line on the palpebral conjunctiva of the lower lid. This line is the edge of the retractors. Also, there is lack of lid retraction on downgaze.

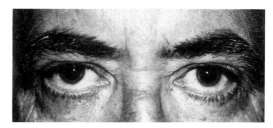

Figure 12.4. Scleral show is a term given to lid positions in which portions of the sclera are abnormally exposed. With the lower lid, as illustrated, this is most often due to lid laxity, which may result in ectropion. Scleral show can also appear with the upper lid and is most often seen with lid retraction in thyroid disease.

5. Scleral Show?

Normally, the lower lid is 1 mm above the limbus. If there is white showing between the lower lid margin and the lower limbus, this may be due to laxity (Fig. 12.4).

ENTROPION

Definition

Entropion is a turning in of either eyelid (Fig. 12.5). The lashes may rub the globe. Chronic irritation and visual loss may occur.

Types

Congenital Entropion

Congenital entropion results from developmental defects of the eyelid retractors.

Acute Spastic Entropion

Acute spastic entropion follows irritation and inflammation of the eyelids. The inflammation makes the lid less pliable and distorts the normal anatomy so that the lid turns in. Acute spastic entropion may also be seen with inflammation after intraocular surgery.

Involutional Entropion

Involutional entropion is usually observed in the lower eyelids; however, the upper eyelids may also be involved. In this condition, a number of factors can contribute: looseness of the eyelid margin or the canthal tendons, a change in the attachments of the eyelid retractors, alteration of the orbicularis muscle position in relationship to the tarsus so that it

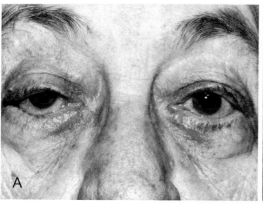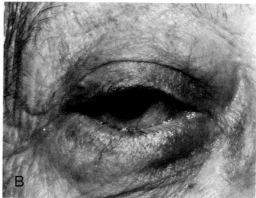

Figure 12.5. Entropion is an inturning of the lid. **A** illustrates lower lid inturning. **B**, The lashes can be seen next to the globe. Irritation and tissue damage from lashes rubbing on the cornea can be a serious complication. (Credit: Ted Wojno, M.D.)

overrides the tarsus, or change in position of the globe, moving posteriorly.

Cicatricial (Scar) Entropion

This may be seen with a number of conditions:

- Pemphigoid (autoimmune) (Fig. 12.6) (see page 335);
- Stevens-Johnson syndrome (see page 368);
- Infectious—trachoma (see page 374);
- Infectious—herpes zoster (see page 298);
- Thermal burns;
- Chemical burns (see page 139);
- Postsurgical.

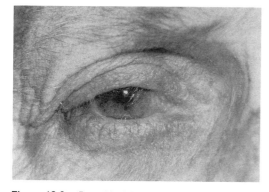

Figure 12.6. Pemphigoid with entropion. Conjunctival scarring caused by ocular pemphigoid can produce inturning of the eyelid, as illustrated (entropion). (Credit: Ted Wojno, M.D.)

BLEPHAROSPASM

Essential Blepharospasm

Essential blepharospasm is bilateral uncontrolled spasm of the eyelids. Although it may start on one side and be asymmetrical, it is a bilateral disease. The spasms can be strong and prolonged enough to make patients functionally blind even though visual potential is normal.

Essential blepharospasm starts in patients 50 years old and older. The spasms are made worse by stress and emotional tension, a feature that has caused the mistaken impression that there might be a psychiatric cause. Spasms disappear during sleep and anesthesia. Patients typically develop mechanisms to relieve the spasms. Touching the forehead, pressing the upper eyelid, or moving certain parts of the face seems to break the spasms early. Characteristically, there is no ocular abnormality. However, trigger mechanisms have been suggested, such as irritation from a staphylococcal chronic ocular infection or the presence of a foreign body. Most physicians think that the cause is in the central nervous system.

Meige's syndrome is a variant of essential blepharospasm. In Meige's syndrome, the muscles of the lower face are also involved with the orbicularis spasm of essential blepharospasm. Tongue, mouth, and jaw movements can be seen in Meige's syndrome.

Hemifacial Spasm

Hemifacial spasm involves one side of the face. The spasms tend to be shorter than those seen with essential blepharospasm. The spasms do not disappear with sleep.

The majority of patients with hemifacial spasm will have vascular compression of the seventh nerve at the brain stem. The spasms are not synchronous, a feature that helps differentiate them from early blepharospasm.

EPICANTHUS

Definition

The epicanthus is a fold of skin covering the medial junction of the upper and lower lids (Fig. 12.7). The epicanthus may originate from either above or below the canthal region.

Types

There are four types:

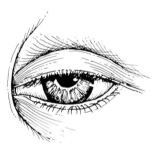

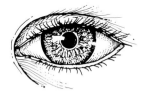

- Epicanthus supraciliaris arises from the eyebrow region and curves downward toward the tear sac.
- Epicanthus palbebralis arises from the upper lid above the tarsal region and extends to the lower margin of the orbit.
- Epicanthus tarsalis arises from the tarsal fold and bends in with the skin around the medial canthal area.
- Epicanthus inversus arises in the lower lid and extends upward in a crescent shape to cover the medial canthus.

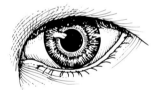

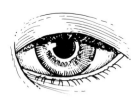

MALIGNANT EYELID LESIONS

Both basal cell carcinomas and squamous cell carcinomas involve the eyelid. They are common enough to require exclusion in a routine examination. Metastatic carcinoma (sebaceous gland carcinoma) may be mistaken for the benign lesion, chalazion. At times, the eyelid can be the initial site of presentation of more general disease. For example, in AIDS patients, Kaposi's sarcoma has been a presenting sign of the more general immune-deficient patient. Melanomas on the eyelid are rare (Fig. 12.8).

Figure 12.7. There are four types of epicanthus. Epicanthus is a skin fold over the inner portion of the eye and is classified according to position: *top to bottom,* epicanthus superciliaris; epicanthus palpebralis; epicanthus tarsalis; epicanthus inversus.

BASAL CELL CARCINOMA

Appearance (Fig. 12.9)

These are nodular lesions, often with central ulceration, and they may have a rolled margin, which is often described as "pearly."

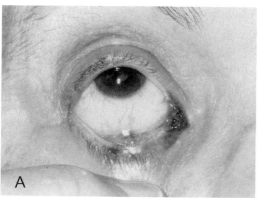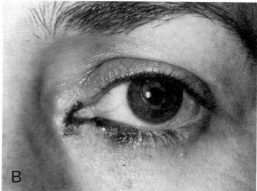

Figure 12.8. Malignant melanoma along the skin of the eyelid is uncommon. These are two examples of malignant melanoma in the lid. (Credit: Ted Wojno, M.D.)

They may be diffusely infiltrative. They may also be cystic and pigmented.

Characteristics

This is a slow-growing tumor. The eyelid is the most common site for basal cell carcinoma. Basal cell carcinoma accounts for 90% of all lid cancers and is 10 times more common than squamous cell carcinoma.

Basal cell carcinoma is related to ultraviolet exposure and damage. It occurs often in fair-skinned individuals with high sun exposure.

The lesion appears most frequently on the lower lid and the medial canthus. It involves the upper lid and lateral canthus less often.

SEBACEOUS CARCINOMA

This is the second most common eyelid malignancy (Fig. 12.10). It may be misdiagnosed because of confusion with chronic chalazion (see page 209) or chronic unilateral blepharoconjunctivitis. There is a greater frequency in women and orientals.

The onset is usually beyond middle age. Tumors arise from meibomian glands or from the glands of Zeiss. The upper eyelid is involved twice as often as the lower lid. Regional metastasis occurs in 25% of cases, and the overall fatality rate is 20%.

Because these are frequently misdiagnosed as recurrent chalazia, a high index of suspi-

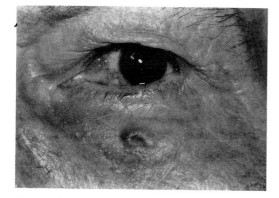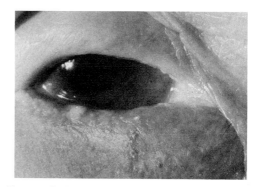

Figure 12.9. This basal cell carcinoma on the lower lid presents with a characteristic central excavation. The lesion itself has a reddish coloration. Notice the surrounding area of swelling, indicating subcutaneous extension.

Figure 12.10. Meibomian gland carcinoma (sebaceous cell carcinoma). This patient has an increase in size of the lower lid due to tumor infiltration. Note the loss of lashes. This is a meibomian gland carcinoma. The patient died from metastasis 6 months after this photograph.

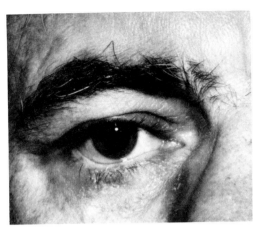

Figure 12.11. Squamous cell carcinoma is a common eyelid lesion. It is locally invasive. (Credit: Ted Wojno, M.D.)

cion is needed. Biopsy materials should be sent when a suspected recurrent chalazion is removed.

SQUAMOUS CELL CARCINOMA

Squamous cell carcinoma is a flesh-colored nodule. Squamous cell carcinoma on the eyelid has a very low probability of metastasis as opposed to such tumors in other sites. These tumors almost always arise from previous actinic keratoses. With enlargement, the tumor tends to form an ulcer in the center of the nodule. There is a flesh-colored border. In the center of the ulceration, a thick crust may form (Fig. 12.11). It may be confused with keratoacanthoma, which also forms a central crust.

METASTATIC CARCINOMA

Metastatic carcinoma of the eyelid is not common and represents less than 1% of eyelid tumors. Breast carcinoma is the most common primary site. Metastatic breast carcinoma appears as diffuse, painless, noninflammatory, full-thickness induration of the lid margin.

Metastatic malignant melanomas, metastatic squamous cell carcinomas from the lung, and adenocarcinomas of the gastrointestinal or genitourinary tracts metastasize to the eyelids primarily as inflamed, nontender subcutaneous nodules or as solitary ulcerated lesions.

KAPOSI'S SARCOMA

Kaposi's sarcoma may present as an isolated eyelid or conjunctival tumor. Kaposi's sarcoma is an angiosarcoma.

Skin lesions may be reddish or brown macules that may become nodular and take on a red to blue coloration. Lesions of the skin have been known to regress completely. When the conjunctiva is involved, it is usually the lid (palpebral) conjunctiva. Periocular involvement is rare. This tumor has a high association with acquired immune deficiency syndrome (AIDS) and may be the first presenting sign of this disease.

BENIGN EYELID LESIONS

There are a number of benign eyelid lesions that occur frequently on the skin of the lids and on the lid margins. Many of these lesions have different causes, and their natural courses vary tremendously. Some are premalignant. It is important to understand basic diagnostic futures to reassure patients and define the physician's diagnostic responsibilities.

Actinic Keratosis

These are lesions directly related to actinic or solar (ultraviolet) radiation damage (exposure) to epidermal cells. Characteristically, they occur in fair-skined and older people, especially those who have had prolonged sun exposure.

The lesions are usually multiple and affect not only the eyelids, but the face, forearm, hands, and bald scalp areas. They are often associated with elastosis, telangiectasias, epidermal atrophy, and lentigo.

The lesions are small, red (erythematous), or yellowish brown. They tend to be oval papules with a rough, adherent, scaly look. To touch, the lesions are gritty, rough spots.

Actinic keratosis, after prolonged periods, can evolve into invasive squamous cell carcinoma. (Actinic neoplasms have a low biologic activity, and less than 1% metastasize.)

Apocrine Hydrocystoma

Other Names

Cystadenoma, sudoriferous cyst, cyst of the gland of Moll

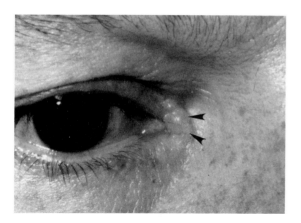

Figure 12.12. Cysts that originate in the glands of Moll are often close to the color of the skin. This cyst *(arrowheads)* is at the inner canthus. (Credit: Ted Wojno, M.D.)

Definition

This is a true adenoma of the secretory cells of the gland. It occurs as a single lesion, and it occurs during the fifth or sixth decade of life. It is a solitary, bluish, cystic lesion. It is usually only a few millimeters in diameter but may be larger. The lesion is compressible. It is characteristically translucent or semitransparent (Fig. 12.12).

Chalazion

Chalazion is a chronic inflammatory reaction in a meibomian gland. It appears as a round, red elevation under the conjunctiva of the lid, or, if more external in the lid, under the skin. Chalazia probably develop most often after an acute focal infection of the gland (sty or hordeolum). As they progress, chalazia can become secondarily infected, causing hyperemia, pain, and edema of surrounding tissues. Later, they resolve, usually completely, but they may leave a dense fibrous nodule (Figures 12.13 and 12.14).

Patients who have chronic recurrent chalazia have been treated with long-term, low-dosage oral tetracyclines. Why patients respond to this therapy is unknown.

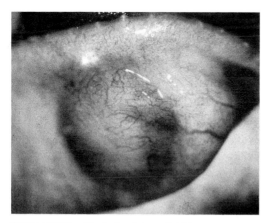

Figure 12.13. Chalazion (internal). This lid swelling is due to granulomatous inflammation starting in a meibomian gland within the tarsal plate. Here the eyelid is everted to show the conjunctival portion of the lid. This chalazion is classified as internal because most of the swelling is on the inside of the lid.

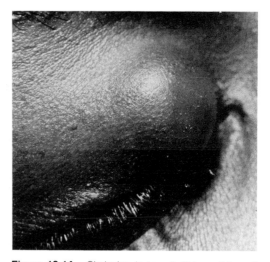

Figure 12.14. Chalazion (external). This eyelid swelling is due to a granulomatous inflammation of the meibomian gland within the tarsal plate. Here the swelling is nasal along the upper eyelid. The lashes can be seen below in this enlarged photograph. The chalazion is called external because the primary swelling is under the skin portion of the lid.

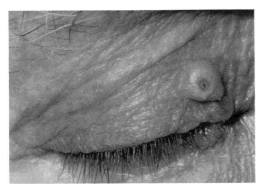

Figure 12.15. Inclusion cyst. (Credit: Ted Wojno, M.D.)

Danger

Recurrent inflammation in the lid is not always a chalazion. Meibomian gland carcinoma, a dangerous tumor that is difficult to manage, can mask as recurrent chalazion. It is wise to send all excised material thought to be a chalazion to the laboratory for pathologic confirmation. This is especially true if the inflammation is recurrent in the same position on the lid.

Infundibular Cyst

Other Names

Epidermal inclusion cyst, sebaceous cyst

Definition

This cyst arises from the infundibulum of the hair follicle. It produces normal keratin (not sebum).

Appearance

The lesion is slow-growing, round, fluxuant, and freely movable as a dermal subcutaneous mass. It is whitish (Fig. 12.15). Secondary infection and rupture of the cyst wall with an inflammatory reaction are frequent.

Keratoacanthoma

Appearance

This is a dome-shaped tumor with a central, keratin-filled crater that may be darkly pigmented. It grows rapidly.

Features

This is a common, benign, asymptomatic tumor that is self-healing. It is an epithelial neoplasm and important because it must be differentiated from squamous cell carcinoma. It is most often solitary.

Keratoacanthoma is most often seen on fair-skinned individuals, usually men, who have had prolonged exposure to sun. It is most common on the face, with the lids being involved in 6% of the cases. The growth is rapid, over a 3- to 6-week period, from a small, flesh-colored papule to a dome-shaped, brownish nodule with a central keratin-filled crater.

Molluscum Contagiosum

Ocular Features

These are small, solid, dome-shaped lesions with a central depression (Fig. 12.16).

Cause

Poxvirus, the largest filterable virus known to infect humans, causes molluscum contagiosum.

Characteristics

The eyelid is one of the most common sites. A tiny pimple enlarges to produce a dome-shaped, pink or ivory papule 1 to 5 mm in diameter. The individual molluscum has a cheesy central core, which is expressed with pressure. Lesions may persist for months or years. The lesion itself can cause a toxic fol-

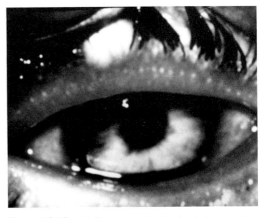

Figure 12.16. Molluscum contagiosum lesions on the eyelids. Their appearance can be variable. Diagnosis is important because expression of the lesions is usually curative. Molluscum may be associated with a conjunctivitis (follicular). (Credit: George Waring, M.D.)

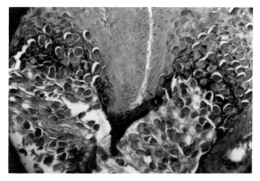

Figure 12.17. Molluscum contagiosum can be diagnosed on histologic features. Large numbers of eosinophilic inclusion bodies and hyperplastic epithelium that forms in lobules are seen. There is a fibrous capsule covered with a normal surface epithelium. (Credit: George Waring, M.D.)

licular conjunctivitis (page 18) and a superficial punctate keratitis (page 26). The histologic appearance is shown in Figure 12.17.

Differential Diagnosis

Warts, keratoacanthoma, sarcoid, trichoepithelioma, and basal cell carcinoma

Pyogenic Granuloma

This lesion is neither granulomatous nor pyogenic. It is composed of fibroblasts, capillaries, and lymphocytes. It is dark red and varies from 2 to 10 mm in size but may become larger (Fig. 12.18). Pyogenic granulomas tend to grow rapidly and may undergo spontaneous regression. Biopsy is often indicated because these lesions may simulate Kaposi's sarcoma.

Seborrheic Keratosis

These are extremely common and asymptomatic lesions. They are proliferations of normal epithelial cells that occur in middle aged to elderly people. They account for approximately 10% of eyelid lesions. They are unrelated to actinic damage.

Seborrheic keratoses tend to be flesh-colored to yellowish tan plaques with a greasy or waxy surface. They are well demarcated with an elevated border. They appear as if they were stuck on the facial skin. In the early stages, they measure 1 to 3 mm and are oval and flat. Later, they are larger and thicker and may be folded. There may be multiple keratin plugs that will give the surface a pitted appearance. Pigmentation from light to deep brown may be seen within the plaque.

Seborrheic keratoses may be confused with nevi, pigmented basal cell carcinomas, or malignant melanomas. These lesions are benign.

Sty (External Hordeolum)

This is a microabscess of the gland of Zeis or of an eyelash follicle. Sties are very tender and usually have a surrounding cellulitis.

Chronic recurrent sties should trigger a search for chronic staphylococcal infection or an underlying systemic illness such as diabetes. An internal hordeolum is an infected meibomian gland (Fig. 12.1).

Trichoepithelioma

Features

This is a dome-shaped papule. It is usually flesh-colored and tends to remain stable.

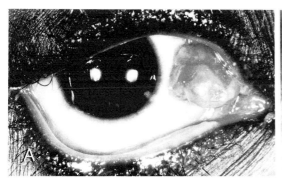
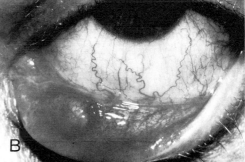

Figure 12.18. Conjunctival or pyogenic granuloma. Conjunctival granulomas appear as fleshy, hyperemic masses. Illustrated are two examples: **A**, near the inner canthus; **B**, on lower lid. (Credit: Ted Wojno, M.D.)

Characteristics

Trichoepithelioma usually appears as a solitary lesion. It is the result of aborted hair follicle formation. These papules consist of horn cyst formed by giant cells and foci of calcification. There are central cords of hypercellular stroma. Trichoepithelioma almost never ulcerates and has little tendency to grow.

Differential Diagnosis

Basal cell carcinoma, intradermal nevus, neurofibroma, sarcoid, adenoma sebaceum

No associated ocular findings are seen with trichoepitheliomas.

(Multiple trichoepitheliomas are present in an autosomal dominant syndrome (epithelioma adenocysticum of Brooke), which starts in the second decade of life. A few to hundreds of small papules or nodules are seen bilaterally and symmetrically. They are most prominent in the nasolabial fold, on the upper lip, on the side of the nose, and on the eyelids. They are also found on the trunk. These lesions are not aggressive and are asymptomatic, but they may cause significant cosmetic disfigurement. No associated ocular findings are found with this syndrome.)

Vitiligo

These are white patches on the skin. They appear as patchy, progressively enlarging areas of depigmentation. The condition may be associated with familial tendencies in 20 to 30% of cases.

Ocular Conditions Commonly Associated with Vitiligo

- Vogt-Koyanagi-Harada syndrome
- Sympathetic ophthalmia
  (Poliosis is also associated with these two ocular syndromes.)

There is a high association with autoimmune diseases and there are frequently circulating antibodies. The condition is thought to be a result of autoimmune activity against melanocytes. There are a number of other diseases associated with vitiligo:

- Alopecia areata
- Thyroid disorders
- Diabetes mellitus
- Pernicious anemia
- Addison's disease
- Candidiasis (mucocutaneous)
- Melanoma

Warts (Verrucae)

Warts are caused by DNA papilloma viruses. Warts on the eyelids may be flat or appear as papillomas (Figs. 12.19 and 12.20). Papilloma types tend to enlarge slowly, are irregular, and are hyperkeratotic. Warts are important in ophthalmology because they can cause secondary ocular irritation (conjunctivitis).

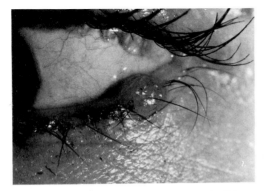

Figure 12.19. This is a verruca (wart) on the lid margin. This may be associated with a conjunctivitis. Removal of the lesion is curative. (Credit: Ted Wojno, M.D.)

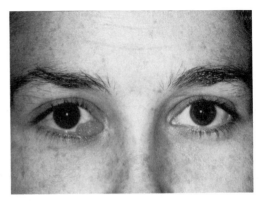

Figure 12.20. Papilloma of viral origin. (Credit: Ted Wojno, M.D.)

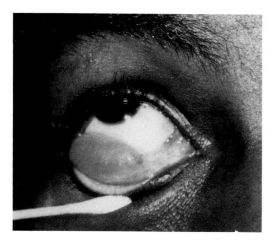

Figure 12.21. Conjunctival cysts are infrequently as large as this example. The cysts are fluid-filled and are easy to diagnose and treat. (Credit: Ted Wojno, M.D.)

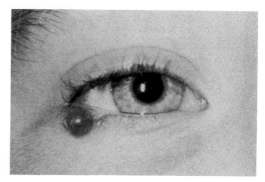

Figure 12.23. Hemangiomas are vascular tumors. This tumor is at the outer portion of the lower eyelid. In color, the tumor is red. (Credit: Ted Wojno, M.D.)

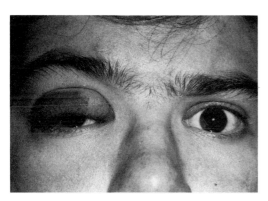

Figure 12.22. Capillary hemangioma. (Credit: Ted Wojno, M.D.)

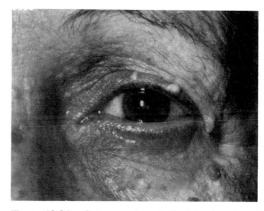

Figure 12.24. Cutaneous horn. In the lateral portion of the upper lid near the junction with the lower lid is an epithelial horn. Also, there are white inclusion cysts along the upper lid margin. (Credit: Ted Wojno, M.D.)

ADDITIONAL LESIONS OF THE EYELID WITH CHARACTERISTIC APPEARANCES

- Conjunctival cyst (Fig. 12.21)
- Hemangioma (Figs. 12.22 and 12.23)
- Cutaneous horn (Fig. 12.24)

GENERAL CONDITIONS THAT MAY INVOLVE THE EYELID

- Pemphigoid (see page 335)
- Erythema multiforme (see page 288)
- Sarcoidosis (see page 175)
- Amyloidosis
- Lupus erythematosus
- Scleroderma
- Neurofibromatosis (see page 168)
- Sturge-Weber syndrome (see page 169)
- Tuberous sclerosis (see page 170)
- Nevus of Ota (see page 328)
- Vitiligo
- Herpes simplex (see page 32)
- Herpes zoster (see page 298)
- Varicella
- Metastatic neuroblastoma

13

Orbit

ANATOMY AND PHYSIOLOGY (FIGS. 13.1 TO 13.4)

Walls of the Orbit

The orbital walls are composed of seven bones: ethmoid, frontal, lacrimal, maxillary, palatine, sphenoid, and zygomatic.

Orbital Fissures

Posteriorly, the superior orbital fissure is the opening between the greater and lesser wings of the sphenoid. The superior orbital fissure transmits the third, fourth, sixth, and first divisions of the fifth cranial nerve together with sympathetic nerve fibers. Most venous drainage from the orbit passes through this fissure by way of the superior ophthalmic vein to the cavernous sinus.

The inferior orbital fissure is surrounded by the sphenoid, maxillary, and palatine bones. It transmits the second (maxillary) division of the fifth cranial nerve, the zygomatic nerve, and branches of the inferior ophthalmic vein.

Optic Canal

The optic canal is 5 to 10 mm long and is located within the lesser wing of the sphenoid bone. The optic nerve, the ophthalmic artery, and sympathetic nerves pass through the canal. The orbital end of the optic canal is the *optic foramen,* which measures less than 6.4 mm in diameter in an adult. Enlargement of the optic foramen occurs with optic nerve gliomas. A diameter greater than 7 mm is abnormal. Also, a difference of more than 1 mm between right and left optic foramen is abnormal.

The volume of the orbit is 30 cc.

Soft Tissue in the Orbit

The optic nerve in the orbit is 25 mm long. It is surrounded by pia, arachnoid, and dural meninges.

The anulus of Zinn is a fibrous ring that is the common origin of the four rectus muscles. It is fused to the optic nerve dural sheath at the optic foramen.

Other soft tissue structures are:

- Extraocular muscles and nerves
- Extraocular vessels
- Orbital fat
- Lacrimal gland

COMMON DISEASES OF THE ORBIT

Inflammatory Orbital Pseudotumor

Definition

Inflammatory orbital pseudotumor is a nonspecific inflammatory lesion of the orbit

214

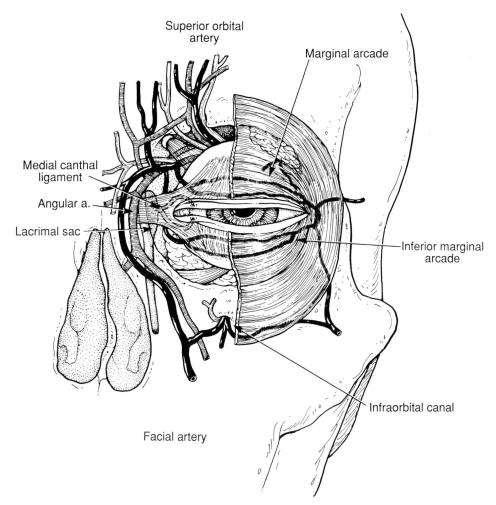

Superior orbital
artery

Marginal arcade

Medial canthal
ligament

Angular a.

Lacrimal sac

Inferior marginal
arcade

Infraorbital canal

Facial artery

Figure 13.1. Anatomy of the orbit: frontal view.

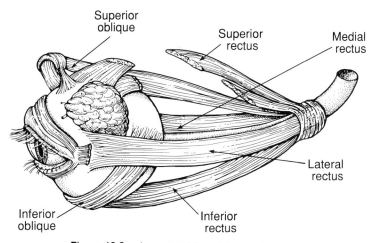

Superior
oblique

Superior
rectus

Medial
rectus

Lateral
rectus

Inferior
oblique

Inferior
rectus

Figure 13.2. Anatomy of the orbit: muscles.

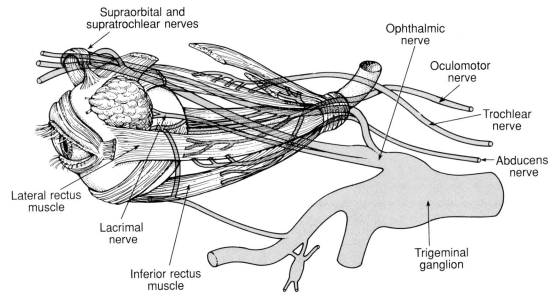

Figure 13.3. Anatomy of the orbit: nerves.

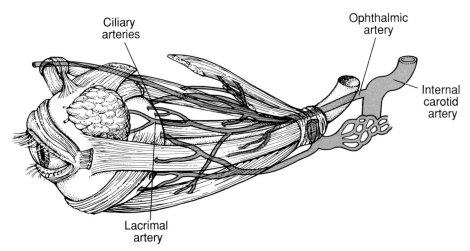

Figure 13.4. Anatomy of the orbit: vessels.

for which no identifiable local or systemic cause can be found.

Histopathology

There is a highly variable cellular infiltrate consisting of small, mature lymphocytes, plasma cells, histiocytes, eosinophils, and neutrophils all set in a hyalinized connective tissue stroma. Lesions are often richly vascularized. Endothelial cells are hypotrophic and large.

Anatomical Classification

- Diffuse
- Localized
  —Myositis
  —Periscleritis
  —Dacryoadenitis
  —Perineuritis

An Immunologic Base

Because of a loose association with various other immunologic disorders such as Crohn's disease, serum sickness, asthma, and upper respiratory infections, immunologic mechanisms are suspected. Cell marker analysis has helped to differentiate benign from malignant features. Polyclonal B cell proliferation represents benign histopathologic features. Monoclonal B cell proliferation represents histologic features of malignant lymphoma.

Clinical Presentation

Diffuse Form. In acute stages, this type of pseudotumor presents with the onset of pain and lid edema. There are varying degrees of chemosis, erythema, and proptosis as well as extraocular muscle dysfunction. It is unilateral in about 90% of cases. There is no sex or age predominance.

When the position of the diffuse pseudotumor is anterior in the orbit, it may be associated with uveitis, papillitis, or exudative retinal detachment. When posteriorly placed in the orbit, it may be associated with optic neuropathy. (Color vision, visual acuity, and visual fields are usually normal in cases of posterior diffuse orbital pseudotumor.)

The subacute or chronic form of diffuse pseudotumor leaves orbital dense collagenous tissue, which causes fibrosis in all orbital structures and eventually results in a fixed globe and visual loss.

Localized Forms.

Myositis. Pseudotumor may affect one or more muscles. It may cause diplopia and elimination of muscle action in certain fields. On computed tomographic (CT) scanning and ultrasound examination, there is enlargement of the muscle. Myositis may more frequently present bilaterally then other forms of pseudotumor. In pseudotumor, the tendon is involved in contrast to thyroid muscle involvement, where the tendon is spared.

Periscleritis. In the posterior portion of the globe affected by this pseudotumor, there is pain, blurred vision, and rare instances of uveitis. A T sign (increased density in posterior sclera and nerve regions, forming an inverted T) may be noted on ultrasound examination. Periscleritis may be clinically difficult to distinguish from posterior scleritis.

Dacryoadenitis. Pseudotumor involving the lacrimal gland presents with lacrimal gland tenderness, swelling of the outer lateral portion of the lid, and localized chemosis. It can be differentiated from lacrimal gland in-

volvement with viral infections, such as mumps or mononucleosis, because in pseudotumor there is a lack of adenopathy and lymphocytosis.

Perineuritis. This presents similar to the presentation of optic neuritis. It is unusual.

Differential Diagnosis of Orbital Pseudotumor

Conditions in Which the Bone or Sinuses Are Involved.

- Acute orbital cellulitis
- Vasculitis—Wegener's granulomatosis, periarteritis nodosa, midline granuloma
- Orbital malignancies
- Ruptured dermoid cyst
- Eosinophilic granuloma
- Fungal infection—aspergillosis and mucormycosis

Conditions in Which Bone and Sinus Involvement Usually Is Not Present.

- Dysthyroid ophthalmopathy (euthyroid Graves' disease)
- Lymphoma/leukemia
- Local causes of orbital inflammation including foreign body, ectopic lacrimal gland, and sclerosing hemangioma with orbital hemorrhage

Lymphangioma of the Orbit

The onset is usually within the first decade of life. The clinical presentations fall into four classifications:

- Visible on the lid or conjunctiva
- Causing variable proptosis but with no visible lesions
- Causing variable proptosis with varicosities that are visible
- Acute orbital hemorrhage

Histology

These tumors are large, serum-filled spaces that are lined by flattened endothelial cells. There are neither pericytes nor smooth muscle in the walls of these spaces. Scattered follicles of lymphoid tissues may be found in the interstitium between the serum-filled spaces. They tend to infiltrate with growth and do not encapsulate. Lymphangiomas do not involute as do capillary hemangiomas in children.

Chocolate Cysts

Hemorrhage into these lymph cavities can produce a cyst that appears the color of chocolate. These resolve spontaneously.

Characteristics

Frequently, proptosis gets worse under certain conditions such as position change, bending over, or upper respiratory infection with coughing or straining occurs. Lymphangiomas show on CT scans as thready material and may appear in grape-like clusters.

Many untreated lymphangiomas have no serious complications.

Osteoma

Osteomas are benign tumors. They are multilobulated and are found in the area of the frontal or ethmoidal sinuses.

Dural Shunts

Cause

Arterial blood flows through meningeal branches to enter the venous circulation near the cavernous sinus. (There is only one cavernous sinus so there is interconnection of infection and blood from one side to the other.)

Symptoms and Signs of Dural Shunts

- Torturous episcleral vessels
- Exophthalmus
- Increased ocular pressure
- Ptosis
- Pain and discomfort
- Bruit
- Retinal changes—specific

Diagnosis

CT scan and arteriography

Demography

Female to male ratio, 9:1. Most often seen in postmenopausal woman 50 to 69 years of age.

Course

Spontaneous improvement is common.

Arteriole Communications (A Panorama of Diseases)

Features

- Nonneoplastic
- Thickening and enlargement of adjacent bony structures (true of both benign and malignant vascular lesions)
- Soft tissue changes—the soft tissues themselves are enlarged, for example, the brow hair area may be enlarged over the enlarged brow bone.

Clinical Course

The clinical course may be progressive.

Meningioma

This tumor is locally destructive. It does not metastasize.

Meningiomas are slow-growing tumors with invasion of the orbit (secondary tumors) from intracranial sources, or they may arise primarily in the orbit.

Sphenoid Wing Meningioma

A classic sign is prominence of the temporal muscle. Most of these patients are women in their 30s to 50s.

Important Points about Orbital Meningiomas

Secondary Meningiomas.

- Exophthalmus
- Eyelid edema
- Visual disturbance, but visual loss only late
- Palpable mass, usually in sphenoid area

Primary Meningiomas.

- Visual defect, often early
- Pale, swollen disk
- Optociliary (cilioretinal) vessels

Graves' Ophthalmopathy

Other Names

Thyroid orbitopathy, Graves' disease, Graves' ophthalmopathy, infiltrative ophthalmopathy, congestive ophthalmopathy, thyroid eye disease, eye changes of Graves' disease, malignant exophthalmos, endocrine exophthalmos, dysthyroid ophthalmopathy

Description

Graves' disease is a multisystem disease of unknown cause. Three clinical entities that are pathognomonic: hyperthyroid associated with hypoplasia of the thyroid gland, infiltrated ophthalmopathy, and infiltrated dermopathy.

Graves' ophthalmopathy has the following clinical features: upper and lower eyelid retraction, proptosis (exophthalmus), limitation of ocular movements, eyelid congestion and edema, and epibulbar vascular enlargement.

Graves' ophthalmopathy may be associated with hyperthyroidism, hypothyroidism, or euthyroidism.

Diagnosis is assisted by ultrasonography, CT scanning that shows extraocular muscles that are enlarged with sparing of the tendons, T_3 and T_4 tests, and the thyrotropin-releasing hormone (TRH) test.

Clinical Findings

Woman are affected 8 times more commonly than men. The onset of the disease is usually between 20 and 45 years of age.

Characteristic Symptoms and Signs

- Unilateral or bilateral proptosis may be present. Graves' ophthalmopathy is the most common cause of unilateral and bilateral exophthalmus in adults.
- Retraction of the upper or lower eyelid may occur. This may result in scleral show and the appearance of a thyroid stare.
- Lid lag on downgaze (Fig. 8.5).
- Double vision (diplopia) is usually related to extraocular muscle involvement or proptosis.
- Eyelid edema.
- Conjunctival vascular congestion.
- Extraocular motility restriction (restrictive myopathy) is secondary to inflammation and edema of the muscles, which eventually results in fibrosis. The inferior rectus is the most common muscle involved. (The forced traction test, a test that mechanically

attempts movement of the globe, is positive when restriction of movement is observed.) The medial rectus is the muscle involved second most commonly.
- Visual acuity loss and pain are usually late occurrences in Graves' ophthalmopathy. Vision may decrease because of optic neuropathy from compression of the optic nerve.

Course

Graves' ophthalmopathy resolves spontaneously within a few months to years. Optic neuropathy is due to compression on the optic nerve at the orbital apex by swollen muscles (as suggested by CT scan).

Although not correlated with the ophthalmopathy, patients with thyrotoxicosis from Graves' disease have been found to have thymic pathology. Thymic medullary lymphoid nodules were found in their highest association with a thymic pathology other than myasthenia gravis.

Blow-out Fractures

Blow-out fracture is a fracture of the orbital wall. These fractures are indirect and are not associated with fractures of the inferior orbital rim. Blow-out fractures result from a compression force at the inferior rim of the orbit, which leads to buckling and fracture of the orbital floor. If increased orbital pressure is present at the time of the fracture, orbital tissues are pushed through the floor of the orbit into the maxillary sinus antrum. A trapping of the inferior rectus muscle may result.

Cause

Almost always, the cause is a direct blow to the orbit by a large object such as a ball, fist, or part of an automobile in an automobile accident. The object is almost always larger than the orbital diameter opening (the approximate entrance opening is 35 mm high and 40 mm wide).

Signs

- *Ecchymosis* and *edema* of the eyelids.
- *Double vision* (diplopia). Usually the double vision is vertical (that is, it

occurs on attempted upgaze or downgaze).

- *Limitation of motion* of the globe. As entrapment of the inferior rectus muscle in the orbital fracture is not uncommon, vertical movements upward may be restricted. Hemorrhage and damage to the extraocular muscles from direct trauma may also limit movement of the globe.
- *Enophthalmus.* The globe may be recessed (enophthalmus). This may be masked by orbital edema and hemorrhage after the injury. The enophthalmus may become more prominently observed as the acute edema and hemorrhage of the trauma subside.
- *Intraorbital nerve dysfunction.* Anesthesia inferior to the orbit in the region of distribution of the sensory intraorbital nerve may indicate orbital fracture.
- *Emphysema.* Emphysema of the orbit and eyelids is due to air escaping into the subcutaneous tissue. This is especially true when a medial wall fracture has occurred, with air escaping from the ethmoid sinus.

Wegener's Granulomatosis

Wegener's granulomatosis is a triad of necrotizing granulomas of the upper and lower respiratory tract, glomerulonephritis, and small vessel vasculitis. Signs appear in the upper respiratory tract in 98% of patients, whereas lung and kidney involvement are less common.

From the ophthalmologist's point of view, Wegener's granulomatosis may mimic other conditions. The eye signs are not common as a presenting sign of Wegener's, yet it occurs often enough to be considered frequently in the differential diagnosis of orbital swelling and uveitis. For example, the proptosis that occurs in Wegener's may be misinterpreted as Graves' ophthalmopathy or pseudotumor. The peripheral keratitis may be confused initially with the marginal keratitis of rheumatoid disease.

The diagnosis is more obvious when granulomas erode tissue surrounding the sinuses and the middle ear. In fact, the most common otologic manifestation is serous otitis media. In addition, nasopharyngeal ulcerations and saddle nose deformity from septal perforations are seen. As a guideline, any unusual sinusitis presenting with atypical eye signs should be considered as a possible presentation of Wegener's granulomatosis.

Some of the eye signs are a result of contiguous sinus involvement. The best way to establish the diagnosis is by CT scan. Bony erosion occurs, and it should be specifically sought.

Scleritis and keratitis can also occur. The scleritis can be painful and unresponsive to therapy. The keratitis is peripheral and is usually unilateral.

Consistent blood findings and a chest x-ray help establish the diagnosis. Test for anemia, leukocytosis, elevated sedimentation rate, and the presence of a mild hyperglobulinemia. On chest x-ray, look for one or more nodules without calcification and, as a rule, without associated mediastinal lymphadenopathy.

Mucocele

Mucocele of the sinus is a cystic structure that is lined with epithelium. The cyst enlarges and erodes the bony walls of the sinuses and frequently invades the orbit. Mucoceles are filled with a thick, mucoid secretion that may become infected and turn to pus (pyocele). Most mucoceles arise from the frontal and ethmoid sinuses.

Diagnosis is made by x-ray or CT scan in a patient with forward displacement of the eye. Bony erosion is a characteristic finding.

DIAGNOSTIC FEATURES OF ORBITAL DISEASE

Differential Diagnosis

Pain

Orbital lesions that are frequently painful:

- Idiopathic inflammatory pseudotumor;
- Orbital cellulitis;
- Orbital hemorrhage;

- Malignant lacrimal gland tumors;
- Nasopharyngeal carcinoma.

Orbital diseases that are usually not painful:

- Metastatic disease;
- Orbital abscess;
- Arteriovenous malformations.

Orbital diseases that are rarely painful:

- Thyroid eye disease;
- Pleomorphic adenoma of the lacrimal gland;
- Rhabdomyosarcoma;
- Basal cell carcinoma;
- Optic nerve tumor;
- Peripheral nerve tumor.

Progression of Signs and Symptoms

Progression characteristics are important in the differential diagnosis of orbital lesions.
Acute onset in days or weeks:

- Idiopathic inflammatory pseudo-tumor;
- Orbital cellulitis;
- Rhabdomyosarcoma;
- Neuroblastoma;
- Metastatic disease;
- Leukemia, especially granulocystic carcinoma.

Conditions with chronic gradual onset over a series of months to years:

- Dermoid cyst;
- Cavernous hemangioma;
- Pleomorphic adenoma of the lacrimal gland;
- Optic nerve tumor;
- Peripheral nerve tumor.

Conditions of the orbit that may have intermittent progression of symptoms and signs:

- Orbital varix;
- Orbital lymphangioma;
- Pseudotumor;
- Mucocele.

Proptosis

Proptosis is an additional sign of orbital disease. The character of the proptosis may help establish a diagnosis.
Axial Proptosis (Forward Displacement).

- Cavernous hemangioma
- Optic nerve tumor
- Arteriolovenous malformations
- Metastatic tumors to the posterior orbit
- Neurilemoma
- Rhabdomyosarcoma

Superior Displacement. This may occur with maxillary sinus tumors.
Inferior Displacement.

- Thyroid eye disease
- Capillary hemangioma
- Neurofibroma
- Lymphoma
- Idiopathic inflammatory pseudotumor

Palpation

Palpation of the orbit and of an orbital mass may assist in diagnosis.

- Superior nasal quadrant
  —Mucocele—fluctuant
  —Pyocele—tenderness of the frontal sinus
  —Dermoid—smooth, firm, and oval in children; may be tender in adults
  —Encephalocele—may be fluctuant and may transilluminate
  —Metastatic—tends to be very hard and is attached to underlying bone
  —Plexiform neuroma—may be palpated and feel like a series of firm worms
  —Neurofibroma—is firm to palpation and often extends medially and interiorly
  —Fibrous histiocytoma—may be cystic, especially when first encountered, but with recurrences may be firm to palpation
- Superior temporal quadrant
  —Pseudotumor
  —Lymphoma

—Lacrimal gland tumor
—Dermoid—usually anterior in children but may extend posteriorly in adults
- Inferior location
  —Pseudotumor (often painful on palpation—see above)
  —Lymphoma, which may be bilateral, tends to be nontender, will move with palpation, and will feel nodular)
- Rise in blood pressure over 200 mm Hg systolic palpation
  —Carcinoid
  —Pheochromocytoma

Pulsation

Pulsation may also occur with or without proptosis. It is an indefinite indication of certain conditions:

- Neurofibromatosis;
- Arteriovenous malformation;
- Choroid-cavernous sinus fistula;
- Dural fistula;
- Encephalocele;
- Surgical or traumatic removal of the orbital roof.

Special Diagnostic Features

There are also periorbital changes that can help establish the diagnosis.

- A salmon-colored mass in the subconjunctival area, especially in the superior cul de sac—think lymphoma.
- Entropion associated with a ptosis—think pseudotumor.
- If lid retraction and lid lag are present—think dysthyroid.
- If there is injection and increase in vascularization over the lateral rectus—think dysthyroid.
- If there is a pseudo-lid retraction caused by a mass in the superior fornix:
  —Contralateral ptosis;
  —Blow-out fracture.

- If corkscrew vessels in the conjunctiva are prominent—think arteriovenous fistula.
- With strawberry marks—think capillary hemangioma.
- With continuous vascular anomalies—think varix or lymphangioma.
- With an S-shaped lid, especially the upper lid—think plexiform neurofibroma of neurofibromatosis.
- If there is associated anterior uveitis with orbital involvement—think pseudotumor or sarcoid.

VASCULAR LESIONS OF THE ORBIT

- Anomalies
  —Arteriovenous communications
  —Malformations of the cavernous sinus
  —Inflammations
  —Wegener's granulomatosis
  —Polyarteritis
- Tumor vascularization
  —Neurofibroma, schwannomma
  —Metastatic (for example, renal carcinoma)
- Blood vessel tumors
  —Capillary hemangiomas
  —Lymphangiomas
  —Cavernous hemangioma of the orbit
  —Cavernous hemangioma of bone (predilection to the lateral portion of the orbit)
  —Hemangiopericytoma (usually benign but may be malignant)

Enlargement of Superior Ophthalmic Vein

Cause

Traumatic carotid-cavernous sinus fistula

Feature

Blood flow from the carotid artery into the cavernous sinus, with backflow into the venous system, causes increased size of the superior ophthalmic vein.

IMPORTANT POINTS ABOUT ORBITAL DISEASE

Dermoids

Dermoid cysts in a child are usually external but on occasion may be inside the orbit. Dermoid cysts are attached to periosteum of the underlying bone.

Dumbbell-shaped dermoid is an extension of dermoid outside the orbit from an interorbital position in which the dermoid goes under the temporalis muscle. On CT scanning, it appears as a dumbbell. Dumbbell-shaped dermoids may pulsate with chewing (use of the temporalis muscle causing dermoid mass to move).

Rhabdomyosarcoma

This is the most common orbital malignancy in children. Ninety percent are diagnosed by the age of 15.

Lymphoma

Lymphoma is the most common orbital malignancy in adults. Presentations include salmon-colored masses in the subconjunctival areas, an orbital soft tissue mass, and a rapidly growing subcutaneous mass.

Metastatic Tumors to the Orbit

In women, breast cancer is most common; in men, lung cancer is most common; in children, neuroblastoma is most common.

Eosinophilic Granuloma

Radiation is usually used to treat eosinophilic granulomas. Complete resolution has been seen on occasion.

Differential Diagnosis of Orbital Disorders in Adults

- Graves' ophthalmopathy
- Cavernous hemangioma, lymphangioma
- Lacrimal gland tumor
- Pseudotumor
- Lymphoma
- Meningioma
- Dermoid and epidermoid cyst

14

Special Considerations
in Children

Congenital Ptosis	Orbital Disorders of Children
Congenital Nystagmus	Ophthalmia Neonatorum
Primary Congenital Glaucoma	

Many ocular abnormalities that appear in adults also appear in children. In this section, only those diseases or conditions that have major importance in the pediatric age group are included.

CONGENITAL PTOSIS

Ptosis is a droop of the upper lid. A poorly developed levator muscle is the most common cause of congenital ptosis.

Diagnosis

It may be difficult to determine the degree of ptosis in infants. The usual technique of measurement in an adult is to hold up a millimeter ruler and measure the distance between the inferior and superior lids at different gaze positions (primary, down, up). This is frequently not possible in infants.

An acceptable way to measure ptosis in infants is to remember that the normal lid position is 3.5 mm above the visual axis in the center of the pupil. The limbus is 5.5 mm above the visual axis. While the infant fixates, an estimation of the degree of ptosis can be determined by remembering these anatomical landmarks.

In infants with congenital ptosis, the presence of amblyopia (page 000) must be determined. There is a danger of amblyopia in in-

fants with ptosis; however, it is unusual, if not rare. When it develops, it may be preventable by early surgery.

Important Observations for Amblyopia

Retraction of the Normal Lid in Unilateral Ptosis

Remembering Herring's law (page 300), lid retraction of the normal eye compared to the eye with congenital ptosis means that the infant is trying to open the eye with ptosis. Excess nerve stimulus is directed to the abnormal lid to attempt opening. Excess stimulus goes also to the normal lid, resulting in a retraction. If the infant is trying to open the eye, amblyopia (decreased vision) is not a problem because a visual stimulus is perceived.

Arched Brow

If there is evidence of brow arch, it means that the accessory muscles normally not used in lid opening are now employed to elevate the eyelid. Arching of the brow is an indication that vision is present and that amblyopia is not a potential problem.

Conditions Associated with Congenital Ptosis That Do Not Do Well Surgically

Third Nerve Palsies and Ptosis

These patients frequently do not do well because of a lack of Bell's phenomenon (page

260), which causes drying and complications to the globe.

Blepharophimosis

The blepharophimosis syndrome, which presents with telecanthus, epicanthus inversus, and severe ptosis, frequently does not respond well to surgical correction.

Marcus Gunn Phenomenon

In the Marcus Gunn phenomenon, which is due to aberrant regeneration of the third nerve with misdirection of third nerve fibers, ptosis is associated with jaw movements. Marcus Gunn patients get well spontaneously. (See Acquired Ptosis, page 202.)

CONGENITAL NYSTAGMUS

Nystagmus (page 112) is a rhythmic oscillation of the eyes. Congenital nystagmus is any nystagmus that occurs shortly after birth or during early childhood.

Characteristics

Congenital nystagmus tends to be almost always horizontal. It can be of many types: pendular, jerk, or latent. Patients are almost never aware of any motion of the image (oscillopsia), in contrast to acquired nystagmus.

Pendular Nystagmus, Congenital

In this type of nystagmus, the eyes oscillate slowly in almost equal rhythm to both sides, as would be seen in the movement of the pendulum of a grandfather's clock. This pendular motion is most often due to loss of vision. The character of the nystagmus changes frequently, for example, when gaze is directed from far to near (convergence). When trying to decrease the effect on vision of this pendular movement of the eyes, head movements (head nodding) may be present.

Jerk Nystagmus, Congenital

This type of congenital nystagmus refers to movements of nystagmus that vary with the oscillations. The motion is fast when the eyes look out (lateral gaze) and slow as the eyes come inward. With positioning of the head, the degree of the oscillations may decrease. The patient may turn the head to find this point of relative decrease in oscillation intensity, which is known as the null point.

Latent Nystagmus, Congenital

When both eyes are fixating on a target, there is no nystagmus. However, when one eye is covered, nystagmus occurs. This is a jerk type of nystagmus where the fast component beats away from the covered eye. For example, if the right eye is covered, the fast component jerks rapidly to the left and returns slowly to the right.

Patients with latent nystagmus often have better visual acuity when they are using both eyes. With one eye covered, visual acuity in the other eye may be decreased.

Sensory Deprivation Nystagmus

Congenital blindness or any other severe loss of vision can result in random wandering of the eye in movements that are slow and widespread. This type of sensory deprivation nystagmus never develops if blindness occurs after the age of 6. It always develops if blindness occurs before the age of 2. The development is variable between the ages of 2 and 6.

Spasm Nutans

Characteristics

This nystagmus, which tends to be fine and very rapid so that the eye appears to be shimmering, occurs during the 1st year of life (between 2 and 12 months). This is frequently associated with a nonpurposeful head nodding, uncorrelated with the nystagmus. The nystagmus is most often monocular. In one-third of patients, there is an abnormal position of the head (head turning or torticollis).

Diagnosis

Spasm nutans has a major triad of diagnostic features: head nodding (approximately 90%), ocular nystagmus (approximately 80%), and torticollis or head turning (approximately 40%).

PRIMARY CONGENITAL GLAUCOMA

Other Names

Primary congenital glaucoma, primary congenital open angle glaucoma, primary infantile glaucoma (juvenile glaucoma is used in glaucoma diagnosed after 3 years of age)

Onset

Primary congenital glaucoma is usually diagnosed at birth or soon after. It represents 70% of the congenital glaucomas.

Clinical Features

There are three classic manifestations that should point to the diagnosis of primary congenital glaucoma in the infant:

- Epiphoria (excessive tearing);
- Photophobia (hypersensitivity to light) due to corneal edema;
- Blepharospasm (tight squeezing of the eyelids).

Ocular Signs

Increasing Corneal Diameter

The normal cornea at birth is less than 10.5 mm in diameter. Because of increased pressure in the globe due to glaucoma, expansion of the globe (buphthalmus) occurs. The diameter of the globe is over 12 mm.

Corneal Edema

This presents as a corneal haze. It is secondary to the rise in intraocular pressure and usually clears when pressure is normalized. In prolonged, advanced cases, the opacification may persist.

Intraocular Pressure

The normal infantile intraocular pressure under anesthesia is 9 to 10 mm Hg and in the unanesthetized newborn is 11 to 12 mm Hg. Any pressure greater than 20 mm Hg is suspicious of congenital glaucoma.

Tears in Descemet's Membrane (Haab's Striae)

These may be multiple and typically are oriented to the horizontal plane. They are associated with corneal edema.

Gonioscopy Findings

The anterior chamber is characteristically deep. In the angle, there is a high insertion of the iris root, which forms a scalloped line. Abnormal tissue can be seen in the angle. A glistening appearance may be seen, or a fine fluffy tissue may be present. The angle is usually avascular; however, loops of vessels from the major arteriole circle can be seen above the iris root.

Ophthalmoscopy

As in adults, there is preferential loss of the neural tissue in the vertical poles of the optic disc. Cupping of the optic nerve proceeds rapidly in infants, even more so than in adults. Tissue loss may be reversed if the pressure is lowered promptly.

Differential Diagnostic Signs of Congenital Glaucoma

Differential Diagnosis of Large Cornea

- Primary congenital glaucoma
- Congenital megalocornea without glaucoma
- Enlarged globe with high myopia

Tears in Descemet's Membrane

- Primary congenital glaucoma
- Birth trauma (usually oblique or vertical)
- Band-like structures in posterior polymorphous dystrophy

Corneal Opacification in Infancy

- Primary congenital glaucoma
- Development anomalies
  —Peters' anomaly
  —Sclerocornea
- Dystrophies
  —Congenital hereditary corneal dystrophy
  —Posterior polymorphous dystrophy
- Choristomas
  —Dermoid
  —Dermis-like choristoma
- Metabolic errors
  —Mucopolysaccharidoses
  —Cystinosis

- Inflammation
  —Congenital syphilis
  —Rubella
  —Edema due to birth trauma

Associated Diseases

Congenital glaucoma is present at birth or during the neonatal period. It can be associated with various diseases:

- Rieger's syndrome
- Peters' anomaly
- Aniridia
- Sturge-Weber syndrome
- Lowe's syndrome
- Marfan's disease
- Neurofibromatosis
- Rubella syndrome

ORBITAL DISORDERS OF CHILDREN

General Classification

- Congenital and developmental
- Infections
- Inflammations
- Tumors
  —Primary
  —Secondary
  —Metastatic

Congenital and Developmental Abnormalities

Anophthalmus

Anophthalmus (lack of development of the globe) is usually unilateral. There is almost always some vestigial remnant of the globe, which closely relates to microphthalmos. In anophthalmus, care by an experienced ophthalmic plastic surgeon is necessary because of soft tissue contraction as well as distortions of the bones of the orbit. The lack of a globe or the lack of a normal size globe affects the normal development of orbital soft and bony structures. An early approach to this problem by appropriate therapies allows better cosmetic possibilities.

Craniofacial Syndromes

Cleft Syndromes. These are failure of a suture closure (see Tessier's Classification, page 372).

Cranial Stenosis Syndromes. These are early closure of suture lines. These include such diseases as Crouzon's disease.

Infections—Orbital Cellulitis

Orbital cellulitis presents as fever, malaise, and increased white blood cell count. This is an acute, active infection that is usually secondary to sinusitis. The ethmoid is most frequently involved. The most frequent organisms are:

- *Influenzavirus;*
- *Staphylococcus aureus;*
- *Streptococcus.*

Diagnosis is especially important because cavernous sinus thrombosis and meningitis can result from orbital cellulitis. The differential diagnosis includes preseptal cellulitis, which is limited to inflammation in front of the orbital septum.

Inflammations

Pseudotumor

Pseudotumor in children is acute and presents with pain. Computed tomographic (CT) scanning is effective for diagnosis. Pseudotumor may involve the lacrimal gland, may involve muscles of the eye, may cause an optic neuritis, or may be diffused throughout the orbit. Histological examination shows an infiltrate composed of lymphocytes and plasma cells.

Myositis

Inflammation of the muscles occurs and responds to steroid therapy.

Tumors of the Orbit

Cystic Tumors of the Orbit—Dermoid Cyst

Dermoid cysts are usually external to the orbit in children. In adults, dermoid cysts tend to be found inside the orbit. Dermoid cyst tumors in children tend to be superotemporal along the brow.

Lipodermoid

This is usually temporal and presents as a yellowish mass in the subconjunctival region. These frequently extend posteriorly.

Vascular Tumors of the Orbit in Children

Capillary Hemangioma. Capillary hemangiomas are found primarily in children. Cavernous hemangiomas are found primarily in adults.

Capillary hemangiomas occur just after birth and during the first few weeks of life tend to increase in size. They are often associated with strawberry nevi elsewhere on the body. These tumors will involute by 4 or 5 years of age.

Lymphangiomas. To assist in diagnosis, examine the hard pallet of the child, where lymphangiomas may occur and may be coexistant with orbital lymphangiomas. With lymphangiomas of the orbit, hemorrhage is a frequent problem. Patients may present with acute forward displacement of the globe (proptosis) secondary to massive hemorrhage in the orbit.

Neural Lesions Presenting as Tumors of the Orbit in Children

Gliomas. Gliomas present with axial proptosis (page 259). Symptoms frequently appear during the first decade of life. Crossed eyes (strabismus) may be associated. There may be an afferent pupillary defect, an optic nerve atrophy, or papilledema. Of these patients, 25% will have signs and symptoms of neurofibromatosis (page 168). CT scan is usually diagnostic with a diffuse pattern.

In glioma (polycystic astrocytoma), Rosenthal fibers (degenerative fibers) are characteristic. Cystic degeneration can occur.

The course of gliomas is variable. Many gliomas do not progress. If there is good vision, the child can be followed for years. However, one must observe carefully and exclude extension into the chiasm, which may require aggressive management. Intracranial extension with increased intracranial pressure does occur.

Neurofibromatosis. An S curve of the upper lid is characteristic of neurofibromatosis. Palpation of the lid demonstrates a wormlike mass in the eyelid.

The pathology of neurofibromatosis is proliferation of Schwann cells. Overgrowth of fibroblasts occurs. Café au lait spots and axillary freckles occur. Fibrosa molluscum may also be present on the skin.

An important clinical finding is pulsation exophthalmus. When dysplasia of the orbital wall results, connection to the intracranial space with temporal lobe herniation occurs, and pulsation of the globe (pulsation exophthalmus) is caused by pressure transmitted from the cranium to the orbit.

Pulsation exophthalmus also occurs with arteriovenous malformations. Bruits are present. In pulsation exophthalmus with neurofibromatosis, no bruits are present.

Neurofibromatosis is autosomal dominant with irregular penetrance. Iris nevi can often help establish the diagnosis.

Muscular Tumor That Is Orbital in Children—Rhabdomyosarcoma

This is the most common primary malignant orbital tumor in children. There are four major types of rhabdomyosarcoma:

- Embryonal;
- Alveolar;
- Botryoid;
- Pleomorphic.

Embryonal and alveolar types tend to occur in younger individuals. Botryoid and pleomorphic types tend to occur in older individuals.

The embryonal type is most often seen in children. It has a predilection for the superior orbit and is associated with bony destruction.

Emergency. Diagnosis of rhabdomyosarcoma is an emergency because of rapid progression, bony destruction, and extension.

Histology. Myoblasts and cross-striations are seen.

Osseous Lesions in the Orbits of Children—Fibrous Dysplasia

This slowly progressive disease process is caused by new bone formation with fibrous tissue in the marrow. Surgical removal is indicated.

Secondary Orbital Tumors in Children— Retinoblastoma

Retinoblastoma can extend from the globe into the orbit. Retinoblastoma is the most common secondary orbital tumor in children. Flexner-Wintersteiner rosettes are characteristic findings in the orbit. The retinoblastoma may extend through the optic nerve or may migrate through the long posterior ciliary nerves. These extensions should be looked for when a globe is removed for retinoblastoma.

Calcium in the tumor assists in making the diagnosis. CT scanning and x-ray films will show calcium; however, magnetic resonance imaging (MRI) scans will not show calcium because of the nature of the scan.

Metastatic Tumors to the Orbit in Children

Neuroblastoma. Neuroblastoma is the most common metastatic tumor to the orbit in children, but it is rare. Of these metastases, 50% are from the adrenal medulla. Hemorrhages in the orbit are a frequent occurrence with neuroblastoma. There is inflammation from necrosis because the tumor outgrows its blood supply.

Leukemia. Leukemic infiltration of the orbit is seen in children.

Dermoid

Dermoid cysts are choristomas (containing both epidermis and skin appendages). Although usually present at birth, they may not become evident until childhood. Characteristically, they are deep in the lateral aspect of the upper eyelid between the frontal and zygomatic sutures.

Dermoid cysts tend to be moderately firm, 2- to 5-cm masses beneath the skin. They are freely mobile in most cases but at times may be adherent to adjacent periosteum. They are not tender.

OPHTHALMIA NEONATORUM

Definition

Ophthalmia neonatorum is inflammation of the conjunctiva (conjunctivitis) during the

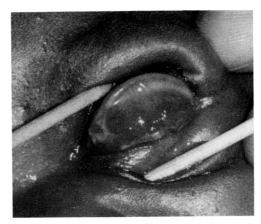

Figure 14.1. Ophthalmia neonatorum is an infection in the neonate. These conjunctival infections may have multiple etiologies, and some can cause severe visual loss. Prompt diagnosis is essential. Illustrated is a child with ophthalmia neonatorum due to inclusion conjunctivitis.

1st month of life (Fig. 14.1). This inflammation can be due to numerous organisms. It has important clinical implications because some organisms can progress with rapid tissue destruction and permanent visual loss. The major considerations for ophthalmia neonatorum are chemical, chlamydial, gonococcal, bacterial, and viral (herpes simplex).

Chemical

Silver nitrate 1% solution has been used as a prophylaxis against ophthalmia neonatorum. It has helped to decrease the incidence of *Neisseria gonorrhoea*. In many states, it is required to be instilled in all newborns. Although effective against gonococcus, it is not effective against chlamydia or viral diseases.

Silver nitrate itself may cause a chemical conjunctivitis. Typically, the conjunctivitis begins a few hours after the delivery and the instillation of drops. Chemical conjunctivitis lasts no longer than 24 to 36 hours. Chemical conjunctivitis occurs in a high percentage of newborns (in some studies, as high as 90%). There is usually no difficulty in differentiating chemical conjunctivitis from more severe causes of ophthalmia neonatorum. Although chemical conjunctivitis is the most common cause of ophthalmia neonatorum, it does not have serious sequelae.

Chlamydial

Other Names

Chlamydia trachomatis or *Chlamydia ocu-logenitalis,* inclusion conjunctivitis, inclusion blennorrhea

Onset

The classic onset of chlamydia conjunctivitis is thought to occur at 5 to 14 days. However, it is now known that chlamydia may occur as early as 24 hours and as late as 3 to 4 weeks after delivery.

Symptoms

There is a mild unilateral or bilateral mucopurulent conjunctivitis. Lid edema, chemosis, and conjuctival injection occur. Follicles are absent because the infant does not develop a follicular response until after 4 months of age. Membranes or pseudomembranes (Fig. 2.16) may occur. Occasionally, corneal opacification can result.

Systemic Complications

Chlamydia can cause a unique neumonitis with eosinophilia. Of infants who have chlamydia pneumonitis, over one-half will have conjunctivitis within the 1st month. Systemic involvement may include otitis media, rhinitis, anorectal infection, and vaginitis.

Diagnosis

Diagnosis is established by conjunctival scrapings. Basophilic intracytoplasmic inclusions are found in conjunctival epithelial cells along with polymorphonuclear leukocytes, lymphocytes, and, at times, Leber cells. The inclusion bodies are known as Halberstaedter-Prowazek.

Gonococcal (*Neisseria gonorrhoea*)

Onset

Classic teaching indicates an early onset between 2 and 4 days. There is a hyperacute conjunctivitis with purulent exudate. Chemosis and injection of the conjunctiva are present. Membranes and pseudomembranes occur. Corneal ulceration and perforation may occur if not appropriately treated.

Systemic involvement of the infant is also common. The central nervous system involvement is especially important to rule out, and a spinal tap is often indicated.

Diagnosis

Diagnosis is initially suggested by Gram stain. Gram-negative diplococci are seen in polymorphonuclear leukocytes. Cultures are important. Thayer-Martin media is best, and chocolate agar is a second choice.

Bacterial

Onset

Bacterial conjunctivitis, other than gonococcal, occurs 1 to 30 days after delivery. There may be predisposing factors. Local trauma to the conjunctiva or cornea with loss of the protective epithelial barrier has an important role in the establishment of bacterial ophthalmia neonatorum. Obstruction of the nasal lacrimal duct may inhibit effective drainage. The onset is usually by the 5th day.

Signs and Symptoms

Lid edema, chemosis, conjunctival injection, and discharge are common signs. Systemic symptoms should be sought because septicemia may occur, especially with *Pseudomonas.*

Causes

Causes of bacterial conjunctivitis are:

- *Staphylococcus aureus*
- *Streptococcus pneumoniae*
- *Haemophilus*
- *Pseudomonas aeruginosa*
- *Escherichia coli*
- *Proteus*
- *Klebsiella pneumoniae*
- *Enterobacter*
- *Serratia marscens*

Diagnosis

Conjunctival scrapings with Gram's stain should be sought to determine the presence of organisms. Blood agar and chocolate agar are used for culture.

Viral

Herpes simplex type I or II, although type II is the most common (genital type), can cause ophthalmia neonatorum.

Onset

The onset is usually within the first 2 weeks of life. The conjunctivitis begins as lid edema, conjunctival injection, mucoid discharge, and chemosis.

Viremia occurs because this is a primary infection. Skin changes, central nervous system involvement, and chorioretinitis are common. The viremia can be fatal.

Conjunctival scraping shows a bacteria, and there is a lack of significant polymorphonuclear leukocytes or lymphocytes. Occasional multinucleated giant cells or eosinophilic intranuclear epithelial inclusions are seen. Viral cultures are useful.

Diagnostic Essentials

Because of the importance of these infections in a newborn, it is essential to do an adequate workup.

1. Detailed Maternal History. Careful history for previous venereal disease or exposure, cervical cultures during pregnancy, or the presence of cervicitis should be sought.

2. History of Delivery. A long, difficult delivery, rupture of membranes before delivery, or trauma to the conjunctival corneal epithelium should be sought.

3. Conjunctival Scrapings. Scrapings should be taken from the conjunctiva, being sure of obtaining cellular material. Gram stain and Giemsa stain should be used to fix the slides.

4. Cultures. Cultures are mandatory. Blood agar, chocolate agar, and Thayer-Martin medium are suggested. Viral and chlamydial cultures should also be done if possible. On bacterial cultures, sensitivities should be requested because resistant organisms, especially in gonococcus, may be present.

15

Refraction

Lens Power	Myopia
Emmetropia	Hyperopia
Ametropia	Astigmatism

LENS POWER

A diopter is a unit of measure of the power of the lens to alter the direction of light rays. It is related to the focal length of the lens. The focal length is the distance from the center of the lens to the point at which parallel rays are refracted (Fig. 15.1).

D = diopter
F = the focal length of the lens in meters
$D = 1/F$

One diopter would have a 1-meter focal distance. A 4-diopter lens would have a 0.25-meter focal distance. A 10-diopter lens would have a 0.1-meter (10-cm) focal distance.

Note the difference between positive lenses and negative lenses. Positive lenses converge parallel rays, and negative lenses diverse parallel rays. With convergent lenses, we speak of plus dioptric power or plus lenses; with divergent lenses, we speak of minus dioptric power or minus lenses.

EMMETROPIA (Fig. 15.2)

An emmetropic eye focuses parallel rays of light directly on the fovea without accommodation. In essence, the refractive power of the lens and cornea correlate exactly with the length of the globe. No glasses are needed for distant vision.

AMETROPIA

In ametropia, there is a refractive error in that the cornea and lens fail to focus the image on the retina. Ametropia includes hyperopia, where the image falls behind the retina, or myopia, where the image falls in front of the retina. Astigmatism, where the image is

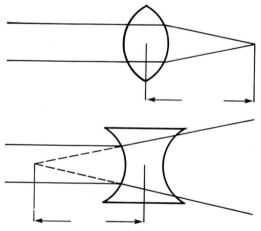

Figure 15.1. A diopter is a measure of lens power. One diopter will focus parallel light rays at a point 1 meter from the lens. There are plus diopters or minus diopters. *Top,* The convex lens converges rays at a distance of 1 meter. Convergent lenses are plus diopters. *Bottom,* A concave lens diverges rays. To determine the point at which parallel rays meet in a divergent lens, imaginary lines project backward to a point in front of the lens. Divergent lines have minus or negative diopters.

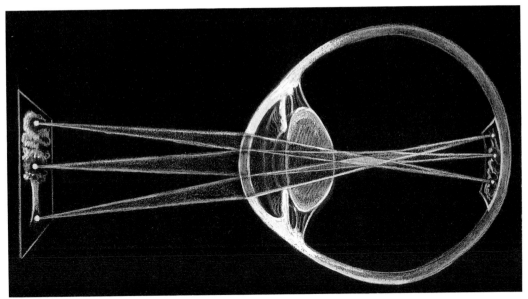

Figure 15.2. Emmetropia is when the light rays from the object are focused on the retina. An object is multiple point light sources that are then focused as multiple light points on the retina as the image. In contrast to emmetropia, ametropia is when the focus is not directly on the retina. In myopia, the multiple point foci are focused in front of the retina and, in hyperopia, the foci are focused behind the retina.

focused in two different planes either in front or behind the retina, is also ametropia.

Myopia

Myopia (Nearsightedness) Types (Figs. 15.3 and 15.4)

Myopia, that condition where the cornea and lens of the eye focus the image in front of the retina, is clinically divided into three types.

Physiologic Myopia. This is the most common myopia and refers to failure of the refractive power to match the length of the globe.

Pathologic Myopia. Pathologic myopia is a term applied to any myopia that causes degenerative changes in the eye. The eye enlarges excessively in all dimensions, especially anteroposteriorly. When the anterior-posterior length of the globe is increased, the myopia is also known as *axial myopia.*

Pathologic myopia is usually associated with more than 6 diopters (see page 232) of myopia. The pathologic myopia tends to increase rapidly during adolescence, when it may also be referred to as progressive or *malignant myopia.*

Ophthalmoscopic Findings in Pathologic Myopia. A myopic crescent appears as a white area (sclera) just adjacent to the temporal side of the optic disc (Fig. 15.5). The optic disc may also be abnormal in shape and color. There is frequently decreased pigmentation of the retinal pigment layer so that the choroidal veins are very distinctly seen in a rather striking pattern (tigroid). The choroid may also be atrophic, and stark white sclera may show through. At times, there is proliferation and migration of the retinal pigment, causing clumps of pigment in the atropic retinal pigment epithelium.

Pigment proliferation in the area of the fovea centralis (Fuchs' spot) occurs between the ages of 30 and 50 years and reduces visual acuity significantly. The fovea centralis may become atrophic, and central vision may be lost.

The vitreous may be more fluid than would be expected in a normal eye. Myopic degeneration of the peripheral retina may lead to retinal holes and retinal detachment.

Comment. There is no scientific evidence to indicate that anything alters the progression of pathologic myopia to its predestined

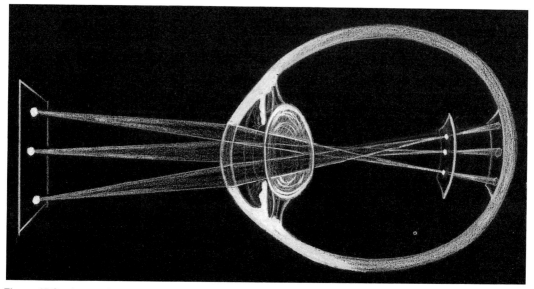

Figure 15.3. In myopia, the multiple point light sources from the object are focused in front of the retina.

end, although the use of glasses, contact lenses, and drops (such as atropine) have all been suggested to change pathologic myopia. Definitive treatment for pathologic myopia is not available.

Lenticular Myopia. In elderly patients who have nuclear sclerotic cataracts, the lens becomes hard and dense, especially in the nuclear portion. This increase in density may produce a myopia. Although such patients still cannot see well at a distance, they suddenly find that they are able to read at close range. This is the "second sight" of progressive cataract. This second sight is limited and

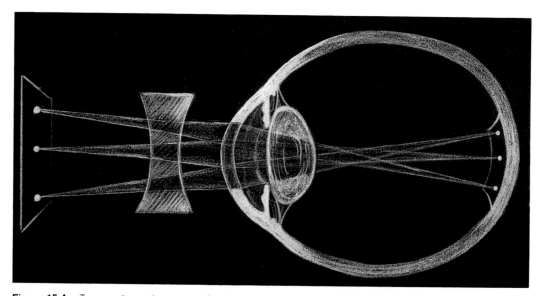

Figure 15.4. To correct myopia, a convex lens is used to move the multiple point light sources back on the retina.

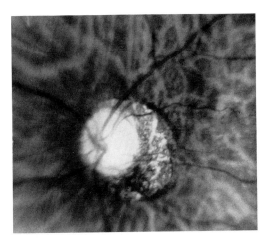

Figure 15.5. Myopic degeneration. The prominent choroidal vessels and the characteristic changes around the disc, sometimes described as a myopic crescent, are typical of high myopia. In the crescent area, there is some increased pigment around the disc. (See color Fig. C.26.)

it may last only a few months before the cataract progresses and vision decreases. Myopia is corrected by the use of a convex lens (or minus lens) that diverges light rays and moves the abnormal focal point back to the retina.

Hyperopia

Hyperopia is a refractive error in which parallel rays of light come to focus behind the retina (Fig. 15.6). Hyperopia can be corrected, to some degree, by adjustment of the natural lens within the eye (accommodation). Normally, accommodation is used for near focusing. In hyperopia, accommodation is used for distant vision and excessive accommodation is needed for near vision. This use of accommodation in hyperopia can cause visual fatigue, discomfort, and headache—symptoms called asthenopia. Hyperopia is corrected by lenses that converge parallel rays of light—called convex or plus lenses—and therefore move the image from behind the retina onto the retina (Fig. 15.7).

Astigmatism

Image Review

An object can be thought of as an infinite number of small points. Each point of the object represents a source of divergent light rays. These light rays are focused by the eye on the retina. The focus of all of the object points forms the image. This assumes that there is no irregularity in the refractive system of the eye.

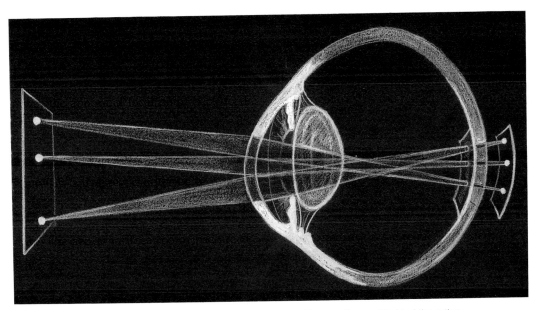

Figure 15.6. In hyperopia, the multiple point sources from an object are focused behind the retina.

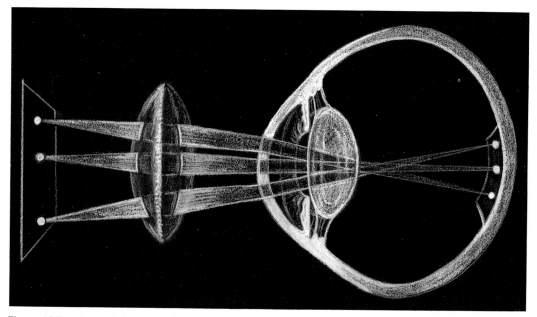

Figure 15.7. Hyperopia is corrected by the use of a convex lens. This lens brings the multiple foci onto the retina.

In a nonastigmatic lens, all points of light from the object are focused on one plane. An astigmatic lens has two focal planes, and in each plane the point object source is focused as a line (Fig. 15.8).

When there is an irregularity or astigmatism, a point of light source from the object is not focused as a point on the retina. Instead, the point is focused as a line. This is because the power of the refractive system differs, depending on where light rays enter the system (Fig. 15.9). Remember, the image of the entire object is not a line—only the point object source is focused as a line.

For most astigmatic systems, each of two lens powers (90° from each other) focuses a

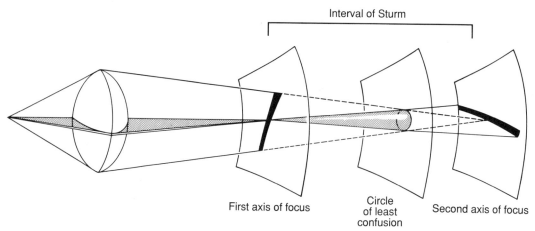

Interval of Sturm

First axis of focus

Circle of least confusion

Second axis of focus

Figure 15.8. Focus of an astigmatic lens, the circle of least confusion. An astigmatic lens, represented at the *left*, focuses in two planes. The point source of an object is focused in one plane, here represented vertically and anteriorly, and then is focused again in another, posterior plane as a horizontal line. That area between, where the point source is represented as a circle, is known as the circle of least confusion. This is where the best possible visual acuity can be obtained in the astigmatic system.

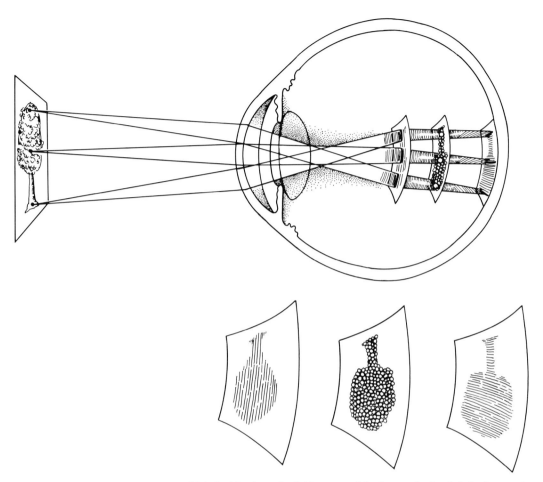

Figure 15.9.   Astigmatism causes multiple foci for the point light source of the image. On the *left,* the image of a tree is actually multiple points of origin of light. In the astigmatic eye, the focus mechanism of the cornea and the lens is not regular. Illustrated is an astigmatism where point light sources are first focused as vertical lines anteriorly. Posteriorly, the same origin points are focused as horizontal lines, illustrated directly on the retina. At a point between the first focal plane and the second focal plane, there is a position known as a circle of least confusion where the best visualization occurs. Correction of astigmatism brings the two focal planes, vertical and horizontal, together. (Illustrated is a simple myopic astigmatism.)

point of light as a line. The two powers of the lens focus two different lines 90° each other.[a]

In an eye with astigmatism, there are powers in both axes of the astigmatic lens. However, the powers differ. Therefore, when one lens axis is focused, there is a line focus of an object point source and, when the other lens axis is focused, there is an additional, different line focus of an object point either in front of or behind the first and rotated 90° from the first. This can be demonstrated by using two spherocylindrical lenses, as found in the trial lens set, and a point light source. Two different lines are focused by these two unequal spherocylindrical lenses.

Although an astigmatic lens or lens system will focus rays from a point source in a line, light rays before they come to that line focus converge and after that the focus will diverge.

---

[a]In the simplest type of astigmatic system (a cylindrical lens, for example), there is no power in one axis and, 90° away from that axis, there is power to the cylinder. In this type of lens, the only possible focus of light rays from a point source is in a line.

The lens converges and diverges rays in elliptical fashion (Fig. 5.8).

The Interval of Sturm

If we imagine an astigmatic eye that focuses a point object as a line in one axis and as a 90°-rotated line further away, we can imagine that light rays in the first line are focused and then begin to diverge and that those in the second line will still be converging as they pass by the first line of focus. Between the first focus and the second focus, light rays are converging and diverging. The distance between the initial line focus and the second line focus is known as the interval of Sturm. For low astigmatism, the interval is short; for high astigmatism, the interval is longer.

Midway between the two lines in the interval of Sturm (i.e., between the first line focus and the second line focus), there is an area where the diverging rays from the first line of focus and the converging rays of the second line of focus superimpose to form a circle. Remember that this is from a single point light source on the object. Although this circle formed from the diverging and converging rays is not the single point of focus that the point object source would be in a nonastigmatic system, the circle does represent the best focus in the astigmatic system. For that reason, the circle is known as the *circle of least confusion* (Fig. 15.9).

The circle of least confusion is an important concept. When the eye has an astigmatic system for which it can accommodate, the eye can adjust the astigmatic system so that the circle of least confusion falls on the retina and provides the best, although not perfect, acuity.

Correction of Astigmatism

The cylindrical lens used in refraction has power in one axis and no power in another axis. By using a cylindrical lens with power in a single axis, we can eliminate the distance between the two line foci in astigmatism. This allows one line of the two focal lines in an astigmatic system to be brought to focus with the other line. When this occurs, the astigmatic eye is corrected and becomes a regular or spherical system. We can then adjust the position of the spherical system so that it finally focuses on the retina. This allows a corrected point light source from an object to be directly focused as a point on the retina.

We can look at this another way. Again imagine a line focus in the vitreous and another line focus oriented 90° to the first and behind the retina. By placing a plus (or convergent) cylindrical lens so that it focuses the line behind the retina at the point where the first line is focused in the vitreous, we have created a point focus rather than two separate line foci. This is known as collapsing the interval of Sturm and will correct the astigmatic system. Once the proper cylindrical lens is placed adjustment of the astigmatic corrective system back to the retina can be done with minus lenses. Collapsing the interval of Sturm and adjusting the resulting point light source for an object point is the basis for refraction for astigmatism.

Clinical Significance

High astigmatisms that are uncorrected from birth can cause decreased vision or amblyopia. Because in astigmatism the point objects are never focused clearly on the macular area, development of the perception of a clear visual image is prevented. If the astigmatism is not corrected early in childhood, permanent amblyopia uncorrectable by lenses can develop.

Astigmatism, because it may produce an overworking of accommodation in order to attempt to focus the image, may be a cause of symptoms associated with eyestrain. These symptoms (asthenopia) may be expressed as tiredness, eye fatigue, headache, brow ache, or pressure in and around the eyes.

High astigmatisms that are seen in such conditions as keratoconus (page 12) or after penetrating keratoplasty may not be completely corrected by lenses. When high astigmatisms exist, they require thick lenses for grinding to obtain the large powers and appropriate cylinders. This creates the possibility of aberration of the image because of the thickness of the glasses alone.

PART

2

16

Essential Topics and Definitions

ABBREVIATIONS

In ophthalmology, abbreviations are used frequently, probably too often. This list is for reference and does not suggest usage. The most important and commonly used abbreviations are in boldface.

AC	anterior chamber
AC/A	accommodative convergence/accommodation ratio
ACT	alternate cover test
AION	anterior ischemic optic neuritis
ALTP	argon laser trabeculoplasty
APD	afferent pupillary defect (see RAPD)
AMD	age-related macular degeneration
AT	**applanation tension**
A/V	artery to vein ratio
BI	base in
BO	base out
BSS	balanced saline solution
C/D	**cup to disc ratio**
C&F	cell and flare
CF	**count fingers**
CL	contact lens
CMD	cystoid macular degeneration
CME	**cystoid macular edema**
COAG	chronic open angle glaucoma
C/R	chorioretinal
CSR	central serous retinopathy
D&C(Q)	deep and clear (quiet)
D&V	ductions and versions
DVD	dissociated vertical deviation
ECCE	**extracapsular cataract extraction**
EKC	**epidemic keratoconjunctivitis**
EOG	electrooculogram
EOM	**extraocular muscles**
ERG	**electroretinogram**
ET	**esotropia**
ET′	esotropia, near
Et	esophoria

EUA	exam under anesthesia
EWCL	extended wear contact lens
FA	fluorescein angiography
FP	fundus photos
FTN	finger tension (normal, hard, soft)
GCA	giant cell arteritis
GPC	giant papillary conjunctivitis
HCL	hard contact lens
HM	**hand motion**
ICCE	**intracapsular cataract extraction**
IO	inferior oblique
IOL	**intraocular lens**
IOP	**intraocular pressure**
I/P	iris and pupil
IR	**inferior rectus**
IVF	intravenous fluorescein
K's	keratometry
KP	**keratitic precipitate**
LLLL	lids, lashes, lacrimals, lymphatics
LP	**light perception**
LR	**lateral rectus**
MF	mutton fat
MG	Marcus Gunn
MR	**medial rectus**
NAG	narrow angle glaucoma
NFL	nerve fiber layer
NI	no improvement
NLP	**no light perception**
NPDR	nonproliferative diabetic retinopathy
NS	nuclear sclerosis
NVD	neovascularization—disc
NVE	neovascularization—elsewhere
NVG	neovascular glaucoma
OAG	open angular glaucoma
OD	**right eye**
OS	**left eye**
OU	**both eyes**
PAS	**peripheral anterior synechiae**
PC	posterior chamber
PD	**prism diopters or pupillary distance**
PDR	proliferative diabetic retinopathy
PERRLA	pupils equal, round, reactive to light, accommodation
PH	**pinhole**
PHNI	pinhole no improvement
PI	peripheral iridectomy
PK	**penetrating keratoplasty**
POAG	primary open angle glaucoma
POH	**presumed ocular histoplasmosis**
PP&P	posterior pole and periphery
PRP	**panretinal photocoagulation**
PSC	**posterior subcapsular cataract**
PVD	**posterior vitreal detachment**
PVR	proliferative vitreoretinopathy
RAPD	**relative afferent pupillary defect**

RD	**retinal detachment**
RK	**radial keratotomy**
RLF	**retrolental fibroplasia**
ROP	**retinopathy of prematurity**
RPE	**retinal pigment epithelium**
S&P	sharp and pink
SCL	soft contact lens
SLE	slitlamp examination
SMD	senile macular degeneration
SO	superior oblique
SPK	**superficial punctate keratopathy**
SR	**superior rectus**
SRM	subretinal (neovascular) membrane
TA	temporal arteritis
TM	trabecular meshwork
TN<	**tensions**
Va	**visual acuity**
VER	**visual evoked response**
VF	**visual fields**
VH	vitreous hemorrhage
VR	vitreoretinal
XT	**exotropia**
X(T)	**intermittent exotropia**

ABSOLUTE SCOTOMA

An absolute scotoma is an area in the visual field where no testing object, regardless of size or brightness, can be seen. An absolute scotoma, except for the one created by the optic nerve (blind spot), is abnormal.

ACANTHAMOEBA KERATITIS

Acanthamoeba keratitis, although unusual, is most often seen in patients who use soft contact lenses. Predisposing factors are the use of homemade saline as a cleansing agent, hydrogen peroxide disinfection, swimming while wearing contact lenses, and a history of improper lens care.

The keratitis may appear as a ring infiltrate of the cornea (Fig. 16.1). The epithelium also shows a ring defect. *Acanthamoeba* keratitis is most frequently associated with moderate to severe pain. The pain can be incapacitating. The course is protracted.

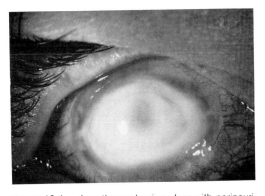

Figure 16.1. *Acanthamoeba* ring ulcer with perineuritis presenting as peripheral infiltrates. *Acanthamoeba* causes an unusual infection that is seen primarily in contact lens wearers. It presents with pain and with a ring ulcer, although the presentation may be variable. In the later stages, typical peripheral infiltrates (here illustrated as reverse wedges) result from perineural inflammation. In the very early stages, inflammation of corneal nerves is characteristic of this inflammation. (Credit: Louis A. Wilson, M.D.)

ACOUSTIC NEUROMA

Eight per cent of all primary intracranial tumors are acoustic neuromas. They account for 80% of all primary tumors of the posterior fossa. This tumor most frequently produces signs and symptoms in patients between the ages of 30 and 40 years.

The most common ophthalmic complaints are diplopia and blurred vision. Examination often reveals decreased corneal reflex, nystagmus, and papilledema. Abnormal extraocular muscle movements and lagophthalmos can occur.

The most frequent nonocular symptom is *unilateral hearing loss.* The patient may note hearing loss in one ear while using the telephone.

The signs and symptoms of acoustic neuroma can be explained by direct tumor involvement of the eighth cranial nerve and brain stem, tumor expansion to adjacent cranial nerves, and increased intracranial pressure from an enlarging tumor mass.

Tumor size correlates with signs and symptoms. Tumors larger than 2.0 cm cause nystagmus (page 112), those larger than 2.5 cm cause decreased corneal sensitivity (Fig. 1.4), and those larger than 4.5 cm cause papilledema (page 98).

Accurate diagnosis and rapid surgical intervention are necessary for good outcome in patients who present with tumors large enough to cause signs and symptoms on ophthalmologic exam.

ACUTE (EPIDEMIC) HEMORRHAGIC CONJUNCTIVITIS

Cause

Picornavirus (usually enterovirus 70, also coxsackievirus A24)

Clinical Characteristics

- *Enlarged lymph nodes* on the face in front of the ears (preauricular adenopathy)
- *Follicular conjunctivitis* (page 18)
- *Hemorrhages* under the conjunctiva, usually on the upper part of the globe, which may be extensive
- Corneal epithelium with very fine, round (punctate), scattered inflammation
- Highly contagious and spreads in *epidemics*
- Course self-limited, lasting 10 days or less

ACUTE HYDROPS

Acute hydrops is associated with keratoconus (page 12). In keratoconus, the normal spherical curvature of the cornea alters into a cone shape. This stretches the anatomical layers of the cornea. Ruptures in the inner layers of the cornea—Descemet's membrane is most important—can occur. When rupture occurs, there is a sudden clouding of the cornea due to the influx of aqueous (edema). Fluid influx occurs as Descemet's membrane ruptures, disrupting the endothelial monocell layer. The dehydrating function of the endothelium is lost, and fluid seeps into the cornea.

Acute hydrops may be associated with rubbing the eye, especially in retarded children with Down's syndrome, who have a higher prevalence of keratoconus. Acute hydrops clears spontaneously over weeks or months. A corneal scar may remain. Often, relatively good vision may return.

ACUTE MACULAR NEURORETINOPATHY

Characteristics

Acute macular neuroretinopathy usually follows a systemic viral illness and is seen primarily in young patients of either sex. Patients experience mild visual decrease with areas of central visual loss (paracentral scotomata).

Diagnosis

Ophthalmoscopy shows retinal lesions, which are usually wedge-shaped, in and around the macular region. These lesions are in the deep neurosensory retina and may involve both eyes. They appear reddish brown. Red-free light may help distinguish the lesions because they are difficult to see with white light.

Fluorescein angiography is usually normal, although hypofluorescence of the areas involved may be seen.

Course

Lesions in the retina disappear, but the areas of central visual loss (scotomata) remain and may be significant enough to cause symptoms.

ACUTE MULTIFOCAL POSTERIOR PLACOID PIGMENT EPITHELIOPATHY (AMPPE)

Acute characteristic inflammatory changes of the retinal pigment epithelium and choroid are seen in AMPPE. In general, the visual acuity recovery is excellent. The condition is bilateral. Long-term follow-up demonstrates progressive pigment epithelial atrophy in some patients, which may cause decreased visual acuity.

The cause is unknown. It has been recognized that some patients with AMPPE have a number of systemic conditions. Of these, cerebral vascular inflammation may have the most serious consequences.

ACUTE RETINAL PIGMENT EPITHELIITIS

Characteristics

Acute retinal pigment epitheliitis starts suddenly with visual decrease in one or both eyes.

Diagnosis

Ophthalmoscopy shows small, grayish, dark lesions, usually two to four, at the level of the retinal pigment epithelium in and around the macula. Fluorescein angiography is normal early but, as lesions regress, hypofluorescence may occur.

Course

The condition resolves in 6 to 12 weeks, and visual recovery is complete.

Complications

Neurosensory retinal separation; rarely, subretinal neovascular membrane

ADAPTOMETRY

Adaptometry is a technique used to measure dark adaptation (page 283). Dark adaptation is adjustment of the retinal neuroreceptors to decreased illumination.

ADIE SYNDROME

Adie syndrome has two features:

- Tonic pupil (Adie's pupil), which responds poorly to light and usually is unilateral; and
- Decreased deep tendon reflexes.

(See Adie's Tonic Pupil, page 94.)

AFTERCATARACT

An aftercataract is not a cataract in the sense of a lens opacity within the crystalline lens. Instead, it is an opacification in the pupillary region behind the iris, which occurs after cataract surgery. This is usually when the lens capsule is left, some lens fibers remain, and scarring (that is, fibrosis) occurs. The aftercataract has become important as extracapsular cataract surgery has become more common. Aftercataracts occur more frequently in children than in adults because of the more active healing powers in children, which result in significant fibrosis.

These aftercataracts can be incised so that the visual opening is clear. Lasers (YAG) may also be used to make holes in the aftercataract membrane without the need for surgery.

AGNOSIA, VISUAL

Visual agnosia is an inability to recognize an object by sight. A patient looks at a piano but does not recognize it. Yet, by touching a piano, hearing a piano played, or seeing the word "piano," the patient is able to know it.

Visual agnosia is associated with lesions of the dominant parietal cortex, Brodmann's area 18, or the corpus callosum. When the corpus callosum is involved, other perceptual abnormalities occur—alexia, symbolic agnosia, and agraphia.

AGR TRIAD

Characteristics

Aniridia, genitourinary abnormalities, and mental retardation

Genetics

When the AGR triad is present, deletion of the short arms of chromosomes 11 and 13 is found. (See Aniridia, page 251.)

AIR-PUFF NONCONTACT TONOMETER

An air-puff, noncontact tonometer applies a 3-ms puff of air against the cornea. The identation pattern produced in the cornea is detected by the tonometer's sensor. The pressure is measured by determining the amount of corneal flattening by the fixed air-puff pressure. The readout is digital.

This tonometer does not touch the eye and does not require anesthesia. These features make it good for mass screening programs.

ALBRIGHT'S SYNDROME

Albright's syndrome is fibrous dysplasia with cutaneous pigmentation and precocious puberty in female patients. When fibrous dysplasia involves the orbit, forward displacement of the globe (proptosis), strabismus, corneal exposure related to the proptosis, and optic atrophy occur.
(See Fibrous Dysplasia, page 228.)

ALOPECIA AREATA

Loss of the eyebrows and lashes may be associated with the more general condition of alopecia areata. To make the diagnosis, look for sharply defined patches where lashes, eyebrows, and hair are lost without signs of inflammation.

ALZHEIMER'S DISEASE AND VISUAL IMPAIRMENT

Patients with Alzheimer's disease may have characteristic visual complaints. Despite normal visual acuity, they may be unable to read. They may complain of spatial deficits or bumping into objects, and they may have difficulty in recognizing faces.

Visual field defects are found along with loss of contrast sensitivity, changes in color vision, and abnormal visual evoked potentials. They may have difficulty initiating eye movements. Optic nerve pallor and an enlarged optic nerve cup are also seen.

AMIODARONE

Use

This benzofuran derivative is used to treat cardiac arrhythmias but most often is used in patients with angina pectoris and particularly the arrhythmias of Wolff-Parkinson-White syndrome.

Corneal Complications

Many patients on this medication will develop small deposits on the basal cell layer of the corneal epithelium. These deposits appear as small dots. They rarely interfere with vision. They *resolve* when treatment is stopped.

Dosage

The corneal changes are very mild at a dose of less than 200 mg per day.

AMSLER GRID

Because the macula is the most sensitive area of visual discrimination, minor changes in the macula are perceived as significant visual distortion. This distortion is called *metamorphopsia.* The Amsler grid is useful in detecting subtle, early changes of metamorphopsia in macular disease.

How to use the Amsler grid: One eye is tested with the other eye occluded. The patient stares at the central dot in the Amsler grid and describes any irregularities in the lines or squares that surround the dot. Metamorphopsia will appear as broken or wavy lines or distorted boxes.

The test is used not only in the office but also by the patient at home to document the progression of disease. The test is particularly helpful in following patients with age-related macular degeneration (page 130).

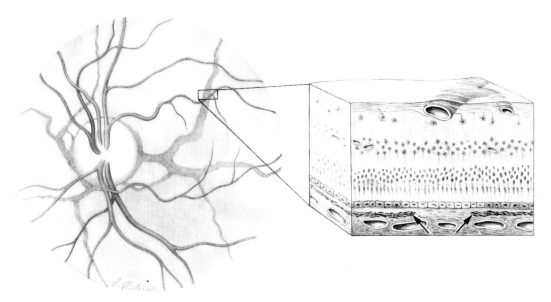

Figure 16.2. Angioid streaks are breaks in Bruch's membrane that appear as reddish or reddish brown radiations from the optic disc. Cursory examination may confuse these with retinal or choroidal vessels. The *arrows* in the histologic drawing indicate the level at which the break occurs. Angioid streaks are associated with pseudoxanthoma elasticum, Paget's disease, and sickle cell disease. (See color Fig. C.35.)

ANGIOID STREAKS

Angioid streaks (Fig. 16.2) are tapering discolorations, resembling retinal vessels, that radiate out from the disc. Most often they are red to orange, but they can also be gray to brown, depending on the fundus pigmentation. Typically, there is a ring around the disc (peripapillary) from which these streaks extend. They are almost always bilateral.

Although they have been reported in isolated association with many diseases, they are most often seen in these three conditions:

- Pseudoxanthoma elasticum (PXE) (Fig. 16.3) (80% of patients with PXE will have streaks);
- Paget's disease (10% of patients will have streaks);
- Sickle hemoglobinopathies (1% of patients will have streaks).

The streaks are breaks in Bruch's membrane (Fig. 4.3). Calcification and thickening are thought to make Bruch's membrane brittle and susceptible to this cracking. In pseudoxanthoma elasticum, the calcification of elastic tissue seen in other parts of the body could also affect Bruch's membrane, which has an elastic tissue component. The calcium deposits of Paget's disease have been linked to PXE, and it is possible that a similar mechanism for developing streaks occurs in these patients.

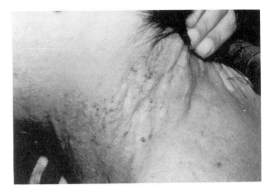

Figure 16.3. Pseudoxanthoma elasticum shows skin changes and can be associated with ocular changes, primarily angioid streaks. (Credit: George Waring, M.D.)

No elastic tissue defects occur with sickle hemoglobinopathies. In these patients, it has been suggested that a brittleness of Bruch's membrane results from the hemolysis of sickled red blood cells and iron deposition in the membrane.

The streaks themselves do not affect vision. Other changes often do, however. Neovascular membrane formation can result in subretinal neovascularization with serous detachment of the macula and subsequent visual loss. Pigmentary disturbances of the macula, choroidal atrophy, and proliferation of connective tissue and pigment can all result in visual disturbances.

Treatment of the streaks is not indicated because neovascular membranes may be stimulated by the laser beam used for treatment. When complicated neovascular membranes occur, however, laser therapy may be required.

Although the *diagnosis* is fairly easy to make by observation of the posterior pole by ophthalmoscopy, it is occasionally useful to use *fluorescein angiography* to confirm the diagnosis. Look for these *characteristics:*

- Increased fluorescence if there is thinning of pigment epithelium over an intact choriocapillaris;
- If the choriocapillaris is separated, very little fluorescence is seen centrally, but there is hyperfluorescence along the edges;
- If fibrovascular ingrowth is present, early fluorescence and then late staining are seen.

A systemic workup is indicated in patients with angioid streaks because a disease will be identified in about half. Thirty-four per cent will have PXE, 10% Paget's disease, and 6% sickle hemoglobinopathies. The most useful tests are:

- X-ray films of skull, abdomen, and lower extremities;
- Biochemical survey including serum alkaline phosphatase;
- Calcium and phosphorus;
- Hemoglobin electrophoresis;
- Skin biopsy.

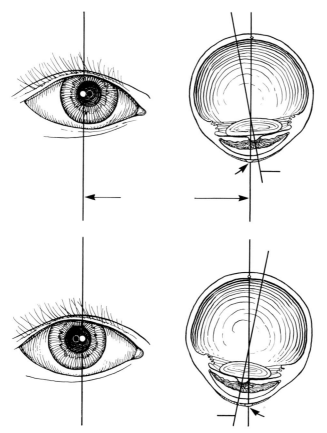

Figure 16.4. The angle kappa is the difference between a line drawn through the center of the pupil (pupillary line) and a corneal light reflex (CLR). To determine the angle kappa, have the patient look directly at a point light source. This reveals the corneal light reflex. The angle kappa is the difference between this and the center of the pupil. In a negative angle kappa, the corneal light reflex is temporal to the pupillary line *(top)*. In a positive angle kappa, the corneal light reflex is nasal to the pupillary line *(bottom)*.

ANGLE KAPPA

The angle kappa is the angle formed by two lines, an imaginary line through the center of the pupil (pupillary line) and another imaginary line along the line of sight (visual axis).

The angle kappa is measured clinically by observing the corneal light reflex. The patient looks at a light. A pinpoint of light is seen by the observer on the superficial cornea. This reflex will be to one side of the center of the pupil. The difference between center of the pupil and the light reflex on the visual axis is the angle kappa (Fig. 16.4).

The angle kappa is called *positive* when the corneal light reflex is nasal to the center of the pupil and *negative* when the corneal light reflex is temporal to the center of the pupil.

Effect on Strabismus

A small positive angle kappa (corneal light reflex nasal to center of the pupil) is common in normal eyes. If it is fairly marked, it may simulate abnormal alignment of the eyes outward (exotropia). In patients with strabismus, the presence of a large positive angle kappa may cause an outward eye deviation (exotropia) to appear greater than it actually is. Where the eyes are turned in (esotropia), the deviation may appear less than it actually is.

A negative angle kappa (central light reflex temporal to the center of the pupil) is not common in a normal eye. It simulates an esotropia. In patients with strabismus, it can cause an esotropia to appear greater than it is or cause an exotropia to appear less than it is.

Eccentric fixation occurs when light focuses off the usual alignment on the fovea. Because eccentric fixation nasal to the fovea occurs commonly in esotropia, eccentric fixation will present as a *negative angle kappa.*

Measurement of the Angle Kappa

A light is held approximately 1 foot from the patient while the eye not being examined is covered. The patient fixates on the light. The difference between the corneal light reflex and the center of the pupil is then measured in millimeters.

Causes of a Negative Angle Kappa

The major cause of negative angle kappa is high *myopia. Retinopathy of prematurity,* by dragging the macula either temporally or nasally, may also cause either a positive or a negative angle kappa. *Diabetic retinopathy* can cause a negative angle kappa.

ANGULAR BLEPHAROCONJUNCTIVITIS

Angular blepharoconjunctivitis is maceration of the tissue at the canthus. It is associated with localized or generalized conjunctivitis and skin changes. It is most commonly caused by staphylococcal organisms but is classically associated with *Moraxella.* On occasion, angular blepharoconjunctivitis can be associated with a superficial corneal punctate keratitis.

ANIRIDIA

Definition

Aniridia is a bilateral condition in which the iris is hypoplastic.

Additional Structures Affected

Aniridia is associated with numerous other defects in the eye: cataract, macular hypoplasia, refractive errors, corneal opacification, strabismus, optic nerve hypoplasia, photophobia, nystagmus, and decreased vision.

Decreased Vision

All patients with aniridia have decreased vision. Most will have less than 20/100 vision in the better eye. This decrease in vision is due to macular hypoplasia or optic nerve hypoplasia. Progressive loss of vision is frequent because of cataract, corneal clouding, and glaucoma.

Important Association with Tumors

Patients with aniridia have a higher prevalence of *Wilms' tumor* than the general population.

Genetics

Aniridia is a phenotypically heterogeneous defect that occurs in many different forms. It has been reported as an autosomal dominant condition and has also been associated with several systemic syndromes. It has been linked with the loci of chromosomes 1 and 2 and with the deletion of a p-13 on chromosome 11.

Gonioscopy

The appearance of the iris can vary considerably. Small portions of tissue can almost always been seen on gonioscopy. The angle structures are usually normal. (See AGR Triad, page 246.)

ANISOCORIA (ESSENTIAL ANISOCORIA)

Anisocoria is a difference in pupillary size. Although it may have various definitions, it is most commonly accepted at 0.4 mm. A 0.4-mm difference approximates the difference that can be detected clinically. The difference remains the same in dim or bright illumination. With anisocoria, the pupillary reflexes are normal. It is important to differentiate anisocoria from other causes of unequal pupils (see Pupil, page 93–96). Anisocoria is not related to a disease process and is thought to be a normal finding.

Important Features of Anisocoria

- At any one time, approximately 21% of individuals will have anisocoria when defined at 0.4 mm.
- In patients who are examined repeatedly, anisocoria does not persist from day to day and, over a 5-day period, only 3% will have persistent anisocoria on every day.
- From day to day, the larger pupil always remains on the same side.
- When measured every day over 5 days, an incidence of anisocoria will be seen at least once in 41% of patients.

Clinical observation usually relates more to area than actual pupillary diameter. When area is considered, the difference becomes more marked when pupils are small than when they are large. Therefore, it is important to measure pupillary size when determining anisocoria.

ANKYLOBLEPHARON

Ankyloblepharon, a congenital defect, refers to fusion of the lid margins, usually laterally. It is an autosomal dominant trait and it is almost always seen with other congenital anomalies.

ANTERIOR CLEAVAGE SYNDROME

Other Name

Mesodermal dysgenesis (no longer recommended)

Terminology

Terminology is confusing in this spectrum of presentations of a developmental anomaly. (For further study, see Shields et al.: Axenfeld-Rieger syndrome: A spectrum of developmental disorders. *Surv Ophthalmol* 29:387, 1985; Waring et al.: Anterior cleavage syndrome: A stepladder classification. *Surv Ophthalmol* 20:3, 1975.)

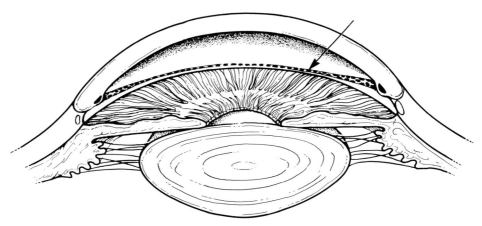

Figure 16.5.   Posterior embryotoxon is an increase in the size of Schwalbe's line, which is also more centrally displaced than usual and which may be visualized, at times, without the use of high magnification. Posterior embryotoxon is part of the anterior cleavage syndrome.

Abnormalities

The anterior cleavage syndrome includes a number of clinically identifiable anterior segment abnormalities that are present from birth:

- Posterior embryotoxon (prominent Schwalbe's ring) (Fig. 16.5);
- Axenfeld's anomaly (Fig. 16.6) (prominent Schwalbe's ring with iris strands to Schwalbe's ring);
- Rieger's anomaly (Fig. 16.7) (prominent Schwalbe's ring with iris strands to Schwalbe's ring and hypoplasia of the anterior iris stroma);
- Iridogoniodysgenesis (iris strands to Schwalbe's ring, which is not prominent, and hypoplasia of the anterior iris with glaucoma);
- Posterior keratoconus (a posterior corneal depression);
- Peters' anomaly (Fig. 16.8) (a posterior corneal defect with a scar, possibly with iris adhesions to the edge of the scar and lens opposed to the scar).

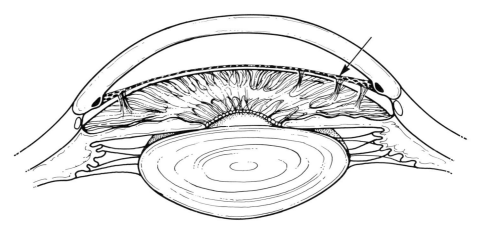

Figure 16.6.   Axenfeld's anomaly is the combination of a prominent Schwalbe's line with iris strands from the iris to Schwalbe's line. Axenfeld's anomaly is part of the anterior cleavage syndrome.

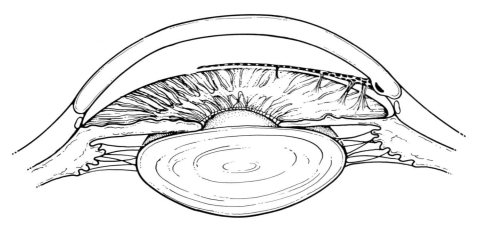

Figure 16.7. Reiger's anomaly is a prominent Schwalbe's line, synechiae and iris strands, and hypoplasia of the iris on the involved side. In the illustration, a normal angle is demonstrated on the *left,* with Reiger's anomalies on the *right,* including a hypoplastic iris. Reiger's anomaly is associated with the anterior cleavage syndrome.

Theories of Origin

Three different developmental pathways have been proposed to result in the anterior chamber cleavage syndrome: (*a*) The mesoderm that forms the cornea, which migrates from the periphery to the center, does not close completely and leaves a posterior corneal defect. (*b*) The lens vesicle in early development, which separates from the surface ectoderm, may not separate properly and may leave a corneal lens adhesion that blocks ingrowth of the corneal mesoderm. (*c*) The intact lens may be anteriorly displaced, contacting the cornea and forming a retrocorneal mass.

Although these concepts are still taught, newer evidence suggests that neural crest cells and not mesoderm are responsible for the spectrum of developmental abnormalities. This theory implicates abnormal retention of endothelial cells (of neural crest origin), which form an abnormal mesoderm on the chamber angle that alters aqueous outflow and results in glaucoma.

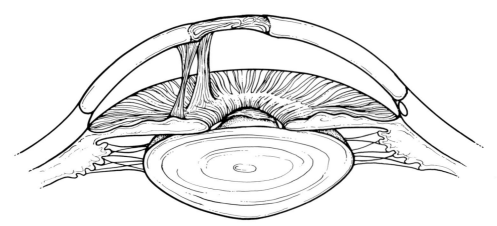

Figure 16.8. Peter's anomaly is the combination of a central corneal defect with iris strands and other cleavage abnormalities. Peter's anomaly is a part of the anterior cleavage syndrome.

ANTON'S SYNDROME

Anton's syndrome is denial of blindness by the patient. The syndrome is occasionally associated with cortical blindness in which there is complete blindness but normal pupillary reflexes.

ANULUS OF ZINN

The anulus of Zinn is a fibrous ring formed in the posterior portion of the orbit near the apex. It is the common origin for the four rectus muscles as well as the levator muscle. The ring is fused to the optic nerve dural sheath at the optic foramen. The orbital pain associated with optic neuritis on globe movement is thought to be due to this attachment.

APERT'S SYNDROME (ACROCEPHALOSYNDACTYLIA)

Apert's syndrome is a craniostenosis syndrome in which there is premature closure of one or more of the cranial sutures. Children with this syndrome have characteristic faces and eye movements. There are *shallow orbits* with *prominent globes.* Ocular muscular imbalance is common, and the eyes are divergent in upgaze but closest together in downgaze *(V syndrome)* (page 258). Patients with Apert's syndrome frequently have underacting superior rectus muscles and also may have underacting superior oblique muscles with overacting inferior oblique muscles. Apert's syndrome is differentiated from a very closely associated syndrome—Crouzon's syndrome—by the presence of syndactyly in Apert's syndrome.
(See Crouzon's Syndrome, page 280.)

APPLANATION TONOMETRY

A tonometer measures tension. An applanation tonometer measures intraocular tension.

Theory

Applanation tonometry is based on the Imbert-Fick principle (page 000). This principle states that measurement of pressure in an intact sphere is related to the pressure that is required on the surface to flatten the sphere divided by the area of the surface causing the flattening. Because the eyeball is a rough sphere and is filled with fluid, this principle is utilized. A 3-mm area is used in applanation tonometry to cause cancellation of two opposing forces, corneal resistance to flattening and capillary attraction between the tonometer and the surface of the eye.

Technique

Topical anesthesia is used. A fluorescein dye is placed in the lower conjunctival sac so that the tear film becomes lightly saturated with the fluorescein. The applanation tonometer is then set against the cornea and tear film. The slitlamp is used to view the tonometer. Readings are taken by approximating the inner edges of two half circles whose position is changed by adjusting the tonometer pressure. Readings are taken directly off a tonometer scale once the end point is reached. These readings are in millimeters of mercury.

This method of measuring intraocular pressure is very accurate and dependable. It requires skill on the part of the examiner. The applanation tonometer may be mounted on the slitlamp. Infrequently, hand-held tonometers that do not require a slitlamp are used. (See Fig. 3.4 on page 41.)

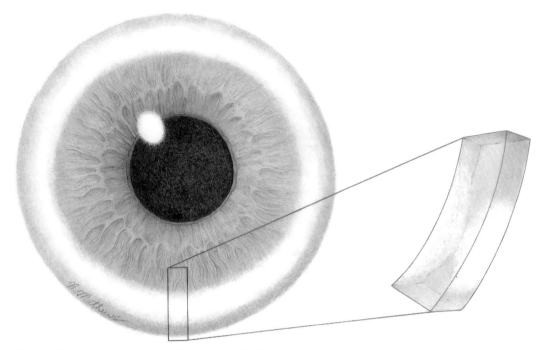

Figure 16.9. Arcus senilis is a white ring deposited in the deep cornea. Characteristically, there is a clear zone between the peripheral edge of the ring and the edge of the cornea. The condition is common, especially in elderly individuals. It is more common in blacks. It is due to deposition of lipids in the cornea.

ARCUS SENILIS

Other Names

Corneal arcus, gerontoxon

Description

Arcus senilis is a gray-white ring around the peripheral cornea (Fig. 16.9). The outer border tends to be distinct while the inner border is indistinct. The ring is 2 to 3 mm wide and is characteristically separated from the limbus by a clear corneal zone.

The ring is deposits of *lipids* (neutral fats, phospholipids, and sterols) in the *corneal stroma*. Lipids are deposited in the cornea in two areas of concentration, one next to Bowman's layer and the other near Descemet's membrane. The epithelium is normal and intact.

Arcus senilis is most often seen in older people, starting in the 40 to 60 age group. After age 80, arcus senilis is almost always present. It occurs more commonly and earlier in blacks than in whites. It is never a threat to vision and is not pathologic.

When it occurs in younger patients, arcus senilis may be associated with hyperlipoproteinemia and elevated serum cholesterol.

ARGYROSIS

Argyrosis is deposition of silver in the cornea, conjunctiva, and lens. In the conjunctiva, silver appears as a slate gray discoloration of the conjunctival surfaces (Fig. 16.10). In the cornea, the silver is seen as fine blue-gray, green, or yellowish deposits in the deep stroma and in Descemet's membrane, primarily inferiorly. There is no visual decrease with the deposition. Cataracts can occur and appear as iridescent changes.

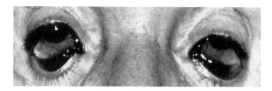

Figure 16.10.   Argyrosis. Silver deposition in the conjunctiva and cornea can occur from topical silver preparations as well as exposure to industrial organic silver salts. The slate gray appearance of the conjunctiva as well as the fine multicolored deposits in the cornea, in the deep stroma, and in Descemet's membrane are seen. There is no visual impairment. (Credit: George Waring, M.D.)

Argyrosis occurs after the use of topical silver protein solutions and after industrial exposure to silver salts. It is a rare condition and has more historic interest than practical differential diagnostic importance in today's practice of ophthalmology.

ARLT'S LINE

Arlt's line is a transverse scar that goes across the superior tarsal conjunctiva (page 19) of the upper lid. The line is found in the later stages of trachoma. (See Trachoma, page 374.)

ASCARIS LUMBRICOIDES

The fluid from a dead *Ascaris lumbricoides* worm, which may get into the eye, produces a painful and severe conjunctivitis. This is also known as Butcher's conjunctivitis.

ASTEROID HYALOSIS (ASTEROID HYALITIS)

Characteristics

This condition is found in older individuals and is most frequently (75%) uniocular. Diagnosis is easily made by slitlamp examination. With the slitlamp focused in the vitreous, the examiner sees small, white spheroid bodies that float in the vitreous gel (Fig. 16.11).

Prognosis

Visual acuity is rarely affected in individuals with asteroid hyalitis. At one time, there was thought to be an association between asteroid hyalosis and diabetes. That is no longer thought to be true.

Cause

The spheroid bodies are calcium soaps. Why these occur in older individuals and are frequently only in one eye is not known.

ASTHENOPIA

Asthenopia is ocular discomfort that the patient may describe, often vaguely, as pain or ache around the eyes, ocular fatigue, or frontal or orbital headaches. Itching, burning, and a general sensation of tiredness around the eyes is also lumped under this term. Asthenopia is caused by *refractive error*.

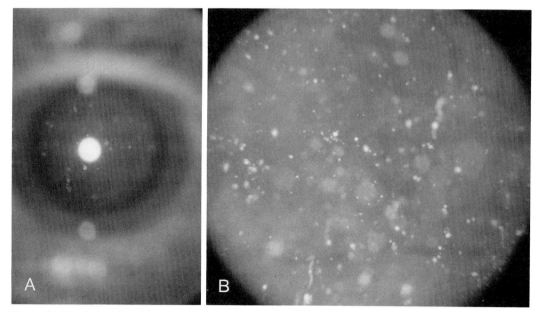

Figure 16.11. Asteroid hyalitis is usually unilateral. It presents as multiple, highly illuminated spots floating in the vitreous. It does not affect vision.

A-V PATTERNS

When looking up and down, most subjects maintain relative parallel alignment of the eyes. A and V patterns refer to changes when looking up and down.

When the eyes are closer together in upgaze and farther apart in downgaze, the edges of the letter A may be imagined. This is called an A pattern. A patterns are not considered clinically significant unless there is a difference of more than 10 prism diopters between up- and downgaze.

V patterns are the opposite of A patterns. If in upgaze the eyes are farther apart and in downgaze they are closer together, the sides of a V can be imagined. V patterns are not clinically significant unless a difference of more than 15 prism diopters between up- and downgaze is measured.

A and V patterns are actually subtypes of horizontal strabismus. Between 15 and 25% of all cases of strabismus also have these patterns. The most common patterns are V pattern esotropia, V pattern exotropia, A pattern exotropia, and A pattern esotropia.

AXENFELD'S ANOMALY

Axenfeld's anomaly is the combination of a prominent Schwalbe's ring and iris strands (see Fig. 16.6). The iris strands are attached to Schwalbe's ring and may be fine, threadlike filaments or broad, thick bands. At times, the iris connections may appear as a confluent membrane with a fenestrated, lattice-like appearance.

Glaucoma

About 50% of patients with a prominent Schwalbe's ring and attached iris strands develop a glaucoma (juvenile type). This is known as Axenfeld's syndrome.

Skeletal Anomalies

Hypoplasia of skeletal structure and facial asymmetry may be present. For further information regarding the spectrum of developmental anomalies, of which Axenfeld's anomaly is only one, see Anterior Cleavage Syndrome (page 252).

AXENFELD'S SYNDROME

The association of glaucoma with a prominent Schwalbe's ring and iris strands is known as Axenfeld's syndrome. Note that a combination of Schwalbe's ring and attached iris strands without glaucoma is Axenfeld's anomaly (previous topic). Axenfeld's syndrome and Axenfeld's anomaly are part of what is most frequently now referred to as the anterior chamber cleavage syndrome (page 252).

AXIAL PROPTOSIS

Axial proptosis is forward displacement of the globe along the axis of the globe. This is seen in patients with certain types of tumors such as gliomas. Other tumors show different types of proptosis: rhabdomyosarcomas, for example, push the globe more frequently down and out.

AXES OF FICK

The axes of Fick are designated to help explain the rotations of the eye around a central point. They are mainly of historic interest.

Basically, there are three rotations that the eye achieves when a central point is considered. The up and down rotation is designated the rotation around the X axis. The left and right rotation is around the line designated the Z axis. There is a rotation around the Y axis that is analogous to a bead rotating on a taut string. This is most easily explained on a diagram (Fig. 16.12).

Listing's is a hypothetical plane that passes through the center of rotation of the eye and includes both the Z and X axis of Fick. The Y axis is perpendicular to Listing's plane. (See Listing's plane, page 314.)

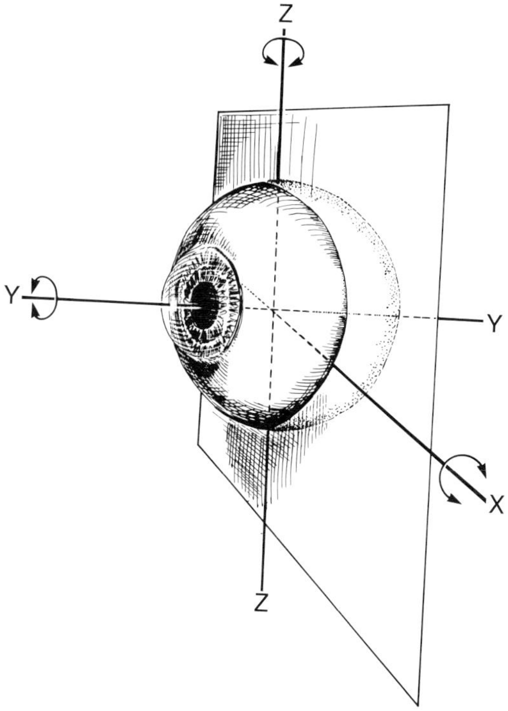

Figure 16.12. Axes of Fick. There are three major axes of eye rotation. These are known as the axes of Fick and are labeled X, Y, and Z.

BAGGY EYELIDS

Other Names

Orbital fat herniation, adipose palpebral bags

Description

Baggy eyelids are a common presentation when orbital fat protrudes into the upper lid through the orbital septum and the levator aponeurosis and into the lower lid be-

tween the orbital septum and the capsulopalpebral fascia. The condition is frequently associated with excessive lid skin, dermatochalasis.
(See Dermatochalasis, page 283.)

BARKAN'S MEMBRANE

Barkan's membrane covers the trabecular meshwork in primary infantile glaucoma. Some think that this membrane blocks the outflow of aqueous and causes the glaucoma.

BASSEN-KORNZWEIG SYNDROME (ACANTHOCYTOSIS)

General Comments

This is an autosomal recessive disorder. The features of the syndrome are crenated red cells, spinal cerebellar degeneration, and serum abetalipoproteinemia.

Ocular Changes

A pigmented retinopathy develops. In the early stages, the pigment retinopathy can be reversed by giving vitamin A.

BELL'S PHENOMENON

When the eyelids shut, the eyes turn upward—a reflex known as Bell's phenomenon. This phenomenon is variable from individual to individual. With normal lid closure, it has little clinical significance.

If deficient lid closure is present, Bell's phenomenon may be an important protective reflex for the cornea, which can dry and scar if exposed. Lid closure is absent or incomplete in nerve palsies, scarred lids, and some patients without pathology who sleep with the lids partially open. In such cases, a vigorous Bell's phenomenon protects the cornea by keeping the eye up and the cornea under the protection of the upper lid.

Bell's phenomenon is absent in patients with nuclear lesions of the seventh nerve.

BERGMEISTER'S PAPILLAE

Bergmeister's papillae is a remnant of the hyaloid vascular system. In embryologic life, the hyaloid vessels extend from the optic nerve through the vitreous and nourish the developing lens. Vessels normally regress completely. However, in some individuals, a remnant remains on the surface of the optic disc. This is known as Bergmeister's papillae. At times, this remnant may extend some distance into the vitreous.

BIELSCHOWSKY HEAD TILT TEST

Bielschowsky's head tilt test, a test for ocular muscle dysfunction, takes advantage of the multiple actions of certain muscles. For example, a muscle that either elevates or depresses the eye also rotates the eye. Rotation keeps the eye straight up when the head is tilted. If a subject is looking at a television set and tilts the head to the right, there are up and down as well as rotary adjusting movements to the eye.

The Bielschowsky head tilt test helps to isolate which vertical-acting muscle might be paretic. For example, the right superior oblique muscle has a function of bringing the right eye down. This action is strongest when the eye is looking inward. This right superior oblique muscle also rotates the eye inward. Thus, the right superior oblique has three functions, two of which are depressing the eye and rotating the eye inward.

If we tilt the head to the right, both eyes make vertical adjustments. Normally there is no deviation, but if the difference in the deviation between the eyes becomes greater when we tilt the head from side to side, it means that a vertical-acting muscle is not functioning. The right superior oblique is implicated on right head tilt because action is greatest for the right superior oblique in right head tilt when it acts to rotate the eye inward. In this position, it also has its downward depression function, which is deficient; therefore, the vertical deviation of the eyes is greater. In left head tilt, however, the inward rotation and depressing actions of the right superior oblique muscle are not used. Only normally functioning muscles of the right eye have taken over, allowing normal alignment of the eyes. Therefore, the vertical deviation of the eyes in right head tilt is not present in left head tilt.

Bielschowsky's head tilt test is often used as the third step of the Three-Step Test for isolating superior oblique palsies.
(See the Three-Step Test, page 153.)

BIRDSHOT CHORIORETINITIS

Characteristics

Birdshot chorioretinitis usually affects women from their 30s to 60s.

Presenting Symptoms and Signs

There is no associated systemic or ocular disease process. These healthy patients present with blurred vision, floaters, and visual distortion (photopsia). As the disease progresses, patients may lose color vision and may have difficulty with night vision.

Diagnosis

Small, multifocal patches of pigment loss are seen in the choroidal pigment epithelium in the posterior portion of the fundus. Retinal and disc edema can be seen, and associated retinal vasculitis is present. Depigmentation of the skin (vitiligo) has been reported.

Course

Although the condition may remain for a prolonged period, it does resolve and is compatible with the recovery of good visual acuity.

Cause

There is no established cause for this syndrome. A genetic predisposition is suspected because an association with HLA-A29 antigen has been reported.

Treatment

No therapy is known to change the disease course.

BITOT'S SPOTS

Bitot's spots are areas of drying and wrinkling of the conjunctiva associated with *vitamin A deficiency*. These are small spots and have a foamy appearance. They do not wet readily after a blink. These spots are found on the conjunctiva that is exposed when the eyelids are open (the interpalpebral fissure).

BLEPHAROPHIMOSIS SYNDROME

Blepharophimosis syndrome is dominantly inherited. It is a congenital eyelid syndrome. It presents with wide spacing between the eyes (telecanthus), skin folds over the inner lids that slant down and out (epicanthus inversus), and severe lid droop (ptosis). In addition, there may be eyelid ectropion, a flat nasal ridge, hypoplasia of the orbital rims, and hypertelorism.

BLUE SCLERA

Blue sclera is caused by a thinning of the sclera and a loss of the water content of the sclera, allowing the dark choroid to be visualized. The dark choroid has a bluish coloration when seen through the sclera.

Blue sclera can be seen in many syndromes. The most common associations are:

- Ehler-Danlos syndrome;
- Osteogenesis imperfecta;
- Paget's syndrome;
- Staphyloma; and
- Others.

BOTULINUM TOXIN

Botulinum toxin has been used in ophthalmology for the treatment of crossed eyes (strabismus) and for the treatment of spasm of the eyelids (essential blepharospasm).

Strabismus

Botulinum toxin is injected into the extraocular muscle. This requires electrophysiologic monitoring to determine when the needle is in the muscle. There is no systemic toxicity at normal dosages. The paralysis lasts for several months. Injections must be repeated because the effect is not permanent. Cases must be carefully selected for this therapy.

Essential Blepharospasm

Injection of botulinum toxin into the orbicularis muscle decreases the spasms in essential blepharospasm (see Essential Blepharospasm, page 205). Although used for the primary treatment of essential blepharospasm, botulinus toxin has also been effective in decreasing residual spasms after surgical removal of the orbicularis muscle. Injection must be repeated every few months.

BOW-TIE ATROPHY

Bow-tie atrophy, a change in the optic nerve that occurs with intracranial lesions, is caused by retrograde degeneration of optic nerve fibers. The changes in the optic nerve where the atrophy characteristically appears are like one side of a bow-tie.

The fibers lost are nasal, macular, and peripheral fibers. The bow-tie atrophy occurs in the eye opposite the side of the lesion. It is associated with the following visual field defects:

- Pregeniculate homonymous hemianopsia or
- Bitemporal hemianopsia.

BOXING AND OCULAR COMPLICATIONS

Boxing is known to produce severe complications in the eye. Approximately two-thirds of boxers will have some ocular injury, and about one-half of these will result in serious sequela. Complications include damage to the chamber angle (causing glaucoma), lens changes (posterior subcapsular and other types), macular lesions, and peripheral retinal tears.

BROWN-McLEAN SYNDROME

Definition

Corneal edema after cateract surgery

Features of This Corneal Change

- Occurs in aphakic eyes
- Occurs in the peripheral cornea with edema
- Is frequently bilateral

There is a high rate of retinal detachment.

Cause

It is suspected that endothelial damage by the iris may be responsible.

BROWN'S SYNDROME

Brown's syndrome is a unilateral inability to raise the inturned (adducted) eye. It is associated with a positive traction test. In congenital Brown's syndrome, the lesion is thought to involve the superior oblique tendon posterior to the trochlea, causing improper function of the superior oblique muscle.

In acquired Brown's syndrome, the following have been reported as causes: operation (tucking) of the superior oblique tendon, involvement of the tendon by the nodules of rheumatoid arthritis, surgery in the area of the trochlea, inflammatory conditions of the superior oblique tendon, and isolated metastatic breast carcinoma in the posterior superior oblique muscle.

BRUCHNER TEST

Use

The Bruchner test screens infants and young children by comparison of fundus reflexes between left and right eyes. Abnormal reflexes are caused by unequal pupils, abnormalities of the posterior pole, opacities of the media of the eye, strabismus, and unequal refractive errors between the eyes.

How to Do the Test

The examiner is at arm's length from the patient using a direct ophthalmoscope. The corneal reflex from the light of the ophthalmoscope (Hirschberg reflex) is observed on the cornea. The light also fills the pupil with a red reflex from the fundus. As a child takes up central fixation, the corneal reflexes are centered and there is brisk constriction of the pupils and dimming of both fundus reflexes. Asymmetrical dimming of fundus reflexes is considered abnormal.

Age of Subjects

The test has limited application. Fundus reflexes are not easily elicited in infants under 2 months of age, and infants between 2 and 8 months of age have an unacceptably high frequency of positive findings not associated with pathology. The test, performed by a skilled examiner, is best used in children over 8 months old.

BUPHTHALMOS

Buphthalmos (Fig. 16.13) is an enlargement of the eye. The corneal diameter, normally 10.5 mm in children, enlarges to 12 mm or more. As the cornea stretches, ruptures in the posterior (Descemet's membrane) can occur, resulting in fluid release into the stroma and corneal edema. The anterior chamber is deeper than normal. As the scleral coat expands, the eye is distorted, which accounts for the name buphthalmos, a derivative from the Greek—ox eye.

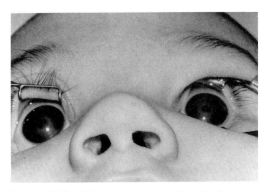

Figure 16.13. This is an example of buphthalmos, enlargement of the globe, usually associated with congenital glaucoma. When the corneal diameters are greater than 12 mm, buphthalmos is diagnosed. This patient with congenital glaucoma has bilaterally enlarged eyes with enlarged corneas. (Credit: George Waring, M.D.)

Buphthalmos is a sign of increased intraocular pressure and is associated with *congenital glaucoma* (page 55). In congenital glaucoma, the trabecular meshwork is defective and blocks aqueous outflow. As a result, pressure builds within the developing eye, causing sclera expansion and buphthalmos. (The sclera does not reach full strength until 3 years of age.) The expansion often takes place in utero; buphthalmos is often present at birth.

After birth, the coexistence of *buphthalmos, tearing, lid spasm,* and *photophobia* are diagnostic of congenital glaucoma.

BUTCHER'S CONJUNCTIVITIS

Butcher's conjunctivitis is a severe, painful conjunctivitis that is associated with marked chemosis of the conjunctiva and lid edema. It is caused by fluids from dead *Ascaris lumbricoides* splashing in the eye. This conjunctivitis is seen most often in butchers or physicians performing autopsies where *Ascaris* may be cut during slicing or examination. The condition is rarely seen and is mainly of historical interest.

C-VALUE

C-value is a measure of the rate at which aqueous leaves the anterior chamber through the trabeculum and other outlets. The normal average total facility of a nonglaucomatous eye is $0.28 + 0.05$ μl per mm Hg per minute. The C-value is measured by tonography.

Tonography is a technique where a tonometer with an indentation plunger is placed on the eye over a period of 4 minutes and the pressure changes are observed. From this pressure change, the facility is calculated in microliters per millimeter Hg per minute.

CAPILLARY HEMANGIOMA OF THE EYELID

Hemangiomas of the eyelid may be small or large. In infants, they should be followed carefully because they may grow and cause amblyopia. Hemangiomas that are present in early life tend to regress spontaneously after a few years.

CARBONIC ANHYDRASE INHIBITORS AND BLOOD DYSCRASIA

Blood dyscrasias are known to occur with the systemic use of carbonic anhydrase inhibitors (Diamox and Neptazane). Aplastic anemia and thrombocytopenia purpura occur. Reactions are idiosyncratic and not dose-related. Although the reactions can occur at any time, the majority occur within the first 4 months after the onset of treatment. Discontinuation of the drug may, in some cases, reverse the dyscrasia, but this is variable.

CAT-SCRATCH DISEASE

Features

- A conjunctival inflammation seen most often in children who have intimate contact with cats
- Low grade fever
- Enlarged lymph nodes in the preauricular area
- Conjunctival granulomas

Course

The disease is self-limited and resolves in 2 to 3 months. Tetracyclines may be used to shorten the course of the disease but should not be used in children under the age of 10. Conjunctival nodules can be excised.

Cause

Pleomorphic Gram-negative bacillus that grows in the blood vessel walls is the cause.

Association

Because of the preauricular node involvement, this is one cause of Parinaud's ocular glandular syndrome (page 256).

CAUSES OF ENOPHTHALMUS

Enophthalmus is a backward displacement of the eye into the orbit. Enophthalmus causes a deep and superiorly displaced upper lid crease. Causes are:

- Bony defect of the orbital wall (due to trauma in most cases but perhaps mucocele);
- Change in the soft tissue (linear scleroderma, usually unilateral);
- Cicatricial changes from metastatic carcinoma (breast most common).

CAVERNOUS HEMANGIOMA OF THE RETINA

Ocular Findings

Cavernous hemangioma of the retina consists of retinal lesions that are dark red saccules filled with venous blood. They have been described as resembling clusters of grapes. They are most often located posterior to the equator of the eye and may occur at the optic disc.

Symptoms

Patients are almost always asymptomatic. The condition is most often unilateral. When symptoms do occur, they usually are related to decreased vision because of hemorrhage, which is rare, or due to lesions involving the macula, which are also rare.

Fluorescein Angiography

In cavernous hemangioma, the blood-retina barrier remains intact. There is no exudate, and with fluorescein angiography there is no leakage of dye. There are no specialized or enlarged feeder vessels or draining vessels, which are seen in von Hippel-Lindau syndrome (also called angiomatosis retinae).

Clinical Course

The lesions of cavernous hemangioma tend to remain stable for years.

Important Associated Systemic Features

Cavernous hemangioma can be associated with hemangioma of the brain and of the skin. The brain lesions can hemorrhage. It is not unusual to have central nervous system symptoms associated with cavernous hemangioma of the retina. Seizures, headaches, intracranial hemorrhages, and focal neurologic signs all occur.

Diagnosis of Intracranial Cavernous Hemangioma

Of the intracranial hemangiomas, 40% have calcification and can be seen radiologically. Computed axial tomography can demonstrate a subcortical nodularity with poor enhancement by contrast agent. Brain scans will show an increase in the uptake of radioisotope. Magnetic imaging may improve the accuracy of intracranial diagnosis.

Inheritance

Although cavernous hemangioma of the retina may occur sporadically, it has also been reported in families. The hereditary pattern is probably autosomal dominant with variable penetrance. For this reason, all direct family members of a patient with cavernous hemangioma should have (a) dilated fundus examination, (b) CT scanning or MRI scanning, and (c) electrocephalography. Intracranial diagnosis is important because lesions that may potentially hemorrhage can be treated surgically or with proton beam therapy.

Phakomatosis

Cavernous hemangioma is a hamartoma (page 168). (A hamartoma is a developmental tumor that comes from cellular elements present in the tissue normally.) Because it occurs in multiple sites—retina, skin, and brain—it has recently been suggested that it be included with the phakomatoses (page 168).

Skin Changes with Cavernous Hemangioma

Vascular lesions of the skin are cutaneous hemangiomas. Because of their appearance, they have been called angioma serpiginosum.

Differential Diagnosis

Cavernous hemangioma is different from retinal telangiectasis (Table 16.1). The two conditions are usually separate and should be differentiated, although on two occasions they have occurred in the same eye. We do not know whether they are related.

Table 16.1.
Cavernous Hemangioma Compared to Retinal Telangiectasis

Cavernous Hemangioma	Retinal Telangiectasis
Multiple lesions	Single lesion
Tend to be independent of retinal circulation	Tend to be along retinal vessels and to stand out at the boundary of ischemic areas
Do not produce exudate	Produce exudate
Not associated with retinal ischemia	Associated with retinal ischemia
Fluorescein angiography: do not leak fluorescein and fill late	Fluorescein angiography: leak fluorescein readily and fill early
Histology: dilated blood vessels with a thin wall of endothelium and stroma; globules are connected small orifices	Histology: Walls are thick with plasmoid and some fibrous material; basement membrane multilaminated; endothelium absent or degenerated

CENTRAL AREOLAR PIGMENT EPITHELIAL (CAPE) DYSTROPHY

Clinical Characteristics

- Autosomal dominant with high penetrance and variable expressivity
- Lack of visual symptoms
- Nonprogressive course

Onset

First decade

Fundus Appearance

A central, depigmented, sharply demarcated macular lesion, this is a dystrophy of the retinal pigment epithelial layer that may progress to produce a confluent retinal pigment epithelial atrophy.

This dystrophy may be the same as, or a variant of, Lefler-Wadswoth-Sidbury foveal dystrophy. The ERG and EOG, dark adaptometry, and color vision testing are normal for this condition.

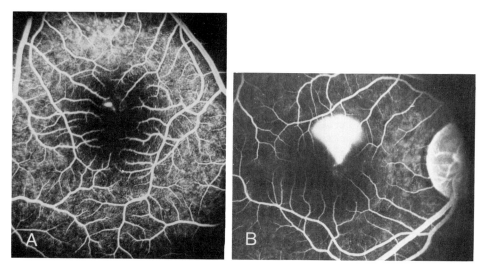

Figure 16.14.   Central serous retinopathy is demonstrated here by fluorescein angiography. **A,** Fluorescein angiography demonstrating an early leak in the macular region. **B,** As time progresses, the leak continues, showing a puff of fluorescein dye. Central serous retinopathy is usually a self-limited condition with transient effects on vision. (Credit: Paul Sternberg, M.D.)

CENTRAL SEROUS CHOROIDOPATHY

Central serous choroidopathy occurs in young male patients who have the symptoms of blurred vision, distortion of the visual image, and a general dimness in one eye.

The condition is due to a focal leak of fluid through a defect of the retinal pigment epithelium. This develops into a serous detachment of the sensory retina. Typical fluorescein angiographic findings show a small focal hyperfluorescent leak in the pigment epithelium (Fig. 16.14).

The condition is usually self-limited. The fluid undergoes spontaneous resorption in 80 to 90% of patients. Some visual symptoms and a mild decrease in vision may persist. Of all patients, 40 to 50% will experience one or more recurrences.

CHARGE SYNDROME

The mnemonic CHARGE stands for **C**oloboma, **H**eart defects, **A**tresia of the choanae, **R**etarded development and growth, **G**enital hypoplasia, and **E**ar anomalies and/or hearing loss.

The CHARGE syndrome has no known cause and is inherited as autosomal dominant, autosomal recessive, and x-linked recessive forms.

Ocular Findings

The ocular finding of coloboma is important because observation may precede diagnosis of the entire syndrome. Coloboma, however, is frequently seen without association with other abnormalities (see pages 268 and 272).

CHERRY-RED SPOT

Clinical Appearance

The retina becomes opaque white around the fovea and the foveolar region, where there is a bright red contrasting spot.

Cause

There are two things that contribute to the cherry-red spot, anatomy and pathology. The *anatomy* of the macula is important because the center of the macula does not contain ganglion cells (Fig. 4.2, page 62). Around the fovea, the retina is very thick because of the high concentration of ganglion cells. In *pathologic* conditions where ganglion cells are opaque and white, the center of the macula with no ganglion cells stays its normal but now contrasting red.

Ophthalmoscopy

This clinical observation is formed by infiltrated ganglion cells which become swollen, white, and opaque. Because there are no ganglion cells directly in the foveola, the normal retinal pigment epithelium and blood in the choroid show through in stark contrast.

Association with Tay-Sachs Disease

The most common association with cherry-red spots is Tay-Sachs disease. In Tay-Sachs disease, the ganglion cells are infiltrated with an accumulation of sphingolipid. However, in Tay-Sachs disease, approximately 10% of patients will not have the cherry-red spot.

Disappearance of Spot

It has also been reported that the presence of the spot reverses in Tay-Sachs disease. This is thought to be due to atrophy of the ganglion cells, which then lose their opaque whiteness.

Association with Other Diseases

This spot is also seen in GM 1 generalized gangliocytosis, Goldberg's syndrome, Niemann-Pick type C disease, and other storage diseases.

CHLAMYDIAL OCULAR INFECTIONS

Chlamydial organisms cause three distinct ocular diseases.

- *Neonatal inclusion conjunctivitis* is an acute conjunctivitis that occurs 5 to 12 days after birth (page 230).
- *Adult inclusion conjunctivitis* is a follicular conjunctivitis often associated with venereal chlamydial infections (page 133).
- *Trachoma* is a chronic follicular conjunctivitis that occurs primarily on the upper tarsal plate and causes conjunctival scarring and corneal changes (page 374).

CHLOROQUINE

Use

Chloroquine is associated most often with antimalarial therapy. In the United States, however, it is frequently used for collagen diseases such as rheumatoid arthritis, systemic lupus erythematosus and discoid lupus erythematosus, and sarcoidosis.

Ocular Changes

Corneal Changes

A diffuse haziness of the epithelium in subepithelial areas occurs in as many as 30% of patients on long-term chloroquine therapy. These changes may cause mild effects. The changes are *reversible* when the drug is stopped.

Retinal Changes

Although not as common as the corneal changes, retinal changes are serious and *irreversible.* Changes occur primarily in the macular region. Pigment migration and edema of the macula occur, and there may be alteration of the retinal vessels. The pigment around the macula forms a ring, which is often called *bull's-eye retinopathy* (Fig. 16.15). Peripheral pigmentary changes are seen also.

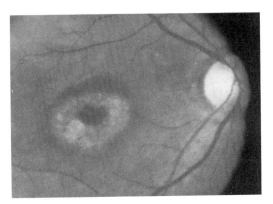

Figure 16.15. Chloroquine retinopathy. Chloroquine, as well as other drugs, can present with a characteristic "bull's-eye" lesion in the macula. The change is irreversible and is caused by pigment migration into the macular region. (Credit: Paul Sternberg, M.D.)

Diagnosis

Early diagnosis is aided by the use of fluorescein angiography. Visual field examination can show peripheral field constriction and central scotomas. Changes are also seen in electroretinographic findings, dark adaptation, and color vision.

Progression

The retinal changes are irreversible and may progress even after the drug is stopped.

Recommended Follow-up for Patients on Chloroquine

Patients on chloroquine should have ophthalmologic examinations after 4 to 6 months, depending upon the dose. Patients on high dosages should be taught to examine their visual acuity and report as soon as they notice any change.

Dosages

Patients on chloroquine dosages of 250 to 750 mg per day administered for a period of months are susceptible to the ocular toxic changes that occur with chloroquine.

CILIOCHOROIDAL EFFUSION

Effusion in the choroid is seen in two major conditions, the uveal effusion syndrome and nanophthalmos. The uveal effusion syndrome occurs most frequently in male patients and is characterized by dilation of episcleral blood vessels, thickened and detached choroid and ciliary body, nonrhegmatogenous retinal detachment with shifting subretinal fluid, and a clinical course characterized by remissions and exacerbation. The intraocular pressure is usually normal.

Ciliochoroidal effusion is also associated with nanophthalmos. Nanophthalmos is a small eye and is not associated with systemic disorders or developmental defects.

It is thought that scleral effusion is caused by a thickened sclera and decreased permeability of this thickened sclera to the passage of protein. The protein builds up, especially albumen, in the superchoroidal space and provides an onconic choroidal tissue pressure, which results in fluid accumulation. The theory is supported by fact; when ciliochoroidal effusion is treated by resecting portions of full-thickness sclera, the effusion subides.

CLIMATIC DROPLET KERATOPATHY

Other Names

Bietti's keratopathy, pearl diver's keratopathy, Labrador keratopathy, spheroid degeneration of the cornea

Clinical Appearance

Climatic droplet keratopathy starts in the early stages as fine, yellow droplets in the edge of the cornea. With time, these small droplets are seen in the central cornea. The cornea eventually clouds, causing blurred vision.

Cause

The condition is seen mainly in men who work out-of-doors. It is thought that climatic droplet keratopathy is due to exposure to ultraviolet light.

COATS' DISEASE

The patient with Coats' disease has retinal hemorrhages, malformed vessels, yellowish exudates beneath the vessels, and microaneurysm. The patient usually experiences a sudden onset of blurred vision. Coats' disease:

• Predominates in males;
• Is unilateral;
• Has onset in teens.

Progression can lead to retinal detachment, cataract, and glaucoma.
The cause is unknown.

COATS' RING (COATS' WHITE RING)

Coats' ring is a small ring, less than 1 mm in diameter, which appears as a gray-white circle in the superficial stroma. It is secondary to a metallic foreign body and is remnants of the iron foreign body that are contained in fibrin. It is not, however, the superficial, round, stromal scars that are frequently residual after foreign body removal.

COCKAYNE'S SYNDROME

Clinical Findings

This autosomal recessive syndrome is characterized by dwarfism and a premature senile appearance. Mental retardation, photosensitive dermal reactions, and early death are characteristic.

Ocular Manifestations

The most common ocular signs are salt and pepper pigmented retinal degeneration associated with optic atrophy and arterial narrowing. Visual loss is common as the disease progresses. A variety of additional changes have been reported, including photophobia, enophthalmos, strabismus, corneal dystrophy, irregular pupils, and a poor response to mydriatic drugs.

COGAN'S SYNDROME

Cogan's syndrome is the occurrence of peripheral subepithelial infiltrates and hearing loss. Ocular symptoms are bilateral tearing, burning, and photophobia. Earaches and dizziness may also be present, although the ocular symptoms start first. Bilateral episcleritis can be observed.

Course

The bilateral subepithelial infiltrates fluctuate in appearance and then resolve. They may recur.

Early Recognition

It is important for the ophthalmologist to recognize that the ocular signs of this syndrome may be accompanied by severe hearing loss that is treatable with systemic doses of steroids. Audiograms are indicated in any patient with peripheral acute keratitis, especially if the peripheral keratitis changes in severity or if ear symptoms are present.

COLLARETTES

Collarettes are desquamated cells at the base of the eyelid lashes (Fig. 16.16). They are frequently associated with ulceration at the base of the lashes. They are described as collarettes because the cells form a circular disk around the lash base, which may be slightly raised above the surface of the lid margin. This change is highly suggestive of the presence of subclinical or clinical blepharoconjunctivitis, most often caused by staphylococcal organisms.

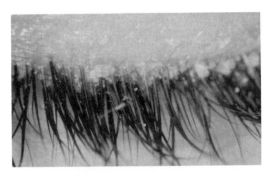

Figure 16.16. Collarettes are desquamated cells at the base of lashes. They are associated with blepharoconjunctivitis, usually due to *Staphylococcus* organisms. (Credit: George Waring, M.D.)

Other debris on the lashes may be confused with collarettes. Scurf is irregular, oily debris associated with seborrhea, and sleves are deposited by *Demodex folliculorum*.

COLOBOMA

The fetal fissure closes during the 2nd month of gestation. Failure of the fissure to close causes a coloboma. Because of the position of the fetal fissure, coloboma presents in the inferior nasal area of the structure involved. Severe colobomas involve many structures—choroid, retina, optic nerve, ciliary body, and iris. Isolated presentations in any of these structures may occur.

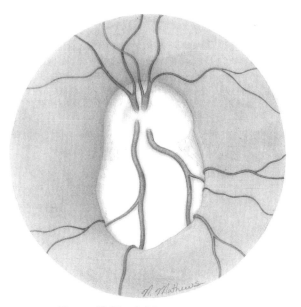

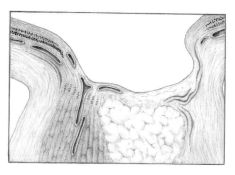

Figure 16.17. Colobomas are congenital defects due to a failure in embryonic closure. They may be variable in their appearance when involving the optic nerve. The inferior position, as illustrated, is characteristic.

Choroidal colobomas (Fig. 16.17) lack pigment epithelium. Usually the retina is present but not visible because of its transparency. Clinically, only the retinal vessels are seen over the background white of the sclera. Iris colobomas (Fig. 16.18) are inferior nasal defects in the pupil with a characteristic frill along the borders.

COLOR VISION

Color vision is the responsibility of visual pigments in the outer segments of the cone receptors in the retina. The rod receptors are not thought to contribute to color vision.

Figure 16.18. Coloboma of the iris is a congenital defect that appears characteristically in the inferior position.

There are three types of pigment within the cone receptors, each of which absorbs in a range of wavelengths centered in the short (blue), middle (green), and long (red) wavelengths. Overall, the eye receives wavelengths of 400 to 700 nm.

The transmission of color image in pattern to the brain depends on an intricate overlapping of regions within the receptive fields. These regions are variously excited or inhibited by shape, motion, patterns, and color. Receptive fields pass on a variety of complex data by stimulation of specific ganglion cells. The data are then integrated and perceived in the cerebral cortex.

Congenital and Acquired Color Defects

Congenital Color Defects

Congenital defects present distinct characteristics. Subjects with congenital defects rarely misname colors. Also, almost always, both eyes are involved equally. Subjects with congenital color defects have a hereditary pattern (X-linked recessive) and have confusion of reds, browns, golds, and olives. Pastel pinks, oranges, greens, and yellows look similar. Purples are confused with blues.

Congenital color defects are constant in type and remain stable throughout life. There is no association of ocular pathology with congenital color defects.

Acquired Color Defects

Patients with acquired color defects frequently name colors incorrectly and report that the color appearance of known familiar objects is now different. The acquired color vision defect is usually in one eye or at least affects one eye more than the other. Acquired color defects are blue/yellow (tritan). Congenital defects are red/green in almost all circumstances. When the red/green defect is acquired, which is rare, it is called protan-deutan.

Any blue/yellow defect should make the examiner suspect an acquired color defect. Acquired color defects vary greatly in type and severity. They are frequently associated with observable ocular pathology.

Classification of Color Defects

Classification of color defects is based on the idea that there are three pigments; red, green, and blue. This principle is the basis of testing defects.

The anomaloscope tests color vision by requiring the subject to match colors (Tables 16.2 and 16.3). Any individual color is matched by the subject using the anomaloscope with a combination of three standard wavelengths of red, green, and blue. Individuals with normal color vision use all three wavelengths to match one color.

Table 16.2.
Color Vision Classification (Tested by Matching a Color with One or More of the Three Primary Colors: Red, Green, Blue)

1. Trichromat: requires all three primary colors for color matching; considered normal; 92% of the population uses this color matching.
2. Anomalous trichromat: uses three primary colors for matching but uses abnormal amounts of one of the primaries.
   a. Protanomalous—uses more red than normal
   b. Deuteranomalous—uses more green than normal
   c. Tritanomalous—uses more blue than normal
3. Dichromat: uses only two of the three primary colors for matching.
   a. Protanope: has loss of the red-sensitive pigment, uses only green and blue
   b. Deuteranope: loss of the green-sensitive pigment, uses only red and blue
   c. Tritanope: loss of the blue-sensitive pigment, uses only red and green
4. Monochromat: requires only one of the three primaries to match any unknown.
   a. Rod monochromat has general cone loss [has low visual acuity, absent color vision, light sensitivity, nystagmus, abnormal photopic ERG, and macular abnormalities (hypoplasia, pigment abnormalities)]. Two types: complete achromatopsia, rod monochromat, which is autosomal recessive, and incomplete achromatopsia, rod monochromat, which is sex-linked recessive or autosomal recessive
   b. Rod monochromat, which has only one type of cone pigment, green, blue, or red; this individual has no color sense but has normal acuity without light sensitivity and without nystagmus and has a normal photopic ERG

Table 16.3.
Classification and Incidence of Color Vision Defects

Color Vision	Inheritance[a]	Incidence in the Male Population
Trichromats		
1. Normal		92.0%
2. Deuteranomalous	X-R	5.0%
3. Protanomalous	X-R	1.0%
4. Tritanomalous	A-D	0.001%
Dichromats		
1. Deuteranopes	X-R	1.0%
2. Protanopes	X-R	1.0%
3. Tritanopes	A-D	0.001%
Monochromats (Achromats)		
1. Typical (rod monochromats)	A-R	0.0001%
2. Atypical (cone monochromats)	X-R	0.000001%

[a]X-R = X-linked recessive
A-D = Autosomal dominant
A-R = Autosomal recessive

They adjust the wavelengths to match the color presented to them. Because they use all three wavelengths, they are called trichromats. The anomaloscope is a research instrument and is rarely used clinically (see "Color Vision Testing," next section).

There are individuals with abnormal color vision who use only two wavelengths to match a color. These are called dichromats. A dichromat may lack red-sensitive pigment, green-sensitive pigment, or blue-sensitive pigment in their cones. (A subject who has a loss of red-sensitive pigment is called a *protanope,* one who has lost green-sensitive pigment is called a *deuteranope,* and one who has lost blue-sensitive pigment is called a *tritanope.*)

There are rare individuals who require only one of the primary wavelengths to match an unknown. These are called monochromats. These do not see any spectral colors and match solely by intensity adjustment. There are two types of monochromats: rod monochromats and cone monochromats.

Rod Monochromats

These patients, who have congenital defects, have generalized cone loss that includes the fovea. They present with poor visual acuity, absent color vision, light sensitivity, and nystagmus. The photopic electroretinogram is abnormal. Macular hypoplasia and macular pigment abnormalities may be present.

There are two forms of rod monochromats: (*a*) complete achromatopsia, which is autosomal recessive; and (*b*) incomplete achromatopsia, which is sex-linked recessive or autosomal recessive. Incomplete achromatopsia rod monochromats tend to have milder visual loss and less color vision disturbance.

Cone Monochromats

These have only one type of cone pigment. There may be a green cone monochromat, a blue cone monochromat, or a red cone monochromat. These subjects have no color sense. However, they have normal visual acuity, no nystagmus, no light sensitivity, and a normal photopic electroretinogram.

Color Vision Testing

There are a number of tests available, many of which detect red/green defects, blue/yellow defects, or both. The tests vary in ease of administration, type of apparatus used, and mode of operation for detecting the defect, color confusion, hue discrimination, matching luminosity, or hue brightness and sensitivity. Color vision tests are:

- AOH-R-R (no longer commercially available);
- Farnsworth-Munsell hundred hue;
- Ishihara;
- Farnsworth's panel-15;
- Nagel's anomaloscope; and
- Sloan's achromatopsia test.

For complete color vision testing, it is suggested that the Farnsworth panel-D15 and the Ishihara test be used in combination.

Color vision testing is recommended for:

- All children as early as they can be tested;
- All patients on the initial office visit;
- Patients with symptoms of difference in color perception between the two eyes;
- All patients with unexplained decreased visual acuity; and
- All patients referred for color vision testing (military, employment situation, school screening test).

COMPUTED TOMOGRAPHY IN OPHTHALMOLOGY

Computed tomographic (CT) scans have greatly enhanced diagnosis in ophthalmology (Fig. 16.19). In the eye, imaging can show:

- Colobomas;
- Persistent hyperplastic primary vitreous;
- Optic disc drusen;
- Astrocytic hamartoma;
- Choroidal osteoma;
- Intraocular foreign bodies; and
- Ocular neoplasms.

In the orbit, CT scans can aid in evaluation of:

- Orbital inflammatory disease;
- Orbital tumors;
- Enlargement of ocular muscles;
- Orbital pseudotumor;
- Lacrimal gland enlargement;
- Optic nerve thickening;
- Evaluation of paranasal sinuses;
- Blow-out fracture;
- Cellulitis.

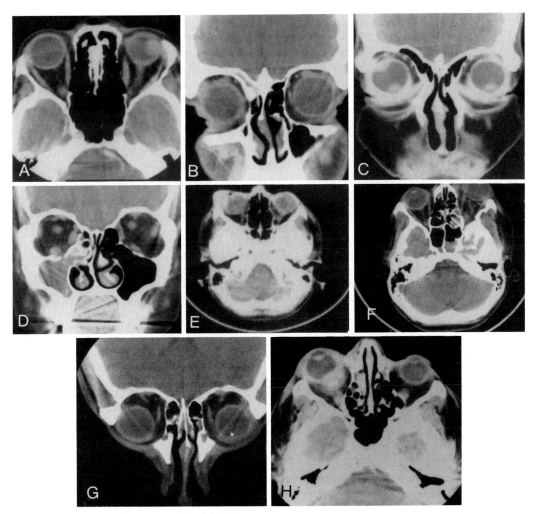

Figure 16.19.   A, Intraocular melanoma on CT scanning showing as a whitish mass inside the left globe. Extension into the orbit is illustrated. **B,** Fibrous dysplasia demonstrated by CT scanning with bony orbital changes illustrated on the patient's right side. **C,** The intraocular melanoma can be seen in the superior portion of the patient's right eye. **D,** Blow-out fracture of the right inferior orbit as demonstrated by CT scan. An inferior defect in the right orbital floor can be seen with prolapse of the contents. The maxillary sinus is also clouded. Blow-out fractures are usually due to large object injury to the orbital area (for example, with a fist or ball). **E,** A hemangioma of the right orbit as demonstrated by CT scanning. In the patient's right eye, swelling next to the globe is demonstrated. **F,** Fracture of the left orbital rim is illustrated. The globe is proptotic, and soft tissue swelling and changes can be noted in the orbit and around the globe. **G,** Intraocular foreign bodies can be demonstrated by CT scanning. Here is illustrated a metallic foreign body in the anterior portion of the globe. **H,** An orbital mass with proptosis is demonstrated in the right orbit of this patient. A retrobulbar mass is pushing the globe forward. The origin of the mass was not determined. (Credit: George Alker, M.D.)

In addition, CT scans have proved helpful in evaluating the cavernous sinus, the optic nerve (glioma), meningioma, metastasis, leukemia, optic neuritis, sarcoidosis, orbital pseudotumor, and the optic chiasm. The postchiasmal visual pathways can also be evaluated for vascular infarctions, arteriovenous malformations, brain abscesses, and demyelination.

CONGENITAL HEREDITARY ENDOTHELIAL DYSTROPHY (CHED)

Clinical Appearance

There is diffuse ground glass opacification of the corneal stroma. The cornea may be 4 times normal thickness. The epithelium has little change despite the presence of gross stromal edema. Corneal sensation is normal. Vascularization is unusual.

Histopathology

There are rare to absent endothelial cells. Descemet's membrane is increased in thickness.

Progression

The vision can be severely affected depending upon the degree of corneal edema and clouding. Results of penetrating keratoplasty are poor in these patients.

Heredity

This dystrophy has been seen as both dominant and recessive inheritance. There is a high risk of disease occurring in offspring, and genetic counseling is important.

CONGENITAL STATIONARY NIGHT BLINDNESS

Congenital stationary night blindness is characterized by the onset of night blindness during infancy. There are five types: (*a*) autosomal dominant type, (*b*) autosomal recessive form, (*c*) X-linked recessive form, (*d*) fundus albipunctatus, and (*e*) Oguchi's disease. Only fundus albipunctatus and Oguchi's disease have abnormal-appearing fundi.

The ERG shows abnormalities (scotopic ERG decreased or not present). Visual fields are normal.

CONJUNCTIVAL PIGMENTED NEVUS

Nevus is a tumor (hamartoma) composed of dermal melanocytes (nevus cells). Conjunctival nevus is the most common conjunctival tumor.

The conjunctival nevus (Fig. 6.20) is congenital, although pigmentation may not occur until late childhood or early adulthood. The nevus is a discrete brown lesion; approximately 50% of the time the nevus is cystic. The pigmentation varies. With conjunctival movement, the lesion also

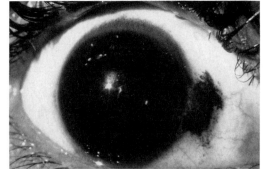

Figure 16.20. Conjunctival pigmented nevus. The darkly pigmented lesion to the outer side of the eye is a pigmented nevus. The diagnosis is suggested by clinical characteristics and is established by biopsy. (Credit: Ted Wojno, M.D.)

moves. These nevi do not grow. The uvea and skin are not involved in conjunctival nevi. Most conjunctival nevi have low or no malignant potential.

In the differential diagnosis, many other conditions must be considered. Congenital ocular melanocytosis (melanosis oculi) is a congenital lesion that shows as diffuse blue or slate-gray sclera. No cysts are present. The lesion will not move with conjunctival movement. When the skin is involved, this lesion is also known as the nevus of Ota. It is most common in blacks and orientals. It is usually unilateral, may be associated with an uveal nevus, and is a differential diagnosis for heterochromia (page 301) for that reason. When the condition occurs in whites, it is potentially malignant.

Primary acquired melanosis (precancerous and cancerous melanosis) occurs in middle age. It has a diffuse brown appearance and moves with conjunctiva movement. This tends to change in appearance as opposed to conjunctival nevi and congenital ocular melanocytosis. Uvea and skin are not involved.

CORECTOPIA

Corectopia is a congenital abnormality of the iris. The pupil is displaced from its normal central location (Fig. 6.21).

CORNEAL STAPHYLOMA (CONGENITAL ANTERIOR STAPHYLOMA)

Posterior corneal defects may present with protrusion of the ectatic cornea with loss of identifiable anterior chamber structures. No Descemet's membrane or endothelium is

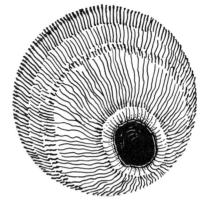

Figure 16.21.   Congenital displacement of the pupil from its normal central position is called corectopia.

seen. The iris is atrophic and is lined on the posterior cornea. The lens is shrunken and abnormal in shape. Vitreous strands and ciliary epithelium are adherent to the lens. This is a part of the anterior chamber cleavage syndrome (page 252).

COTTON-WOOL SPOTS: DIAGNOSTIC FEATURES[a]

Aids

- Clustered in the posterior pole
- Transient; resolve over a period of 4 to 6 weeks
- Correspond to capillary dropout as seen by fluorescein angiography
- Well demarcated
- Superficially located

Cytomegalovirus Retinitis

- Fluffy edges
- Lie deep
- Increase in size on repeated observations

---

[a]Adapted from Mansour, A. M., et al.: Arch Ophthalmol 106:1074–1077, 1988.

Diabetes

- Commonly seen in as many as 44% of patients
- Uncommon once proliferative retinopathy starts
- Concentrated in the posterior pole
- Usually within 3 disc diameters of the optic disc
- Size from .1 to 1 mm
- Average about five per eye with a range of 1 to 20
- Associated with early finding
- Cause—capillary occlusion at sight of formation of microaneurysm

Hypertension

- Close to arteries
- Clear rapidly in 4 to 6 weeks
- Antihypertensive treatment decreases the duration of cotton-wool spots.
- All cotton-wool spots and hypertension disappear within 6 months.

Central Retinal Vein Occlusion

- Large cotton-wool spots
- Spots tend to be confluent

COWS

COWS is a mnemonic for remembering how water, when irrigated into the ear canal, produces certain types of oscillatory eye movements (nystagmus). The response differs when cold water or warm water is used. When warm or cold water is instilled, the oscillations have a fast phase to one side and a returning slow phase. With cold water, the fast phase is to the side opposite the irrigation. With warm water, the fast phase is to the side of irrigation. To remember this, COWS is used (**C**old—**O**pposite, **W**arm—**S**ame).

CREUTZFELDT-JAKOB DISEASE

Creutzfeldt-Jakob disease is due to a slow virus with a long incubation period. It is a rapidly progressive disease that is fatal. It is a disease of gray matter and is characterized by dementia, myoclonus, ataxia, and variable neurologic signs.

Creutzfeldt-Jakob disease is of interest in ophthalmology because it has been known to be transmitted in corneal tissue used for corneal transplantation.

CROUZON'S SYNDROME (CRANIOFACIAL DYSOSTOSIS)

This craniofacial dysostosis (craniostenosis) syndrome is due to early closure of cranial sutures. The cranial facial deformities produce *shallow orbits* with *proptotic globes. Optic atrophy* may be seen secondary to hydrocephalus.

Muscle imbalance is regularly seen in these patients. They have V syndromes (page 258) where the pupil axes are farther apart (divergent) in upgaze and closer (convergent) in downgaze. Crouzon's syndrome is closely related to Apert's syndrome (page 255) but does not have the syndactyly associated with Apert's syndrome.

CUSHING'S SYNDROME OF THE OPTIC CHIASM

Cushing's syndrome of the optic chiasm is characterized by:

- Bitemporal hemianopsia;
- Bilateral optic atrophy;
- Normal skull films.

Causes:

- Suprasellar meningioma;
- Aneurysm;
- Craniopharyngioma.

CYSTICERCOSIS

Diagnosis

The diagnosis is suggested by a cyst either in the vitreous or in the posterior pole of the eye. Hemorrhages, as well as detachment, may occur in the retina around the cyst. A definite diagnosis is made by microscopic examination of the involved area.

Cause

Cysticercosis is caused by *Taenia solium* or by the pork tapeworm, *Cysticercus cellulosae.* There is a systemic infection when the ovum is ingested. Larvi penetrate the intestinal wall and then migrate to the orbit and eye. The larvi change into worms. Worms in the vitreous remain alive and mobile for a time and have been observed in motion in the eye.

CYSTINOSIS

Cystinosis is an autosomal recessive disease. Cystinosis occurs in childhood and is associated with Panconis' syndrome (renal tubular dysfunction with glucosuria, amino acid aminoaciduria, phosphaturia, and renal tubular acidosis). Death usually occurs during childhood.

Ocular Changes

Cystine crystals may be deposited in the cornea and conjunctiva. They are glistening, needle-like to rectangular crystals in the anterior stroma. They tend to be deposited more toward the periphery. They are associated with intense light sensitivity.

Cause

Cystinosis is due to an ineffective lysosomal cystine transport system.

CYSTOID MACULAR EDEMA (CME)

Cystoid macular edema is a nonspecific phenomenon. It may be associated with occlusive, degenerative, inflammatory, or infiltrative disease. It occurs relatively frequently after operations.

Classification

Angiographic cystoid macular edema refers to patients who exhibit no significant visual acuity reduction or symptoms but show fluorescein leakage on a fluorescein angiogram (Fig. 16.22). This has most often been observed after cataract extraction and may occur in as many as 40 to 70% of patients after intracapsular extraction. Extracapsular extraction has a lower prevalence of angiographic CME, approximately 10 to 20%.

Clinical CME causes a significant reduction in vision. It occurs in approximately 1 to 3% of patients more than 1 year after cataract surgery.

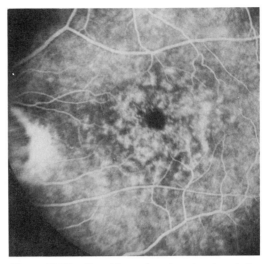

Figure 16.22. Cystoid macular edema is edema in the macular region. It occurs with many types of inflammation and after surgery. A fluorescein angiogram, demonstrated here, has a pattern of a flower petal. Limited cystoid macular edema changes may be demonstrable only by fluorescein angiography. (Credit: Paul Sternberg, M.D.)

Diagnosis

Clinical cystoid macular edema is diagnosed using the slitlamp with a Hruby, Volk, or fundus contact lens. Prominent cyst or perifoveal thickening is seen. Loss of the normal foveal depression and a yellow spot can be seen deep in the retina within the foveal area. The transparent cystic spaces around the fovea are separated by semitranslucent walls. As CME resolves, there may be residual thickening and grayish discoloration of the retina.

The CME following cataract extraction may be associated with iritis, a cloudy vitreous, corneal edema, and glaucoma. CME is thought to be more severe in patients with systemic vascular diseases such as hypertension and diabetes mellitus. It is also thought that people with blue eyes and those who are young are more susceptible.

CYTOMEGALOVIRUS RETINITIS

Cause

This retinitis is caused by the cytomegalovirus, a DNA virus of the herpesvirus group.

Characteristics

Ophthalmoscopy shows a clear separation between involved and uninvolved areas of the retina. Involved areas have opaque white coloration with multiple intraretinal hemorrhages. After the acute phase, a diffuse atrophy occurs and migration affects pigment epithelium and retina.

Prognosis

Loss of vision results from retinal degeneration and macular changes. Retinal breaks occur, and retinal detachment may result.

Laboratory Diagnosis

The virus can be cultured from the urine, from serum, and from tears. It can also be cultured from intraocular specimens—aqueous and subretinal fluid.
(See also AIDS, page 134.)

DACRYOGRAM (DACRYOCYSTOGRAPHY)

Use

This is an x-ray technique with radiopaque dye that is injected into the nasal lacrimal system (page 194). It is a test for an open tear duct and normal drainage.

Technique

The patient is placed in front of an x-ray unit, and the eye is anesthetized with a topical anesthetic. Each punctum is widened with a punctum dilater and irrigated with saline. After an initial baseline x-ray film, radiopaque dye is injected through the punctum into the lacrimal system. Both the involved side and then the normal side receive injections.

Positive Test

If there is retention of contrast medium in the nasal lacrimal system after 30 minutes, a functional blockage is present.

DANTROLENE SODIUM

Dantrolene sodium is used in the treatment of malignant hyperthermia (page 316). It completely inhibits the abnormal rigidity induced in malignant hyperthermia by halothane and succinylcholine. Because it has a high lipid solubility, dantrolene sodium crosses cell membranes easily and then lowers calcium levels. It has no effect on cardiac or smooth muscles at therapeutic levels.

The drug is important in ophthalmology because there is a higher incidence of malignant hyperthermia in patients with strabismus (crossed eyes) who need general anesthesia for surgery.

DARK ADAPTATION

The eye is capable of amazing adjustments (10 to 11 logarithmic units) to changes in light intensity. The photoreceptors in the retina, the rods and cones (page 63), both adapt; however, the sensitivity of the cones is 1000 times less than that of the rods. The process of these cells adjusting when illumination is changed from an intense bleaching light to total darkness can be measured. The process is called adaptometry, and the instrument used is a dark adaptometer.

There are well-known conditions associated with abnormalities in dark adaptation:

- Retinitis pigmentosa;
- Macular edema associated with diabetic retinopathy;
- Progressive cone-rod dystrophies (advanced).

DERMATOCHALASIS

Dermatochalasis, an excess of eyelid skin, causes the baggy lids often associated with old or late middle age (Fig. 16.23). The lid crease becomes indistinct, the brow droops, and the lid drops (ptosis). The appearance of protrusion or bags is caused by normal orbital fat bulging forward through a weakened orbital septum.

Patients may have symptoms. The

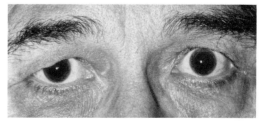

Figure 16.23.   Dermatochalasis is excessive skin, usually on the upper lid. The skin may become so redundant as to hang down in folds. The superior visual field may be obscured. (Credit: Ted Wojno, M.D.)

visual field decreases as the lid falls over vision, and lashes may be present in the line of vision. Patients may also feel heaviness of the lids and ache in the brow.

DERMOIDS

Dermoids are congenital tumors (choristomas) usually located at the inferior temporal limbus (Fig. 16.24). They can involve the cornea, sclera, and bulbar conjunctiva.

Dermoids vary in appearance. They are white to yellow, raised growths. They may appear as multiple masses and may be large enough to obscure the entire cornea. When limited to the cornea, the masses are keratinized epithelium with fatty tissue that contains hair follicles and sebaceous and sweat glands. At times, dermoids may have visible hair.

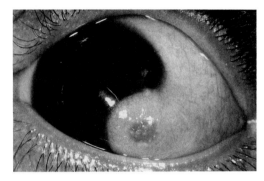

Figure 16.24. This dermoid, which is at the limbus, is in the inferior temporal quadrant, a common position. Centrally, the dermoid contains hair follicles.

Limbal dermoids are associated with developmental anomalies in one-third of patients. The most common anomaly is Goldenhar's syndrome (page 296).

DISTICHIASIS (DISTICHIA)

Distichiasis is a second row of lashes closer to the eye on the lid surface than normal lashes. The second row of lashes is about where the meibomian gland openings are usually found. Most patients are asymptomatic. When the lashes touch the cornea, however, irritation and eventually ulceration can occur.

DOLL'S HEAD MANEUVER (OCULOCEPHALIC MANEUVER)

Doll's head maneuver is used in patients with gaze palsy. If the eyes can be made to deviate into the paretic field of gaze, a supranuclear lesion is present.

To perform a doll's head maneuver, the patient fixates on an object and the head is rotated opposite the paretic field of gaze. A positive test is when, with head rotation, the eyes move to a position not possible on command.

DRUG ABUSE AND EYE SIGNS

Any addictive drugs affect the central nervous system and the eye. For that reason, ocular changes can suggest drug abuse. The following are signs associated with specific drugs:

- Conjunctival and episcleral vessel congestion—marijuana, alcohol, benzodiazepines;
- Miotic pupil—heroin;
- Dilated pupil—cocaine and amphetamines;
- Nystagmus—marijuana, alcohol, and phencyclidine.

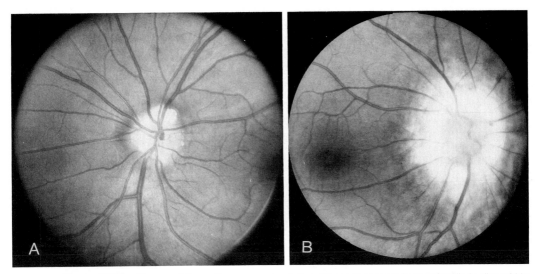

Figure 16.25. Drusen of the optic nerve are common. They are seen as hyperrefractile bodies within the nerve tissue. Drusen may be buried or may be visible, as illustrated in **A.** Optic nerve drusen may be multiple. In **B,** the optic nerve appears enlarged. This is one of the reasons that optic nerve drusen may be mistaken for papilledema, and they are therefore part of the differential diagnosis of pseudopapilledema. (Credit: Paul Sternberg, M.D.)

DRUSEN OF THE OPTIC NERVE

Appearance

These are found before the scleral lamina cribrosa. They vary in size and shape and may be buried beneath the nerve tissue or may be visible. They sometimes present as pseudopapilledema. Optic nerve drusen may be associated with field defects, although loss of central visual acuity is rare. For the most part, these drusen are asymptomatic and without secondary complications, although hemorrhage has been reported.

Differential Diagnosis

Giant drusen of the optic nerve (Fig. 16.25) are astrocytic hamartomas, which are most often associated with tuberous sclerosis. Clinically, drusen at the optic disc are fairly common. Most patients with drusen do not have the giant drusen associated with tuberous sclerosis (page 170).

DUOCHROME TEST

Principle

A white light source focused directly on the retina is actually not a distinct point but a slightly blurred point because of the various color components that make up white light. For example, the shorter wavelengths in the green spectrum of the white light source focus in front of the retina, and the longer wavelengths, such as red, focus behind the retina.

Use of the Principle

The accuracy of the spherical correction can be tested by using this principle of wavelengths focused at different points. By placing a Snellen chart in a half red field on one side and a half green field on the other, the patient can be asked to determine when the letters in the red and those in the green are of equal clarity. This provides endpoints to indicate that the refracted rays in the middle of the spectrum (that is, those wavelengths between the red and green) are focused on the retina.

If the patient sees letters in the red part of the chart clearer, minus lenses are added until there is a balance. If the patient sees letters clearer in the green, plus lenses are added until there is a balance.

Disadvantages of the Test

1. The test does not relax accommodation. Therefore, if accommodation is in play, as it might be in hyperopia, the test may be inaccurate. The test is most useful in myopes.

2. Visual acuity must be better than 20/40 to use the test. At poorer visual acuities, the differences between the red and the green become indistinguishable.

Interesting Aspects of the Test

As the duochrome test depends upon a chromatic aberration of the human lens system, it is not dependent upon color discrimination of the retina. The test can be used in the color-blind eye.

The difference between the red focus and the green focus on the duochrome test as clinically applied is about 0.75 diopters. The midpoint between these two is approximately 0.36 diopters either from the red or the green.

EATON-LAMBERT SYNDROME (MYASTHENIA SYNDROME)

This general syndrome occurs in patients with bronchiogenic carcinoma. Ocular signs are infrequent and consist of *ptosis* and *ophthalmoplegia* when present. In general, there is a weakness of skeletal muscles. Electromyographic findings are diagnostic.

ECTOPIA LENTIS (LENS DISLOCATION)

Mechanism

The lens is normally held in position by zonules. Destruction or absence of the zonules may cause the lens to move from its normal position behind the pupil.

Two Types of Ectopia Lentis

Congenital Dislocation

Congenital dislocation of the lens is most often associated with either Marfan's syndrome or homocystinuria. The position of the lens aids in diagnosis.

- Marfan's syndrome—Lens is typically dislocated up and out (superior and temporal).
- Homocystinuria—Lens is typically dislocated down and in (medially and inferiorly).

Acquired Dislocation

The most common cause of acquired dislocation of the lens is trauma. Syphilis is a rare cause for acquired dislocation.

EHLERS-DANLOS SYNDROME

Ehlers-Danlos syndrome results from a defect in the organization of collagen fibers. Patients have hyperextensibility of joints, flat feet, and kyphoscoliosis.

Ocular manifestations are variable: *blue sclera, keratoconus,* and *angioid streaks* are the most important. Microcornea and myopia also occur (Fig. 16.26).

ELSCHNIG'S PEARLS

When the lens capsule is disrupted and left within the eye, as is common after extracapsular cataract surgery, the lens fibers that remain proliferate. At times, they may form pearl-

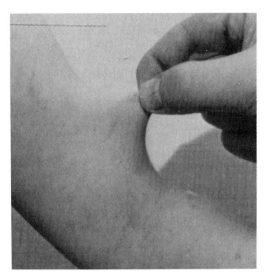

Figure 16.26. The hyperelasticity of the skin seen in Erhlos-Danlos syndrome. (Credit: George Waring, M.D.)

like excrescences, which are known as Elschnig's pearls. Pearls are usually seen on the thick and fibrotic posterior capsule. Although seen in the periphery, they are much more commonly seen toward the center of an intact posterior lens capsule.

ENDOTHELIAL CELL COUNT AND SPECULAR MICROSCOPY

Specular microscopy is a technique where a light source is directed through the cornea and a microscope is used to focus on the endothelium. This allows illumination of the endothelium (Fig. 16.27).

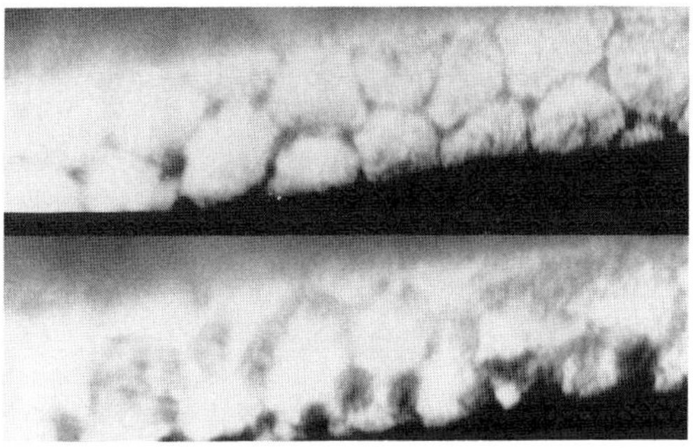

The normal endothelial cell count in the young person is 3000 to 3500 cells per mm^2. In old age, this decreases to approximately 2000 cells per mm^2. With age, the size and shape of the endothelial cell change. In youth, cells tend to be uniform and five-sided in appearance.

In general, function does not cor-

Figure 16.27. The endothelium as seen by spectromicroscopy. The endothelial cells show as multisided, usually pentagonal, cells. In healthy individuals, they have a uniform size and the shape varies little. These rabbit cells have been stressed in the laboratory and show intercellular changes with vacuolization. In humans, the number of cells per unit area also changes with age, after surgical procedures, and with ocular stresses such as trauma and inflammation.

relate well with the number of cells. For example, 400 cells per mm^2 have been seen with clear corneal grafts. Still the technique is useful, especially in surgical decisions. It is thought that a cell count of less than 1000 cells per mm^2 represents an increased risk of corneal decompensation after surgery.

Surgical results can also be monitored by specular microscopy. For example, after intracapsular cataract extraction, the cell loss is between 4 and 21%. The technique of phacoemulsification tends to have higher cell count loss than other techniques. Specular microscopy is used to monitor certain types of techniques and adjust surgical procedures.

Specular microscopy has also been used to evaluate donor tissue endothelium for corneal transplantation.

EPINEPHRINE COMPLICATIONS

Topical epinephrine, used primarily to treat glaucoma, can result in four significant complications:

- *Pigment deposits*—Oxidation products of epinephrine can result in pigmented conjunctival and corneal deposits.
- Epinephrine can cause *canalicular obstruction.*
- *Cystoid macular edema* in patients without the crystalline lens (aphakic). Cystoid macular edema is reversible when the epinephrine is stopped.
- Cardiovascular effects—Epinephrine can cause *palpitation, tachycardia,* and *faintness.* However, serious cardiovascular complications are not caused by topical administration.

EPSTEIN-BARR VIRUS INFECTIONS

Serologic confirmation of Epstein-Barr virus antibodies approaches 100% by the end of the 3rd decade. The Epstein-Barr virus has recently been implicated in a number of ocular infections. It has been associated with stromal keratitis and has been cultured from conjunctival and tear samples. In acute systemic Epstein-Barr virus infections, a follicular conjunctivitis (page 21) is seen in up to one-third of cases.

Posterior ocular involvement associated with Epstein-Barr virus antibodies has been reported as multifocal choroiditis, pigment epithelial disturbances, and vitreous cellular infiltrate.

ERYTHEMA MULTIFORME

Cause

This is an acute hypersensitivity reaction that frequently follows the administration of drugs such as sulphonamides but also occurs after bacterial and viral infections.

Characteristics

The onset is acute. The entire condition lasts 2 to 3 weeks. It tends to be a disease of the young, rarely occurring after the age of 35.

Skin Lesions

Erythema multiforme starts on the arms and legs (extensor surfaces) and spreads to involve the trunk. The lesions are red (erythema) surrounding a pale center. The center may ulcerate, giving a target appearance. The skin lesions heal without scarring.

Ocular Changes

There is an associated conjunctivitis that is bilateral and causes pain and irritation. Patients are light-sensitive. There is a discharge from the ocular surface.

The cornea may be affected secondary to the conjunctival involvement. In late stages, the cornea may vascularize and scar, with severe reduction of vision. Pseudo-membranes (page 22) may occur with this condition.

Mucous Membrane Involvement in the Mouth

Extensive oral ulcerations can occur on the upper and lower lips.

Conjunctival Ulcerations

When pseudomembranes form, there may be ulcerative changes in the conjunctiva. These ulcerative changes are followed by scar formation. The scarring causes a number of complications, including dry eye, because the scarred conjunctiva does not contribute normal amounts of mucus to the tear film, because of abnormal lash growth (trichiasis), and because of inturning of lid (entropion) due to scarring.

Symblepharon is also seen with this condition. Symblepharon is a fibrous band bridging the conjunctiva on the lid to the conjunctiva on the globe. Symblepharon near the nasal portion of the eye can involve the tear drainage system (lower punctum). The conjunctival smears in this condition show polymorphonuclear cells.

ESTHESIOMETER

An esthesiometer is a device that measures the degree of pressure required for a small, thin hair to produce sensation on the cornea. Most clinicians simply use a cotton-tipped applicator pulled up in a wisp and touched to the cornea to observe clinically the degree of corneal sensation present (page 5). The esthesiometer provides quantitation of the response and therefore a more accurate measure of corneal sensitivity.

EXFOLIATION SYNDROME (PSEUDOEXFOLIATION)

Characteristics

Exfoliation affects elderly individuals and may be either unilateral or bilateral. It is found in 3 to 12% of patients with glaucoma.

Most patients with exfoliation do not have glaucoma. However, most patients with the syndrome will demonstrate some elevation of intraocular pressure.

Diagnosis

- *Exfoliation material.* Dandruff-like flakes are seen on the edge of the pupillary margin. Small flakes are deposited on the zonules, on the ciliary processes, and in the chamber angle.
- Disk on the lens. Diagnosis of *lens changes* is best made with a dilated pupil, which reveals an irregular, translucent disk on the lens about the size of the undilated pupil. This central zone is surrounded by a clear zone and then there is a more peripheral, granular zone, giving the appearance of a disk.
- Gonioscopy. By gonioscopy, flakes of exfoliative material are seen and there is a general *increase in pigmentation* of the angle, especially on or around Schwalbe's line.
- *Sampaolesi's line.* A pigmented line near Schwalbe's line is characteristic but not exclusively diagnostic.

EXOPHTHALMOMETER

Forward displacement of the globe (proptosis) can indicate the presence or, more importantly, the progression of a disease process such as Graves' opthalmopathy or tumor. To measure the position of the eye, one uses the lateral orbital rim as a constant reference point for the measurement of the most forward plane of the open eye, the cornea.

The instrument most often used to measure forward displacement is the exophthalmometer (Fig. 16.28). This is an expandable metal bar with a grove on each end that fits on the lateral bony ridges of the orbits. By use of multiple mirrors, the examiner can see and measure on a superimposed scale (Fig. 16.29) the distance of the forward projection of each eye. The examiner stands in front of the patient, although the mirrors will provide a side view image of each eye.

There is both considerable racial and slight sex variation in the absolute measurement of forward eye position. Consider these guidelines. Measurements higher than those noted should suggest abnormal forward displacement of the globe.

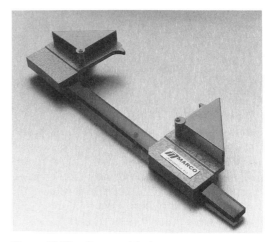

Figure 16.28. The exophthalmometer is used to determine the degree of forward displacement of the eyes. The bony orbital rim is used as a reference point. The instrument is especially useful in following Graves' ophthalmopathy, which often coexists with thyroid disease.

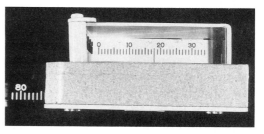

Figure 16.29. Exophthalmometer scale reading. A white card has been inserted to show the scale. Normally, with the card removed, the eye, by a system of mirrors, would be superimposed so that the displacement could be read by determining where the front edge of cornea reflects on the mirror.

Average Measurements

- White males—above 22 mm
- White females—above 20 mm
- Black males—above 25 mm
- Black females—above 23 mm

More important are *differences of 2 mm or more* between eyes or a *progressive increase* in the displacement of an eye as measured at different times, usually over a period of months.

EXUDATES, RETINAL

Retinal exudates are deposits containing fatty components and lipid-filled macrophages. These deposits are associated with chronic edema, which is caused by leakage from abnormal capillaries.

Exudates appear yellow-white against the orange-red background of the pigment epithelium and choroid. They are usually small, discrete spots of varying sizes and shapes. They form in patterns—circinate (ring-like), scattered (diffuse), or radiating to form a macular star. These patterns are caused by both the difference in anatomy between the macula and retina and the varying causes and positions of the edema. No pattern, however, is unique to any one disease process.

Exudates tend to form at the junction of normal and abnormal capillaries. Normal capillaries are impermeable, but abnormal capillaries freely transfer plasma through their walls. Normal capillaries absorb water but not the other plasma constituents that have been released through abnormal capillary walls. Fatty plasma deposits remain. The concentration of these plasma constituents appears as retinal exudates.

Retinal vein occlusion, diabetes, and telangiectasia cause retinal edema adjacent to normal capillaries forming exudates. However, as might be expected, the edema that forms with inflammation of the retina is formed by a different mechanism and is not associated with exudates.

Most exudates will not affect vision. However, exudates in the macula, especially when they appear as solid plaques, are frequently associated with loss of central vision. Exudates will resolve if the recovery of the capillary endothelium is complete. Retinal exudates are also called fatty exudates, hard exudates, and chronic retinal edema. [See also Cotton-wool spots (page 158); Cytoid bodies (page 162); Cystoid macular edema (page 281).]

(Exudates can be seen in Figs. C.9 and C.10.)

FABRY'S DISEASE

Other names

Angiokeratoma corporis diffusum, Anderson-Fabry disease

Ophthalmic Characteristics

Very specific *subepithelial corneal deposits* occur at the level of Bowman's membrane in Fabry's disease. They appear as whorl-like corneal opacities that radiate from the center of the cornea. They are most often in the *lower portions of the cornea.* They range in color from cream to white to golden brown. Vision is usually not affected in these patients.

Lens changes are also characteristic. There is a *posterior subcapsular cataract* that is linear and radiates in spoke-like deposits often along the posterior sutures of the lens. These finely granular deposits may be white to translucent. They can be missed by direct view and are best seen by retroillumination.

Anterior subcapsular lens deposits are also seen in Fabry's disease. They are most often inferior, wedge-shaped, and near the equator. The wedge is positioned with the base at the equator and the apex near the center of the anterior capsule. These deposits have been described as looking like a "propeller."

Retinal involvement also occurs. The vessels, especially veins, appear tortuous. Crossing changes are also seen where veins may be dilated. These changes may or may not be associated with renal hypertension.

General Changes

Patients have cerebral vascular accidents, renal vascular hypertension, and characteristic angiokeratomas. The angiokeratomas are macular punctate lesions that may be red, blue, or black. They first occur in the bathing trunk area, most densely around the umbilicus. Symptoms of fever, painful extremities, and irregular sweating start in late childhood or early adolescence.

Heredity

Fabry's disease is a *recessive X-linked disorder.*

Cause

Fabry's disease is caused by a deficiency of alpha-galactosidase A, which is a lysosomal hydrolase. The lack of this enzyme causes accumulation of ceramide trihexoside.

FACTITIOUS CONJUNCTIVITIS

Factitious conjunctivitis is self-induced. Patients, usually with obvious psychiatric disturbances, cause ocular tissue inflammation by the insertion of chemicals or foreign matter such as small foreign bodies or organic material to produce the conjunctival reaction. This unusual occurrence should be considered in the differential diagnosis of persistent, unexplained unilateral or bilateral conjunctivitis.

FERRY'S LINE

Ferry's line is a deposition of iron in the superficial corneal epithelium at the edge of filtering blebs after glaucoma filtration surgery (see Iron Lines, page 15).

FIBERS OF HENLE

The fibers of Henle are extensions of the cone cells in the fovea. These fibers run from the cone nuclei to the bipolar cells, where they synapse. The fibers of Henle are unique, creating the distinct histology of the fovea (see page 62).

FISHER'S SYNDROME (MILLER-FISHER SYNDROME)

Guillain-Barré syndrome may present as paresis of vertical or horizontal gaze, ataxia, and areflexia. This presentation is without the weakness or respiratory symptoms that often accompany the Guillain-Barré syndrome. The variant of the Guillain-Barré syndrome is known as Fisher's syndrome.

The ophthalmoparesis may involve either vertical or horizontal gaze but also may present as an internuclear ophthalmoplegia (page 117). The pupils may be normal or dilated. Evidence of denervation hypersensitivity to ⅛% pilocarpine may suggest parasympathetic involvement.

Pathophysiology

This variant of Guillain-Barré syndrome is presumed to be a postviral lymphocyte-mediated demyelination of the nerve roots.

Additional Testing Results

CT and MRI scans are normal. The cerebrospinal fluid protein is often elevated, with little cellular reaction.

FLEISCHER'S RING

Fleischer's ring is a deposit of iron in the superficial corneal epithelium around the base of a keratoconus cone. It has no clinical significance (see Iron Lines, page 15).

FLOPPY EYELID SYNDROME

Patients with the floppy eyelid syndrome are most often obese males in the 2nd or 3rd decade. They complain of a swollen eyelid, irritation of the eye, and blurred vision. Examination shows papillary conjunctivitis and keratinization of the conjunctival surface. The upper tarsus is loose and rubbery and is easily everted (Fig. 16.30).

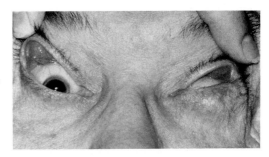

Figure 16.30. Floppy lid is a syndrome primarily found in obese males. It is frequently one-sided and results in inflammatory changes of the conjunctiva due to the excess laxity of the lid. The involved side is usually the one on which the patient sleeps. The condition may be bilateral. (Credit: Ted Wojno, M.D.)

The condition is usually unilateral, and the side involved is the side on which the patient sleeps. Symptoms are worse in the morning.

The fact that it has been reported mostly in males suggests an X-linked inheritance. Although usually associated with obesity, it has generally not been associated with biochemical or inherited disorders.

FOLLICULOSIS

Folliculosis (Fig. 16.31) is a condition where follicles are seen in the conjunctiva with absence of other inflammatory signs such as hyperemia and discharge. This is a form of lymphoid hyperplasia. It may be marked in some children with large follicles on the conjunctival surfaces. The condition is most common from age 4 to 13. No infectious agent has been identified.

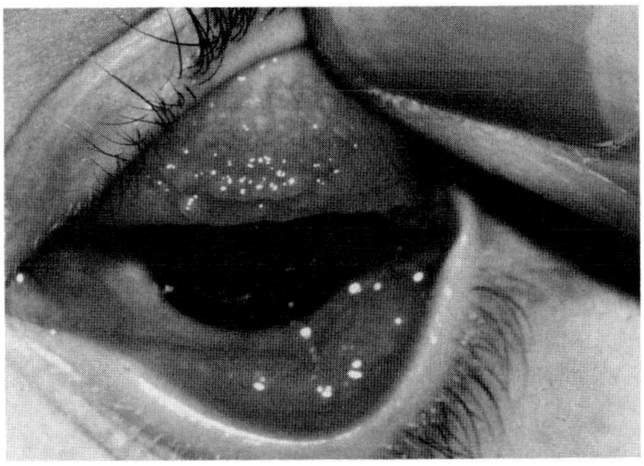

Figure 16.31. Folliculosis occurs in childhood. Follicles are seen on the inferior and superior conjunctival surfaces. This is thought to be a lymphoid hypoplasia. Follicles may become relatively large with minimal symptoms. (Credit: George Waring, M.D.)

FORCED DUCTION TEST

This test is used to evaluate the difference between muscle entrapment (or other restriction) and a paretic muscle. There are different ways of performing the test. In general, a topical or local anesthesia is used. The eye is then grasped with forceps either near the limbus or over the muscle itself. The eye is pushed into the paretic area of gaze. If this can be done easily, the muscle probably has a neurogenic defect. If marked resistance is found, however, the problem is restrictive or mechanical.

FORCED GENERATION TEST

This is a test to judge the amount of contractive force in a muscle. The eye is anesthetized with local or topical anesthesia. The eye is then grasped at the limbus or muscle insertion with forceps. The patient is asked to look in the direction of paretic gaze. The test allows a quantitative judgment of muscle contraction in paretic muscles and also allows determination of normal generated muscle forces when a restriction is present.

FOUR-MIRROR LENS (ZEISS)

This is a gonioscopy (page 44) lens that is unique because there are four viewing mirrors that provide a panoramic view of the chamber angle. This lens is especially useful in the technique of gonioscopy called indentation gonioscopy (page 304).

FOVEOMACULAR VITELLIFORM DYSTROPHY, ADULT TYPE

This is an adult-onset dystrophy that presents with round or oval elevated subfoveal lesions that are approximately one-third disc diameter in size. The color is yellowish. In contrast to a similar-appearing condition described as Best's vitelliform dystrophy, which occurs at an early age, a patient with foveomacular vitelliform dystrophy does not show any abnormalities on the electrooculogram or the electroretinogram and maintains normal color vision.

This dystrophy is caused by atrophy of the outer retina and retinal pigment epithelium in the fovea with accumulation of lipofuscin in the retinal pigment epithelium.

FOVILLE'S SYNDROME

Clinical Signs

Signs are on the same side as the lesion—inability to turn eye out (abduction paralysis), peripheral seventh nerve palsy, Horner's syndrome (page 93), facial hypesthesia, and peripheral deafness.

Cause

Lesion of the pontine tegmentum

FRESNEL PRISMS

A prism has two nonparallel surfaces that form an apical angle. Light entering a prism is deflected toward the base. Prisms are used to deviate light rays or images. Normal prisms tend to be thick and bulky.

A Fresnel prism is a special adaptation of a prism. The Fresnel prism concept is that many small plastic prisms are laid adjacent to each other on a thin platform of plastic. This provides deviation of the image similar to that of a regular prism. However, Fresnel prisms are thin and light. They are made to be pasted on glasses, a feature that makes them widely used.

Fresnel prisms do have disadvantages. They are not as stable as conventional prisms. Contrast may be lost, especially as the prism ages. There is some light scatter, and visual acuity may decrease due to such scattering. Reflections occur in the multiple grooves created by the prisms lying side by side. This is especially true with a prism power of 15 diopters or more.

GALILEAN TELESCOPE

The Galilean telescope has importance in ophthalmology because the magnification produced by this telescope is used in therapy. Principles of Galilean telescopes are also used in the discussion of lens replacement after cataract surgery.

The Galilean telescope has a positive lens (plus lens) and a negative lens (minus lens). The second focal point of the positive lens coincides with the first focal point of the negative lens. The Galilean telescope takes parallel light from a distant object, changes the magnification, and reimages the object at a point in infinity. To obtain a $2\times$ magnification, the focal length of the plus lens must be 10 cm and the focal length of the minus lens must be 5 cm.

GHOST VESSELS IN THE CORNEA

Ghost vessels are vessels that remain in the cornea after inflammation. Although they may be seen directly with the slitlamp, they are best seen by retroillumination using the red reflex. With retroillumination, the vessels appear as hyperreflective, irregular lines in the posterior portion of the stroma or, less frequently, in other parts of the stroma.

Causes of ghost vessels:

- Syphilis;
- Tuberculosis;
- Hansen's disease;
- Cogan's disease;
- Herpes simplex;
- Herpes zoster;
- Mumps;
- Vaccinia;
- Rubeola;
- Variola;
- Chemical burns;
- Onchocerciasis;
- Trypanosomiasis.

GIANT CELLS

Giant cells are large cells with multiple nuclei. They are a sign of granulomatous inflammation. They are also seen with epithelioid cells, plasma cells, and lymphocytes. There are three types of giant cells:

- Langhans' cells (granulomatous processes);
- Foreign body cells; and
- Touton (juvenile xanthogranuloma) cells.

GLAUCOMATOCYCLITIC CRISIS (POSNER-SCHLOSSMAN SYNDROME)

Clinical Presentation

Glaucomatocyclitic crisis presents as *unilateral glaucoma*. The patient has mild discomfort, and there is usually only slight injection of the conjunctiva.

The inflammation in the anterior chamber is also subtle. There are mild flare, occasional cells, and KPs (keratitic precipitates).

The glaucoma that is associated with this mild inflammation may be out of proportion to that which might be expected. Subepithelial corneal edema (microcystic edema) may occur from the increases in intraocular pressure.

Gonioscopy

Gonioscopy shows an open angle, although KPs and precipitates can be seen on the trabecular meshwork. The pupil may be in mid-dilation, in contrast to many other types of anterior chamber inflammation (uveitis), which are associated with small pupils.

Clinical Course

Both the inflammation and the glaucoma are self-limited. The attack resolves spontaneously in a few days to a few weeks. Repeated attacks may occur later in the same eye. Treatment is directed toward control of the inflammation and of the intraocular pressure.

Cause

Unknown

GLAUKOMFLECKEN

Glaukomflecken are irregular white opacities that occur in the anterior portion of the lens in the subcapsular region. These whitish opacities are a diagnostic sign of *angle closure glaucoma.* Additional features of angle closure that may be visible on slitlamp examination when glaukomflecken are present are sector atrophy of the iris, pigment dispersion, and aqueous flare.

GOLDENHAR'S SYNDROME (OCULOAURICULOVERTEBRAL DYSPLASIA)

Ocular features are limbal corneal dermoids, orbital lipodermoids, and notching of the superior lid. Preauricular skin tags are the most prominent childhood feature. Frequent vertebral abnormalities include fused cervical vertebrae, spina bifida, and associated systemic abnormalities (Fig. 16.32).

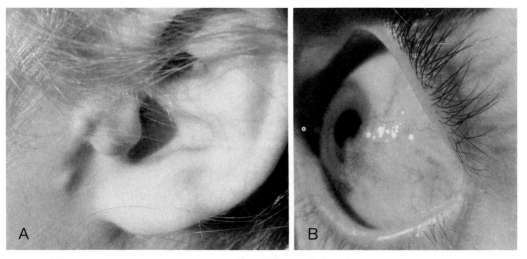

Figure 16.32. Goldenhar's syndrome includes ocular changes of limbal corneal dermoids and orbital ectodermoids and is associated with preauricular tags and vertebral abnormalities. **A,** Preauricular tags are characteristic of Goldenhar's syndrome. **B,** a limbal dermoid that has been partially excised but is in the characteristic inferior temporal position.

GONIOSCOPY—INTERNAL REFLECTION

Definition

Gonioscopy is a technique to examine the anterior chamber angle. It requires a special lens (see page 45).

Explanation

The illuminated chamber angle sends light rays to the cornea. The aqueous/cornea index of refraction is approximately the same so little refraction occurs (see Fig. 3.6). However, at the cornea/air interface, the chamber angle rays are at an angle that is less than the critical angle. Therefore, all rays are internally reflected. The critical angle equals the angle of incidence where the angle of refraction is 90°. Any light rays entering at an angle less than the critical angle will be totally internally reflected (Fig. 16.33).

Gonioscopy lenses, both Goldmann and Koeppe, change the index of refraction of the substance on the cornea from air to glass. This changes the critical angle and prevents total internal reflection of the rays from the chamber angle.

See Snell's law (page 366) and critical angle (Fig. 3.6).

GRADENIGO'S SYNDROME

Gradenigo's syndrome is abducens (sixth cranial nerve) palsy with facial pain. It is caused by petrositis or septic thrombosis of the inferior petrosal sinus.

GUNN'S DOTS

Müller cells are the supporting cells of the retina. They form both the internal limiting membrane and the external limiting membrane. As the inner portion of the cell approaches the vitreous, it forms a foot-

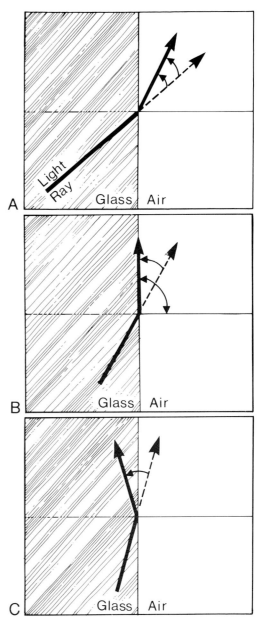

Figure 16.33. Total internal reflection, a principle important in understanding gonioscopy (see page 44). **A,** Snell's law states that, by traveling from a denser to a less dense medium, a new direction occurs. **B,** A critical angle is reached when the angle at which the light ray enters is so acute that the reflected ray follows the interface between the denser and the less dense media. This is the critical angle. When the angle of incidence becomes smaller than the critical angle, total internal reflection occurs. **C,** When total internal reflection is present, no image is seen and it is impossible for light rays to pass the interface between the denser and less dense media.

plate. These footplates can be seen with a direct ophthalmoscope as minute white dots in the posterior pole. These white dots are known as Gunn's dots.

GUNN'S SIGN

When looking at the retinal vessels, one can usually visualize the dark blood in the venous column under the brighter blood of the arterial column. When the arterial wall becomes hyalinized, the wall loses its transparency. The result is a change in the appearance of the vein as it passes underneath the artery. Now the vein appears to taper toward the artery on each side.

Hyalinization of the artery occurs with arteriosclerosis and vascular hypertension. Gunn's sign, therefore, is associated with long-standing hypertension.

Gunn's sign is best seen with the direct ophthalmoscope in the posterior part of the eye but in an area away from where the vessels emerge from the optic disc.

GYRATE ATROPHY

Heredity

Autosomal recessive

Enzyme Deficiency

Gyrate atrophy is due to a deficiency of ornithine aminotransferase. Ornithine plasma levels are 6 to 10 times normal.

Clinical Characteristics

In the retina, large areas with scalloped borders develop because of loss of the retinal pigment epithelium and the choriocapillaris. The retinal pigment epithelium that remains intact shows hyperpigmentation. Both cataracts and myopia are common associations with the retinal changes. The ERG is abnormal.

Patients suffer progressive visual field loss and night blindness. The changes due to this enzyme deficiency are normally restricted to the eye. Only mild systemic effects have been noted, and the lifespan is normal.

HAAB'S STRIAE

Haab's striae are breaks in Descemet's membrane that are seen in primary infantile (congenital) glaucoma (page 55). They are associated with corneal edema, enlarged globe (buphthalmos), and optic nerve cupping.

HARADA'S SYNDROME

See Vogt-Koyanagi-Harada syndrome.

HERPES ZOSTER OPHTHALMICUS

Cause

Herpes zoster is a recurrent varicella virus infection. There are two types: endogenous, which is reactivation of a latent virus from a sensory ganglion, and exogenous, which is caused by direct contact with someone who has an active virus infection.

Predisposing factors include age and immunosuppression. Fifty per cent of people living to age 85 will have had one attack of herpes zoster (dermatologic). Ten per cent will have had two attacks. Herpes zoster is also seen in patients immunosuppressed

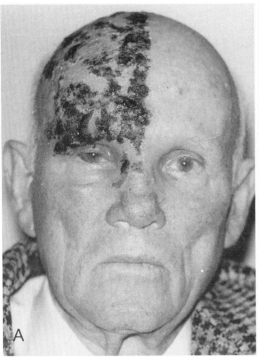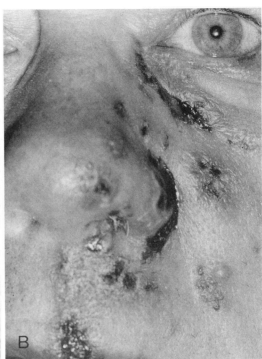

Figure 16.34. Herpes zoster ophthalmicus. Herpes zoster dermatologic changes may be associated with intraocular changes. It is much more common to have intraocular and ocular changes when the nasal ciliary branch is involved. Herpes zoster has characteristic vascular lesions, usually in the distribution of the fifth cranial nerve (**A**). These lesions, which show scaling, are healing. There is one vesicular lesion on the tip of the nose (**B**). Involvement of the tip of the nose, which shows involvement of the nasociliary nerve, is clinically important because there is a higher association of intraocular involvement when this area is involved.

from the acquired immune deficiency syndrome (AIDS), organ transplantation, and blood dyscrasias.

Skin Changes

Skin changes are preceded by malaise and fever. Blisters crust over with hemorrhagic scabs. Pitted scars may be left.

Ocular Changes

Ocular changes are usually related to endogenous reactivation from the trigeminal ganglion. Chicken pox gains access to this sensory ganglion during the primary infection. The fifth cranial nerve and its first division are the most frequently involved.

Ocular involvement is related to the nasal ciliary branch of the fifth nerve (Fig. 16.34). This is the primary sensory nerve to the eyeball. It also provides innervation to the tip of the nose. Dermatologic vesicular involvement of the tip of the nose is often related to ocular inflammation.

Conjunctivitis

Conjunctivitis is secondary to involvement of the lids with a vesicular rash. A follicular reaction may occur.

Keratitis

Keratitis may precede, follow, or occur during the disease process. A diffuse punctate keratitis and at times dendritic ulcers may occur. Corneal sensation may be markedly diminished. Disciform scars may occur. Herpes zoster keratitis has also been associated with Wessely immune rings (page 381). Necrotizing interstitial keratitis with deep neovascularization also occurs. Epithelial breakdown with diffuse stromal edema and inflammation is a destructive complication in some patients.

Iridocyclitis

Intraocular inflammation may occur as in the cornea before, after, or during the dermatologic changes. Intraocular inflammation is characterized by pain, decreased vision, and fine keratotic precipitates. Synechiae may occur.

The iritis with herpes zoster is different than that with herpes simplex. Herpes zoster is a lymphocytic vasculitis whereas herpes simplex is a diffuse lymphocytic infiltrate of the iris.

Glaucoma

Glaucoma occurs from debris clogging the trabecular meshwork. Inflammation of the angle and trabeculitis can also contribute to glaucoma.

HERBERT'S PITS

Herbert's pits are associated with trachoma (page 374). They are depressions in the superior limbal corneal area. The pits are formed by limbal follicular swellings, which then scar to cause the depressions.

HERRING'S LAW (HERRING'S LAW OF MOTOR CORRESPONDENCE)

Concept of Paired Muscles (Yoke Muscles)

In understanding the movement of both eyes together, it becomes obvious that, when one muscle is working to move the eye in one direction, there is another muscle in the opposite eye that works to keep the eye aligned with its fellow. For example, in left downgaze, the right eye is looking down because of the work of the right superior oblique. The left eye is also looking down but because of the work of the left inferior rectus (Table 7.1, page 143).

Herring's Law states that nerve stimulus is equal and simultaneous to those muscles that are paired for movement of both eyes in certain fields of gaze.

Importance of Herring's Law

Herring's law applies to clinical signs when one muscle is paralyzed. With the eyes looking down to the left, the right superior oblique and the left inferior rectus are acting. Nerve stimulus is equal and simultaneous to both muscles. If the right superior oblique is paralyzed, there is an excessive stimulus to compensate both to the paralyzed muscle and its fellow, yoke muscle, the left inferior rectus. The paralyzed muscle does not respond and the normal muscle overresponds, creating vertical imbalance between the eyes.

Herring's law is also important in the understanding of inhibitional palsy of the contralateral antagonist (page 304).

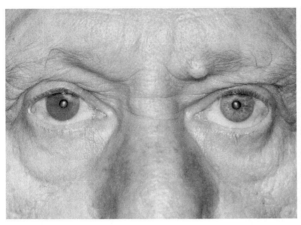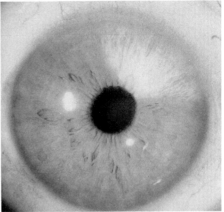

Figure 16.35. Heterochromia and segmental heterochromia. Heterochromia is unequal pigmentation between the two eyes. Heterochromia has multiple causes. For example, the darker eye may have a tumor, such as a melanoma, or, in contrast, the light eye may have Fuchs' heterochromic iridocyclitis or be congenitally depigmented, as is seen with unilateral Horner's syndrome. Segmental heterochromia *(right)* may also occur within the iris. Illustrated is a congenital change, although there are other causes of segmental heterochromia, such as iris tumors.

HETEROCHROMIC IRIDOCYCLITIS (FUCHS' HETEROCHROMIC IRIDOCYCLITIS)

Clinical Presentation

Most typically, the observed signs are heavy keratic precipitates (Fig. C.6) on the posterior portion of the cornea. A hypochromia of the iris (light color to iris) (Fig. 16.35) is seen in the involved eye when compared to the normal side. The light color is due to defects in a posterior iris pigment epithelium. A cataract, which starts in the posterior capsular region of the lens, also occurs in about 70% of patients.

Cause

The exact cause is unknown. It is now thought, however, that this is an immunologic process that may have either (or both) hereditary or infectious precursors.

Complications

Cataract and glaucoma are the most important complications of Fuchs' heterochromic iridocyclitis. The glaucoma is often difficult to manage and may result in significant visual loss.

Corticosteroids

For unknown reasons, corticosteroids are not effective in treating iridocyclitis. For this reason, their use should be restricted if no other indications are present.

HIPPUS

The pupil, when in constant illumination, maintains the same diameter in most patients. However, in some people, wide, rhythmic fluctuations of the pupillary diameter occur when the illumination is unchanged. Both pupils are involved. This phenomenon is known as hippus, and it is not associated with any disease process.

HOLLENHORST PLAQUES

Hollenhorst plaques are small cholesterol emboli that arise from an atheromatous plaque in the carotid artery (Fig. 16.36). These cholesterol emboli, once in the retinal circulation, can lodge at bifurcations of the retinal arterioles. They have a characteristic refractive appearance and may seem to be larger than the vessel in which they are lodged.

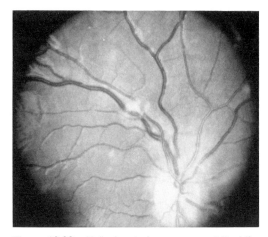

Figure 16.36. Hollenhorst plaques occur at the bifurcations of retinal arterioles. They are cholesterol emboli that arise from atheroma in the carotid artery. (Credit: Paul Sternberg, M.D.)

HRUBY LENS

A Hruby lens is used for focusing the slitlamp into the deeper vitreous, retina, and optic nerve. The Hruby lens is a -40 diopter lens allowing high magnification of the posterior pole. It usually requires dilation of the pupil for use.

HUDSON-STAHLI LINE

The Hudson-Stahli line is a horizontal line due to *iron* deposition in the *corneal epithelium*. It is in the *lower one-third* of the cornea, approximately at the level where the lids close. It is common in elderly individuals (see Iron Lines, page 15).

HUTCHINSON'S TRIAD

Hutchinson's triad is a feature of congenital syphilis that includes *interstitial keratitis* (corneal inflammation), *deafness,* and *notched teeth.*

HYDROPS

See Acute Hydrops (page 13).

ICHTHYOSIS—CORNEAL CHANGES

Definition

Ichthyosis is an inherited X-linked autosomal dominant, recessive, or autosomal hyperkeratotic skin disorder.

Skin

Area of dry and scaly skin cover the entire body (Fig. 16.37). There may be a grayish-brown discoloration in the neck area.

Corneal Changes

Corneal changes occur more often in the X-linked type of ichthyosis. Corneal changes are at the level of pre-Descemet's membrane. They are linear or punctate opacities that appear gray. They are best seen with broad slitlamp illumination. Prominant corneal nerves can be seen.

IDIOPATHIC MACULAR CYST AND HOLE

Characteristics

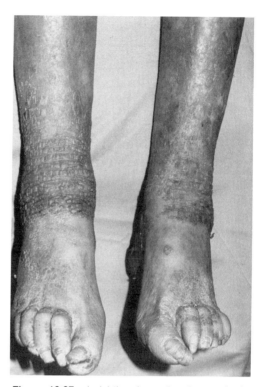

Figure 16.37. In ichthyosis, ocular changes in the cornea are associated with general skin changes. Illustrated are skin changes of ichthyosis in the pretibial area. (Credit: George Waring, M.D.)

Idiopathic macular cyst and hole appear primarily in women aged 60 to 80. The condition is bilateral in 25 to 30% of patients. Patients who have a hole in one eye and a cystic abnormality in the fellow eye have an increased risk of bilateral central vision loss from hole formation.

Cause

The cause of cysts and holes is unknown. Separation of the posterior vitreous has been associated with progression of the cyst to a hole. With rare exceptions, holes do not result in retinal detachment.

Associated Findings

Patients may have associated systemic hypertension. There has also been an association with systemic estrogen therapy.

IDIOPATHIC PRERETINAL MEMBRANE

Symptoms

Patients with idiopathic preretinal membrane experience visual distortion (metamorphopsia) and variable losses of visual acuity.

Characteristics

Idiopathic preretinal membranes can occur secondary to a number of conditions: trauma, intraocular inflammation (uveitis), intraocular surgery, and retinal vascular occlusion. Most membranes do not have clear evidence of a cause. These membranes occur in patients over 50 years of age, with an equal distribution between males and females. Twenty percent are bilateral.

The most important association is posterior vitreous detachment. It is probable that this vitreous detachment dehisces the internal limiting membrane, allowing retinal cells (glial cells) to proliferate along the retinal surface. Contracture of the cellular membrane causes wrinkling and a characteristic "cellophane" appearance of the macula.

Prognosis

Most patients retain useful visual acuity. Only a small percentage (around 25%) will lose more than two lines of vision. Most patients will maintain visual acuity better than 20/50 in the involved eye.

IMBERT-FICK PRINCIPLE

Importance

Applanation tonometry (page 41), the most widely used technique to measure intraocular pressure, is based on the Imbert-Fick principle.

Principle

For an ideal dry, thin-walled sphere, the pressure inside the sphere equals a force necessary to flatten a portion of the sphere divided by the area that is flattened.

Note

The eye does not represent the ideal sphere stated in the principle. There are two major opposing forces. (*a*) The cornea resists flattening, and (*b*) there is a capillary attraction created by the tear film. These two counterforces cancel one another when the applanating surface is 3.06 mm in diameter. The Goldmann applanation tonometer is 3.06 mm in diameter for this reason.

INDENTATION GONIOSCOPY

Indentation gonioscopy is a special technique used to see the chamber angle. Using a gonioprism (usually a four-mirror lens) to see the angle, one applies a gentle pressure against the cornea. This pressure moves the iris back, allowing indentation of the lens iris diaphragm. In the periphery, the iris angle opens, and anatomical structures can be better evaluated.

INHIBITIONAL PALSY OF THE CONTRALATERAL ANTAGONIST

When our eyes move, multiple muscles work. As one muscle increases pull, another muscle relaxes, like two teams in a tug of war.

At any time, the muscles holding both eyes in a certain position of gaze have equal and simultaneous nerve impulses from the central nervous system (see Herring's Law for more detail). To understand the inhibitional palsy of the contralateral antagonist, think of a single muscle that is paretic. The muscle pulling against it requires less nerve stimulus to cause action.

The right superior oblique muscle acts against the right inferior oblique. The right superior oblique pulls the right eye down, and the right inferior oblique pulls it up. When the right superior oblique is paretic, it doesn't take as much central nervous system stimulation to the right inferior oblique to pull the eye up and in. The right inferior oblique has less muscle tone pulling against it. This relates to one eye, the right eye.

Ocular muscles also act in pairs. Because the nonparalyzed muscle does not need as much innervation when the muscle acting opposite to it is paralyzed, the muscle in the other eye acting as a pair with the nonparalyzed muscle will also be affected.

In the example, the left superior rectus is now acting with less innervation because the right superior oblique is paralyzed and less innervation is received by the left inferior oblique. This may make the left superior rectus appear to be nonfunctioning, not because it actually has a paralysis but because its paired muscle in the right eye (inferior oblique) is not receiving the same amount of innervation that it would if the right superior oblique were not paretic.

In essence, muscles have a pull and tug relationship in one eye. Muscles also have a paired function with the opposite eye. If paralysis affects the pull and tug balance, it also affects the paired function. This results in inhibitional palsy of the contralateral antagonist.

INTERNUCLEAR OPHTHALMOPLEGIA

Signs

On gaze to one side, the eye looking toward the nose (adduction) moves slowly or not at all. The eye moving away from the nose has a horizontal to-and-fro motion (nystagmus). Internuclear ophthalmoplegia signs occur when the gaze is away from the side of the lesion.

Location of Abnormality

Injury to the medial longitudinal fasciculus produces internuclear ophthalmoplegia.

Cause

Bilateral internuclear ophthalmoplegia is most often related to the demyelinating disease, multiple sclerosis. However, vascular accidents as well as tumors may occasionally cause internuclear ophthalmoplegia.

IRIDECTOMY

Iridectomies are surgically created defects in the iris. A sector iridectomy is a cut in the iris that involves the stroma as well as the fifth sphincter. Peripheral iridectomies are round or oval homes in the periphery of the iris created by surgery (Fig. 16.38). These iridectomies are usually created by bringing the iris out through a peripheral wound and cutting with scissors.

IRIDOCORNEOENDOTHELIAL SYNDROME

Other Terms

ICE syndrome, essential iris atrophy, iris nevus syndrome, Chandler's syndrome, Cogan-Reese syndrome

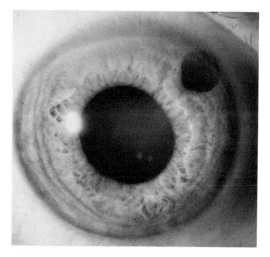

Figure 16.38. An iridectomy is a surgically created hole in the iris. Here the iridectomy shows near the periphery of the iris at the two o'clock position. (Credit: George Waring, M.D.)

Description

A number of individually described and named syndromes are now thought to be part of the iridocorneoendothelial syndrome. In this syndrome, there is progressive atrophy of the iris tissue. Synechiae (peripheral anterior synechiae) scar the areas around the trabecular meshwork, creating glaucoma. There is also endothelial degeneration. Edema of the cornea may occur in the presence of low intraocular pressures. Uncommonly, iris nodules may be a late finding.

IRIDODIALYSIS

An iridodialysis is a tear at the peripheral iris secondary to injury. The pupil may become irregular. Because of the laxity of the iris from a large defect, portions of the iris may fall over the visual axis and occlude vision.

These defects in the iris are almost always related to moderate or severe trauma. They almost always are accompanied by hyphema immediately after the injury (Fig. 16.39).

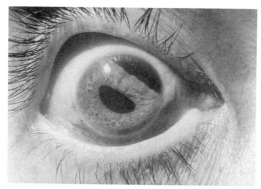

Figure 16.39. Iridodialysis is a tear at the peripheral iris. It is secondary to traumatic injury, usually blunt trauma to the eye. Here the iridodialysis has occurred superiorly and the pupil is irregular because of it.

IRIDOGONIODYSGENESIS

Iridogoniodysgenesis is defined as iris strands in the angle and a hypoplastic anterior iris stroma. All of these eyes have glaucoma. The condition is inherited as an autosomal dominant disorder.

Affected patients may have large corneas (megalocornea), abnormal positioning of the pupil (correctopia), and an indistinct limbus. In general, these are very close to Reiger's anomaly but without the prominent Schwalbe's ring. Most diagnosticians consider this to be a part of the anterior cleavage syndrome (see page 252).

IRIDOTOMY, LASER

An iridotomy is a hole created in the iris. An iridotomy can be created by either the YAG laser or the argon laser. This hole is usually created to relieve the buildup of aqueous (pupillary block) that causes glaucoma. Multiple bursts of the laser destroy tissue until the iris is completely perforated. Laser iridotomies are used to treat narrow angle glaucoma (page 50) as well as pupillary block glaucoma (page 53).

IRIS ABNORMALITIES

Anatomy

The iris tissue forms a diaphragm that opens and closes according to degrees of illumination. Neurologically, the iris is under the control of the sympathetic and parasympathetic systems (page 90–91). Around the pupil is a sphincter muscle. The iris stroma has various pigmentation. Posterior to the iris is a densely pigmented cell layer.

There are a number of iris defects that can be important diagnostically. These have been divided into four categories. They do not represent all possible pupillary abnormalities (see neurologic pupillary abnormalities such as Horner's syndrome, Adie's tonic pupil, and Argyll Robertson pupil).

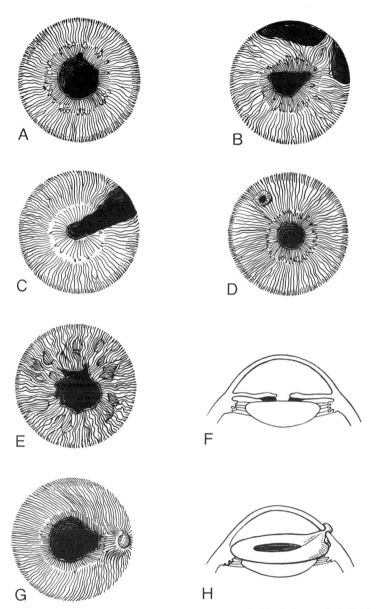

Figure 16.40.   Pupillary abnormalities. Illustrated are certain irregularities in the pupil. **A,** Sphincter tear at the 12 o'clock position. **B,** Iridodialysis with the iris detached at the base. **C,** Sector iridectomy, a surgically created cut in the iris. **D,** Iridotomy, a small, peripheral hole, usually made with a surgical cut or a laser. **E** and **F,** Posterior synechiae secondary to inflammation or trauma. **G** and **H,** Iris prolapse. The iris plugs a corneal perforation. A pear-shaped pupil points toward the perforation. For coloboma and corectopia, see Figures 16.18 and 16.21, respectively.

Traumatic Changes

Sphincter Tear

Figure 16.40A shows a sphincter tear at 12 o'clock. Sphincter tears are usually a result of blunt trauma. They are often associated with hyphema or with traumatic glaucoma, and their presence may help establish a diagnosis when traumatic injury has occurred years before the evaluation.

Iridodialysis

Iridodialysis is a hole or holes created in the pheripheral iris secondary to blunt trauma (Fig. 16.40**B**). Iridodialysis may cause poor pupillary function and may also disrupt the shape and the size of the pupil, affecting vision. Under these circumstances, the defects in the iris may need to be closed. Iridodialysis is almost always associated with hyphema (page 138) and represents moderate to severe injury to the eye.

Surgically Created Abnormalities

Sector Iridectomy

During surgery, especially for cataract, a sector iridectomy may be created. A sector iridectomy (Fig. 16.40**C**) is a cut in the iris that involves the sphincter as well as the iris stroma. These iridectomies have become less common as surgical techniques for cataract removal have changed. Round iridectomies, usually peripheral, do not involve the sphincter and appear similar to laser iridotomies.

Laser Iridotomy

A laser is used to create a hole in the iris. This is known as laser iridotomy (Fig. 16.40**D**). This is most often used to prevent pupillary block glaucoma (page 53). Laser iridotomy can be done with the YAG laser or the argon laser.

Inflammatory Changes

Posterior Synechiae

Posterior synechiae (Fig. 16.40**E**) may result from inflammation due to infection or unknown causes, from disease processes such as sarcoid, or from injury. These posterior synechiae are actually scar tissue between the iris and the lens (Fig. 16.40**F**). The pupil becomes immobile and will not dilate with neurologic or pharmacologic stimulus. The pupillary margins are irregular. If the scar tissue is extensive at the pupillary margin, the aqueous may be trapped behind the iris, causing pupillary block glaucoma (page 53).

Iris Prolapse through a Corneal Defect

When the cornea perforates, either from a ulcer that has eaten through the corneal stroma or from trauma, the iris may draw up and plug the opening. Illustrated is a corneal ulcer with a plug of iris (Fig. 16.40**G** and **H**). This will cause pupillary irregularity with a peaking of the pupil toward the area of perforation. Without magnification, this can be diagnosed as a black or light spot on the cornea with a pear-shaped or peaked pupil.

Congenital Defects

Corectopia

Irregular placement of the pupil is called corectopia (see Fig. 16.21). In the condition, the pupil is off the normal central orientation.

Coloboma

This is a congenital failure of closure of the fetal fissure. The position is typically inferior. Iris colobomas may also be associated with colobomas of other parts of the eye, including the choroid and at times the lens (see Coloboma, Fig. 16.18).

IRIS CYSTS

Iris cysts arise from the epithelial layers of the iris and ciliary body or less often from the stroma. The majority of cysts remain stationary. However, progres-

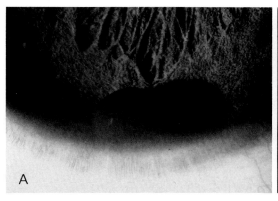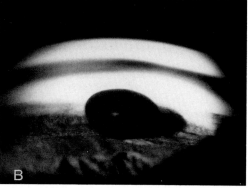

Figure 16.41.   A, This is a cyst of the iris, which may grow and cause glaucoma. **B,** By gonioscopy, the iris cyst can be seen to be between the iris and the cornea.

sion is known, and multiple cysts of the iris and ciliary body can occur in the same eye.

Iris cyst can cause glaucoma. There is a mechanical blockage of the chamber angle preventing the outflow of aqueous (Fig. 16.41).

IRIS PROLAPSE

Iris prolapse occurs when there is a defect in the cornea. The defect in the cornea may be caused by trauma or an ulceration due to infection or stromal melt. Once the cornea is completely perforated, the iris may plug the opening, preventing the exit of aqueous. This plug may be seen as a small spot on the cornea, either black or light-colored depending upon iris color (Fig. 16.42). The pupil is also peaked (or pearshaped), with the point directed toward the area of prolapse.

IRMA (INTRARETINAL MICROVASCULAR ABNORMALITIES)

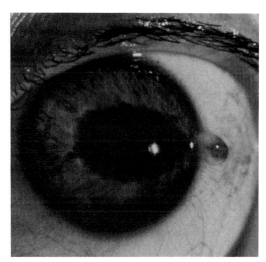

Figure 16.42.   Prolapse of the iris occurs when there is a defect in the cornea. The iris plugs the opening, preventing the exit of aqueous. The pupil is peaked toward the area of prolapse. (See Fig. 16.40, **G** and **H.**)

IRMA are vascular abnormalities seen in diabetic retinopathy adjacent to nonperfused zones in the retina. They are arteriole and venous shunts that appear as dilated, tortuous vessels. IRMA are best seen in red-free (green filter) light (see Diabetic Retinopathy).

THE JONES TEST (JONES I AND JONES II)

Use

The Jones test is used to determine whether tear drainage from the eye into the nose is normal.

Technique

The test is done in two stages.

Jones I Test

Technique. A fluorescein solution of 1% is placed in the patient's conjunctival sac. Both sides are tested. Two cotton-tipped applicators are then moistened with an anesthetic such as 5% cocaine and placed into the left and right nostrils (inferior meatus). After 5 minutes, the applicators are removed.

Results. If dye is noted on the cotton-tipped applicators, it can be assumed that the tear drainage system is normal. However, if no dye is present, the Jones II test should be done.

Jones II Test

Technique. The inferior punctum of the lid is anesthetized with proparacaine, tetracaine, or 5% cocaine. The conjunctival sac is washed with saline to remove all of the fluorescein dye that might remain. The patient is then placed over a sink that is stoppered or over a small basin. Drainage from the nose will run into the sink or basin. A blunt lacrimal irrigating needle on a syringe is used to irrigate 1 mm of saline solution through the lacrimal system.

Results. If fluid runs from the nose and is tinged with fluorescein, the test is positive. A positive test means that fluorescein dye passed from the conjunctiva through the canaliculus and punctum to the lacrimal sac and then was irrigated from the sac. This indicates that the system is open but with some functional blockage. If no dye is retrieved from the nose, the canaliculus or sac is probably obstructed.

Use. This test is used to distinguish between a functional and an anatomical block in the tear drainage system. Functional block is one in which the system is open, but flow does not occur.

Comment

This test is most useful when positive. False-negative tests are not uncommon. Approximately 10 to 20% of normal patients will not have a positive Jones I and Jones II test, indicating a high false-negative rate. If there is a question of functional or anatomical blockage, use additional tests such as dacryograms (page 283).

JUNCTIONAL SCOTOMA

Characteristics

A junctional scotoma shows bilateral visual field changes with a central scotoma in one eye and a superotemporal defect in the opposite eye (Fig. 16.43).

Localization

This sign localizes the lesion to compression of the optic nerve posteriorly. The bilateral defect is related to the special anatomy of the crossing fibers in the chiasm. Some fibers sweep back into the opposite optic nerve (the cause of the superotemporal defect). This fiber sweep is called Willbrandt's knee.

A common cause of a junctional scotoma is meningioma. A patient will have decreased vision in the eye with a central scotoma, abnormal color vision in the eye with the scotoma, and relative afferent pupillary defects (page 92) in the involved eye.

KEYHOLE PUPIL

See Sector Iridectomy, Fig. 16.40C, page 307.

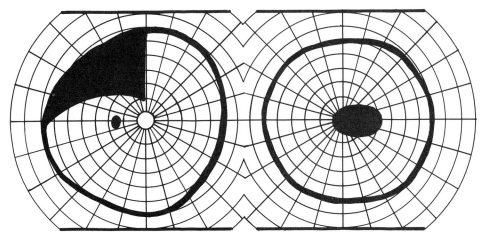

Figure 16.43.   A junctional scotoma is characterized by a central scotoma in one eye and a superotemporal field defect in the opposite eye. A posterior optic nerve lesion is responsible for this characteristic field defect.

KHADADOUST LINE

Khadadoust line is associated with endothelial cell rejection in penetrating keratoplasty. It appears as a gray, irregular line on the posterior, inner surface of the cornea.

KRABBE'S DISEASE (GLOBOID CELL LEUKODYSTROPHY)

Krabbe's disease is a recessively inherited disease. Galactocerebroside accumulates because of a deficiency in beta-galactosidase. Death usually occurs within the first 2 years. There is rapidly progressive CNS degeneration to optic atrophy with blindness. It is important to know that the cherry-red spot (see page 268) is not a feature of Krabbe's disease (compare Tay-Sachs disease).

LACRIMAL PROBING

Probing of the lacrimal system may be either diagnostic or therapeutic. A probe placed into the lacrimal system helps to determine the level of obstruction. Obstruction, of course, can occur anywhere, including the punctum, the canaliculus, the sac, or the nasal lacrimal duct.

A probe is metal, about the diameter of heavy wire, and has a blunt tip. Knowledge of anatomical structure is essential so the probing will not be traumatic to tissue.

Irrigation of the lacrimal system can be a part of the probing. Fluid irrigated into the lacrimal system through the punctum and ampullae should pass into the nose. One can place a cotton-tipped applicator into the nose, insert dye into the fluid to be irrigated, and demonstrate lacrimal patency by showing the passage of dye fluid into the nose (seen on the applicator tip). Lacrimal fluid injected into an inferior punctum that reflexes through a superior punctum indicates obstruction in the ductal system.

LEBER CELL

A Leber cell is an enlarged macrophage that has engulfed cellular debris. It is seen in cells infected with trachoma.
(See Fig. 2.22H.)

LEFLER-WADSWORTH-SIDBURY FOVEAL DYSTROPHY

Inheritance

Autosomal dominant

Clinical Characteristics

This foveal dystrophy develops during the first decade of life. Foveal lesions progress throughout childhood. There is wide variation in the clinical end stage reached by individuals.

Ophthalmoscopy shows three fairly distinct stages, all of which relate to the severity of the effect on visual acuity.

Stage 1

Scattered drusen, pigment dispersion in the fovea, and good vision are characteristic.

Stage 2

Confluent drusen, with or without pigment in the central macular region are seen. There are retinal pigment epithelial atrophy and partial choroidal atrophy. Vision is decreased. Central and paracentral scotomas may be present.

Stage 3

There is choroidal atrophy. Total retinal pigmental epithelial and choriocapillary atrophy is seen in the fovea and the perifoveal region. The central vision is poor. The scotomas, which in stage 2 are small, are now large and may be central or paracentral.

The ERG, EOG, dark adaptometry, and color vision are normal.

LEFORT'S CLASSIFICATION

LeFort's classification of midfacial fractures is important in ophthalmology because midfacial trauma often involves the orbit. Orbital hemorrhage, foreign bodies, and soft tissue injuries result. Loss of visual acuity, strabismus, and ptosis are often present.

LeFort's classification is as follows (Fig. 16.44):

LeFort I

This is a low transverse maxillary fracture above the teeth—there is no orbital involvement.

LeFort II

Pyramid-shaped fractures involve the nasal, lacrimal, and maxillary bones. These fractures involve the orbital floors.

LeFort III

This is a severe fracture causing craniofacial dysjunction. It involves not only the orbital floor but also the medial and lateral orbital walls. The facial skeleton may be detached from the skull. Suspension of the lower face may be by soft tissues only.

LEUKOCORIA (WHITE PUPIL)

Leukocoria, a white or grayish white pupil, is most often seen with mature and hypermature cataracts. The term is also applied to white pupils caused by scarring, tumors, or degenerative processes.

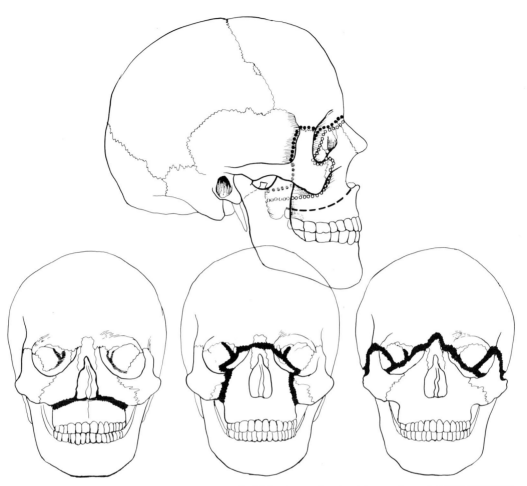

Figure 16.44.   LeFort fractures are midfacial fractures often involving ocular and orbital structures. LeFort I: *bottom left* and *dashed line* in *top drawing;* LeFort II: *bottom center* and *line of open circles* in *top drawing;* LeFort III: *bottom right* and *line of closed circles* in *top drawing.*

LID CREASE

The lid crease occurs in the upper lid where the tendon of the levator muscle pulls the lid. It is normal. The absence of a lid crease means that there is severe ptosis without levator function.

A lid crease is formed by the levator aponeurosis attachment to the lid tarsus and skin surface. A lid crease is different in males and in females—the lid crease is 10 mm above the lashes in women and 7 to 8 mm above the lashes in men. This is important when surgically creating a new lid crease. Upper lid folds refer to the skin that hangs over the crease.

LIGNEOUS CONJUNCTIVITIS

Characteristics

The onset is acute. It most often occurs in children. There is massive collection of granulation tissue on the conjunctiva, usually on the upper tarsal conjunctiva. Both the lower tarsal conjunctiva and bulbar conjunctiva can be involved, however. Excessive amounts of mucus are produced.

Cause

Unknown

LIMBAL GIRDLE OF VOGT

Clinical Appearance

This extremely common finding in older individuals occurs at the edge of the corneal stroma. It is seen both nasally and temporally in the area between the lids. There are small, white deposits with needle-like ends that give a crystalline appearance. Unlike arcus senilis, which usually has a clear zone between the opacification and the edge of the cornea, the limbal girdle may or may not have a clear interval. The opacity is at the level of Bowman's layer. Limbal girdle is seen in middle-aged and elderly people.

A limbal girdle is formed by subepithelial collagen degeneration, sometimes with calcium particles. It has no clinical significance.

LIPOGRANULOMATOSIS (FARBER'S DISEASE)

Ocular Manifestations

Cherry-red spots on the fovea are surrounded by gray macula. The optic disc may be atrophic, and the fundi may have a diffuse peppery pigmentation.

General Manifestations

This autosomal recessive disease occurs with *excess ceramide* accumulations due to *deficient ceramidase* activity. These patients die of chronic respiratory insufficiency during the 1st year of life. They have painful periarticular and tendon swellings that cause flexion contractures. Nodules are seen in the skin and under the skin, characteristically over the wrists and ankles. As cranial nerves and the spinal cord become involved, there is motor weakness, hypotonia, amyotrophia, and loss of reflexes.

LISTING'S PLANE

Listing's plane is a hypothetical equatorial plane and is used to explain the rotation of the globe. Listing's plane passes through the center of the eye near the equator. Listing's plane rotating around the center of the eye would rotate up or down or to the left and right. Listing's plane is illustrated and further discussed under the topic Axes of Fick (page 259). It has mostly historical interest and is not clinically useful.

LOA LOA

Description

This worm, found in Africa, lives in the connective tissue of humans and monkeys. It is transported by the horse fly or mangrove fly.

The worm can migrate into the eye and surrounding tissues. It has been seen in the orbit, under the conjunctiva, in the lid, in the anterior chamber, in the vitreous, and in the retina.

Diagnosis

There is a 60 to 80% eosinophilia. Microfilaria can also be found in the blood when examined at midday.

Quite often the diagnosis is made by the characteristic appearance of the worm on direct visualization or on immediate removal from subcutaneous or subconjunctival tissues.

LOCKWOOD'S LIGAMENT

In the lower lid, the terminal muscle fibers and tendon of the inferior rectus muscle contribute to a fascia called the capsulopalpebral head. The capsulopalpebral head divides into two superior portions as it encircles and eventually fuses with the sheath of the oblique muscle. Anterior to the inferior oblique muscle, portions of the capsulopalpebral head join to form a suspensory ligament known as Lockwood's ligament. Lockwood's ligament is also called the capsulopalpebral fascia. This capsulopalpebral fascia fuses with the orbital septum and also inserts on the lower lid tarsus.

LOW VISION

Low vision is subnormal visual acuity. Low vision is also an abnormal visual field. In general, low vision is an acuity of 20/70 or less.

Low vision aids are necessary when visual changes, either visual field or visual acuity, affect the patient's performance. Low vision aids include spectacles that magnify, hand magnifiers for magnification at near, telescopes for near work and far, nonoptical devices that provide large print (large type books and magazines), masking devices, and control of illumination.

Electronic aids such as television readers may be useful for certain patients to provide magnification for reading. These newer aids provide a more convenient viewing and more rapid reading.

Patients who require low vision aids usually require training in the use of these aids.

LYME DISEASE
General

Lyme disease is a tick-borne spirochetal infection. The general findings include skin rash, arthritis, and cardiac and neurologic findings.

Ophthalmic Findings

Conjunctivitis, most often a follicular conjunctivitis, is seen in approximately 10% of patients with Lyme disease. Additional ophthalmologic changes include stromal subepithelial hazy opacity. Inflammation of the cornea (interstitial keratitis) has also been reported.

LYMPHOID INFILTRATION OF THE UVEA
Other Names

Lymphoid neoplasia, reactive lymphoid hypoplasia

Ophthalmologic Signs

Lymphoid infiltration of the uvea, although rare, may present with ocular signs that can suggest the diagnosis. Multifocal, creamy choroidal infiltrates may be seen. These are nonconfluent. They have indistinct edges and are 1 to 2 disc diameters wide. The differential diagnosis is diffuse choroidal melanoma. The retinal detachment or disturbances of the retinal pigment epithelium that occur with choroidal melanoma are generally not seen with lymphoid infiltration of the uvea.

After initial observation, the lesions, in general, remain unchanged.

Diagnosis

Fluorescein angiography, ultrasonography, and CT scanning all help establish the diagnosis. Thickening of the choroid, the ciliary body, and retrobulbar tissues is seen.

Histopathology

Lesions are diffuse collections of lymphocytes and lymphoplasmacytoid cells. Some cells can possess intranuclear Dutcher bodies. Multinuclear giant cells are seen.

The majority of patients with lymphoid infiltrates of the uvea show no evidence of systemic disease. When systemic changes are present (approximately 10 to 20%), Waldenström's macroglobulinemia or extranodal deposits are usually found.

MACCALLAN CLASSIFICATION

MacCallan described a classification for the progressive conjunctival changes that occur in trachoma (page 374). The classification has four stages:

- Stage 1: Immature follicles are found on upper palpebral conjunctiva, but there is no scarring.
- Stage 2: Follicles are mature on the upper palpebral conjunctiva, and papillary hypertrophy may be present; there is no scarring.
- Stage 3: Follicles and scarring of the upper palpebral conjunctiva are present.
- Stage 4: No follicles are present, but often extensive scarring is seen. Trachoma is inactive.

THE MACKAY-MARG TONOMETER

Description

This tonometer is electronic and measures pressure on the anesthetized cornea by direct contact. The pressure is calculated in the change of scale readings from a baseline and a noncontact curve to the increase after a touch flattening of the cornea.

Use

In severely scarred corneas or in corneas that have irregular surfaces, the Mackay-Marg tonometer provides more accurate pressure readings than those obtained by Schiotz tonometry or applanation tonometry.

MALIGNANT HYPERTHERMIA

Malignant hyperthermia, a dangerous complication of anesthesia, is a generalized muscle membrane disorder that results in acidosis, high fever, and death. The ophthalmologist has a special interest in learning to recognize this condition because susceptible patients have ptosis and strabismus more than do nonsusceptible patients. These patients, while under anesthesia for ophthalmologic surgery, may have their first episode of malignant hyperthermia.

When the muscle membranes of these patients are exposed to triggering agents such as succinylcholine and halothane, there is a rapid release of large amounts of calcium into the cell. This leads quickly to acidosis and fever. The patient becomes rigid. Ventricular ectopy and death soon follow. To save the patient, one must know early signs and start treatment.

Early Signs

- Muscle rigidity after the injection of succinylcholine. Rigidity first occurs in the masseter muscles and may cause difficulty with intubation.
- Cardiac irregularities. Tachycardia is the most consistent early sign. However, it can be easily mistaken for "light anesthesia." Ventricular arrhythmias and fibrillation may follow.
- Skin changes. A generalized erythema occurs. The skin feels warm even though the body temperature may be normal.

Late Signs

- Fever
- Generalized muscle rigidity

Changes in Blood Chemistries

- pH decreases
- pCO increases
- Serum calcium decreases
- Serum potassium increases

Course

Malignant hyperthermia is fatal if not treated promptly. One must lower the intracellular calcium level quickly. Give dantrolene sodium promptly (see page 283). Stop anesthetic agents.

MARCUS GUNN PHENOMENON (JAW WINKING)

In the acquired type, the involved lid droops (ptosis). When the jaw moves, such as in chewing or yawning, the drooping lid is elevated. This phenomenon results from abnormal third nerve (oculomotor nerve) misdirection.

Most Marcus Gunn phenomena are secondary to improper afferent regeneration of the third nerve after injury or damage. Congenital Marcus Gunn phenomenon is extremely rare.

MARE'S TAIL LINES

Mare's tail lines are bundles of superficial corneal lines. They arise from a single point and radiate outward. These lines are coarser than the somewhat similar fingerprint lines. They also may be seen in direct illumination, whereas fingerprint lines are seen with retroillumination.

Mare's tail lines are rarely, if ever, seen with epithelial basement membrane dystrophy (page 10) and should not be confused with the fingerprint lines seen in that condition.

MARFAN'S SYNDROME

Other Names

Arachnodactyly, dolichostenomelia

Eye Changes

The most characteristic change in Marfan's syndrome is an upward dislocation of the lens that occurs in both eyes (ectopia lentis). The lenses may be smaller than normal (microspherophakia).

Moderate to high myopia is often present. Retinal detachment is also more frequent than expected in the normal population and is variably reported from 9 to 54%.

Systemic Changes

The skeletal system shows excess length of the distal limbs, loose jointedness, and scoliosis. The anterior chest is deformed. These patients are frequently tall and gangly due to changes in the distal limbs.

Cardiovascular changes including dilation of the aorta, dissecting aortic aneurysm, and floppy mitral valve are all seen in Marfan's syndrome. Complications from the aortic dilation account for 80% of deaths.

Early Death

Most patients die in middle age, with 50% of all male patients dying by the age 41 and 50% of all female patients dying by the age of 49.

Heredity

This is a familial disorder with autosomal dominant inheritance. Males and females are affected with equal frequency.

MARGIN REFLEX DISTANCE

When measuring lid droop (see Ptosis, page 202), the degree of ptosis can be measured by taking the central corneal light reflex from a light source such as a pen light and measuring from that light reflex to the level of the upper lid margin while the eye is looking straight ahead. The margin reflex distance is a way to evaluate ptosis in addition to those discussed on page 202.

MASQUERADE SYNDROME (IRIDOCYCLITIS MASQUERADE SYNDROME)

Tumors, especially lung tumors such as carcinoma, can present as inflammation in the anterior portion of the eye without other ocular or systemic signs. A high index of suspicion should be maintained in elderly patients presenting with any ocular anterior segment inflammation (see Iridocyclitis, page 172).

MEGALOCORNEA

Megalocornea is an enlarged cornea. If the horizontal diameter of the cornea is greater than 12.5 mm, megalocornea is diagnosed.

Megalocornea can be seen in congenital glaucoma when the eye is stretched from increased intraocular pressure before term or just after birth. This stretching with enlargement of the globe structures is *buphthalmos* (page 264).

MEIBOMITIS

Meibomitis is a noninfectious change of the lid margins (Fig. 16.45) that may result in a relatively severe blepharitis (compare Seborrheic Blepharitis, page 358). Occasionally, a keratitis may be present.

Meibomian secretions are thickened. Meibomian gland orifices have inflammation, and the glands are inspissated. Bulbar conjunctival injection is common. Patients are

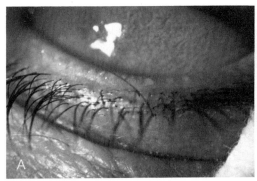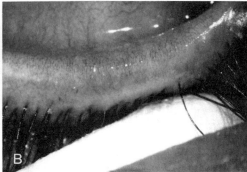

Figure 16.45. Meibomitis—lid margin changes. This illustrates changes in the meibomian gland orifices. **A,** Thickened meibomian gland secretions can be seen as small bubbles over the meibomian gland orifices. **B,** Hyperemia of the lid margin. To the *left*, the small, white dots are inspissated lipid material in the meibomian gland orifices.

frequently symptomatic. Tear film becomes abnormal due to meibomian gland dysfunction, and punctate epithelial erosions of the cornea occur.

Two-thirds of these patients have acne rosacea. Microbial studies show no associated bacterial infection in this process.

MELANOCYTIC NEVI OF PALPEBRAL CONJUNCTIVA

Nevi of the conjunctiva generally develop during the first 2 decades of life. They are almost entirely restricted to the epibulbar conjunctival surface, plica, caruncle and the lid margin.

In contrast, an elevated pigmented lesion of the fornix or tarsal conjunctiva that is acquired in later life must be suspected to be a melanoma or melanoma precursor. These should be biopsied.

Approximately 70% of all conjunctival nevi are pigmented, whereas 30% are not.

MELKERSSON-ROSENTHAL SYNDROME

The Melkersson-Rosenthal syndrome is a recurrent facial paralysis, either unilateral or bilateral, which is associated with chronic facial swelling and furrowing of the tongue (lingua plicata). The onset is in childhood and the cause is unknown. Involvement of the facial nerve and inability to close the lid normally result in secondary eye complications, particularly on the cornea, where blink is needed for tear distribution.

METAMORPHOPSIA

Metamorphopsia refers to the *distortion* of the viewed object and is associated with *macular disease*. The Amsler grid (see page 247) is excellent for detecting metamorphopsia. Patients with aging macular degeneration, for example, can follow changes in their condition by viewing an Amsler grid at home to detect metamorphopsia.

METASTATIC NEUROBLASTOMA

These are the most common tumors metastatic to the orbit in children. Metastasis is frequently the presenting manifestation accompanied by only small occult tumors in the retroperitoneal space, in the adrenal medulla, or in the sympathetic chain. Onset is usually before 3 years of age. Periocular metastasis occurs in up to 25% of cases.

Presenting Ocular Symptom

Unilateral or bilateral eyelid ecchymosis, which may frequently present without proptosis, is often present. This is characterized by discoloration of the lids in the periorbital and orbital regions. This ecchymosis simulates that seen with child abuse.

Anemia is often present at the time of presentation of ocular signs.

Differential Diagnosis

- Leukemia
- Lymphoma and lymphosarcoma

MICROCORNEA

Any horizontal corneal diameter of less than 11.0 mm is microcornea. The normal corneal diameter is 11.0 to 12.5 mm.

MICROSPHEROPHAKIA

Definition

Microspherophakia is a developmental anomaly of the lens in which the lens is small in diameter and also round in shape.

Conditions in Which Microspherophakia Is Found

- Most often associated with Weill-Marchesain syndrome.
- May occur as an isolated finding.
- Occasionally seen in Marfan's syndrome.

Important Clinical Associations

- *Angle closure glaucoma* may occur if the round lens of microspherophakia blocks the pupil and prevents the forward flow of aqueous.
- High refractive *myopia* is associated with microspherophakia because of the increased power of the round lens.
- Chamber angle development may be abnormal in a few patients with microspherophakia and produce a glaucoma that is not narrow angle.

MIKULICZ' SYNDROME

Characteristics

This is enlargement of the lacrimal glands and the parotid (salivary) glands. The enlargement of the lacrimal gland is usually accompanied by dry eye (keratoconjunctivitis sicca).

Causes

There are a number of causes. The most common are leukemia, sarcoidosis, Hodgkin's disease, and tuberculosis.

MILLARD-GUBLER SYNDROME

This is due to a lesion in the ventral paramedian pons. Clinical signs are (a) on the same side as the lesion, a sixth nerve palsy and a peripheral facial nerve palsy; and (b) on the side opposite the lesion, a hemiplegia. This syndrome is caused by ischemia, tumor infiltration or compression, infection, and inflammation, particularly demyelination.

MIOSIS

Miosis is a small pupil.

MITTENDORF DOT

This is a remnant of the hyaloid vascular system, which regresses completely under most circumstances. The dot appears as a small opacity at the posterior surface of the lens. It does not affect vision (see Bergmeister's Papillae, page 260).

MIZUO'S PHENOMENON

Mizuo's phenomenon is the return of normal fundus coloration after complete darkness for 2 to 3 hours in a patient with a rare type of night blindness, Oguchi's disease (page 330).

MÖBIUS' SYNDROME (CONGENITAL BULBAR PARALYSIS)

Clinical Appearance

There is a mask-like facies with poor eyelid closure. There is increased lacrimation and epiphora.

General Symptoms and Signs

In infants, there is poor sucking with tongue atrophy, deafness, mental retardation, webbed fingers and toes, and extra digits. Esotropia also is present. The pathology is hypoplasia or atrophy of the cranial nerve nuclei (sixth, seventh, eighth, and twelfth nerves).

MOLLUSCUM CONTAGIOSUM

Clinical Signs

- Nodules that are elevated, have a pearly surface, and have a central depression occur on the eyelids (Figure 12.16). The appearance may be atypical, and nodules may be small or large.
- There is a chronic follicular conjunctivitis.
- The corneal epithelium may show round defects that may be small or relatively coarse.

Cause

Virus—molluscum

Importance

Although molluscum is not common, recognition can be important because incision of the lesion removes all signs and symptoms.

MOOREN'S ULCER

Mooren's ulcer is an inflammatory ulcerating disease of the marginal cornea. Characteristically, it is painful and progressive.

Clinical characteristics can help make the diagnosis. There is an overhanging, advancing edge of the epithelial defect with vascularization of the ulcer base.

Two Forms

One form is a benign unilateral condition of older males. A second form is a bilateral ulceration that tends to progress and is found in younger patients.

Progression

Advancement of the ulceration occurs centrally and peripherally and may extend into the sclera in severe cases. Perforation is uncommon.

MORNING GLORY DISC

Morning glory disc is a congenital deformity that is a more advanced variation of a coloboma (page 272). The ophthalmoscope shows a whitish-yellowish central mass of glial tissue around the disc. Blood vessels radiate from the mass, and there is atrophy around the disc. Vision is always decreased, usually severely.

MUCOPOLYSACCHARIDOSIS

Mucopolysaccharidoses are a group of diseases due to inborn errors of metabolism. Excessive storage of mucopolysaccharides occurs due to deficiencies in lysosomal acid hydrolases.

The normal cornea contains 4.0 to 4.5% mucopolysaccharides, of which 50% are keratin sulfate, 25% are chondroitin, and 25% are chondroitin 4-sulfate. In mucopolysaccharidosis, dermatan and keratan sulfate appear in the cornea. Heparin sulfate accumulates in the retina and central nervous system.

Hurler's Syndrome

There is moderate dwarfism with grotesque facial features. The abdomen is protruberant. Joint contractures are present. Hands are broad with short, stubby fingers. Mental retardation is severe.

Corneal clouding is a prominent feature of Hurler's syndrome (this helps to differentiate it from Hunter's syndrome). The corneal opacities are in the anterior stroma initially and present as fine, gray punctate opacities. Later, the posterior stroma and endothelium become involved.

Histologically, there are ballooned macrophages in the cornea. Pigmentary retinopathy and optic atrophy are commonly seen.

Scheie's Syndrome

Scheie's syndrome is a variant of Hurler's syndrome. There is early corneal clouding with accumulation of acid mucopolysaccharides. Although the cornea is involved, the other features of Hurler's syndrome are not present. Mental retardation is minimal or absent. The facial features, although they may be characteristic, are not marked. Pigmentary retinal changes and optic nerve atrophy may occur.

Hunter's Syndrome

Hunter's syndrome has both clinical and biochemical features similar to those of Hurler's syndrome. Gross facial features, dwarfism, hernias, and skin changes occur. Deafness is a common feature of Hunter's syndrome. Corneal opacities may occur later in life but are very mild compared to those in Hurler's and Scheie's syndromes.

Sanfilippo's Syndrome

Corneal cloudiness does not occur in Sanfilippo's syndrome. Retinal pigmentary degeneration and optic atrophy have been observed, however.

Morquio's Syndrome

Morquio's syndrome may include corneal cloudiness. However, pigmentary retinopathy and optic nerve changes do not occur.

Maroteaux-Lamy Syndrome

Corneal opacities occur in all cases. Diagnosis usually requires a slitlamp. Optic atrophy and pigmented retinopathy do not occur.

MULTIPLE SCLEROSIS

The most common visual manifestation of multiple sclerosis in the eye is optic neuritis, which occurs in 20 to 83% of patients, depending on the population reviewed. Lesions occur throughout the visual pathways, however, and are seen in optic tracks and optic radiations.

Although CT scanning can demonstrate plaques in the central nervous system, MRI is highly sensitive. Computed tomography identifies definite cases in less than 50%, whereas MRI may show 80 to 100%. MRI most often demonstrates lesions during active disease and is especially useful when multiple lesions are noted clinically and when the cerebrum is involved. In spite of the plaques commonly observed with MRI, homonymous hemianopsia is unusual (1%).

MUCORMYCOSIS

Mucormycosis is one of the phycomycoses. Similar features can be produced by the fungi *Mucor* and *Rhizopus.* Both of these fungi belong to the class Phycomycetes.

Features

Mucormycosis is the most common and most virulent of orbital fungal diseases. Extension is almost always from a sinus or nasal cavity contiguous with the orbit. *Mucor* can invade blood vessel walls, resulting in thrombosis.

Predisposing Factors

Patients are frequently debilitated with metabolic acidosis, associated most frequently with diabetes but also with malignant tumors, treatment with antimetabolites, or treatment with steroids.

Diagnosis

Patients may present with proptosis and an orbital apex syndrome (page 333). Diagnosis is made by biopsy. Nonseptate, large, branching hyphae that stain with hematoxylin and eosin help establish the diagnosis.

MUNSON'S SIGN

Munson's sign is seen in keratoconus (page 13). In keratoconus, the cornea loses its spherical shape and takes on the shape of a cone. This corneal cone distorts the lower lid from its normal curve, which is known as Munson's sign.

To observe this sign, one stands above the eye level of the patient. The observer has the patient look down. As the eye turns down, the cornea moves behind the lower lid and the smooth curve of the lid is distorted into a cone shape.

MYASTHENIC SYNDROME

Also called the Eaton-Lambert syndrome (see page 286).

MYDRIASIS

Mydriasis is a large pupil.

MYELINATED NERVE FIBERS

Normally, retinal fibers are not myelinated. On occasion, they are myelinated and appear as patches of white. These patches may be near the disc and rarely surround the disc completely. Myelinated nerve fibers, however, may also occur as patches of white in the posterior pole, not touching the disc.

In general, myelinated fibers are white and glistening (Fig. 16.46). The borders are characteristically fluffy. On careful examination with high magnification, however, the fluffiness, paradoxically, turns out to be the tapering of individual myelinated fibers, giving a brush-like appearance.

Vessels may be slightly less clear as they course through myelinated fibers, but they are never obscured. Myelinated nerve fibers have no pathologic significance.

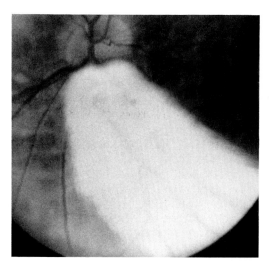

Figure 16.46. Normally, the nerve fibers of the retina are not myelinated. When myelination occurs, it is characteristic in its appearance. The borders are at first glance fluffy in appearance, but on closer evaluation show the distinct termination of myelination along the nerve fibers. Vessels are usually visible underneath the myelination. Myelination may occur around the disc or more peripherally without being adjacent to the disc. Myelination is important to recognize, even though uncommon, because it may be confused with papilledema. (See also color Fig. C.24.)

MYOPIA

Myopia is a refractive error in which parallel rays of light come into focus in front of the retina (Fig. 15.3, page 234).

MYOPIC CRESCENT

In high myopia (nearsightedness), a disc may appear vertically elongated and somewhat larger. The physiologic cup may be flattened temporally. The central vessels enter nasally and often bend sharply.

Peripapillary retinal and choroidal changes show a crescent around the disc—a myopic crescent. This is caused by a failure of the retina and choroid to extend to the edge of the disc. Most often, the crescent is on the temporal aspect of the disc, but it may also be inferior or superior. It is rarely seen nasally. Choroidal vessels may appear sharply delineated in the crescent because they are not covered by the retinal pigment epithelium. Crescents are most often seen in myope's with greater than minus 8 diopters of refractive error.

NANOPHTHALMOS

Nanophthalmos is characterized by a small eye and is not associated with systemic disorders or developmental defects. Signs are a shallow anterior chamber, a narrow angle, a large lens in comparison to eye volume, and severe hyperopia. Nanophthalmos is associated with ciliochoroidal effusion (page 270).

NEONATAL INCLUSION CONJUNCTIVITIS

Other names

Inclusion blennorrhea, ophthalmia neonatorum (page 229), *Chlamydia*

Onset

Neonatal inclusion conjunctivitis classically occurs 5 to 12 days after birth. However, it can occur from 1 day up to 3 to 4 weeks after birth.

Clinical Signs

There is an acute conjunctivitis with a purulent discharge.

Epidemiology

The infant is infected from the mother's cervix during passage through the birth canal. As the parents are infected, one should consider treating them.

Laboratory Diagnosis

Conjunctival scrapings of infected areas should be stained with Giemsa stain. Intracytoplasmic inclusion bodies can be seen in the epithelial cells and are diagnostic. The inclusion bodies are large basophilic inclusions; at times, smaller eosinophilic opacities can be seen (see Fig. 2.22).

Differential Diagnosis

Inclusion conjunctivitis is one of the conditions that must be differentiated from other diseases that cause ophthalmia neonatorum (page 229). Other causes of ophthalmia neonatorum are *Neisseria gonorrhea,* chemical conjunctivitis due to silver nitrate (both of which occur in 24 to 72 hours), and staphylococcal or pneumococcal conjunctivitis, which develops 5 to 7 days after birth.

Lack of Follicles

Although follicles are characteristic of inclusion conjunctivitis in the adult, follicles do not occur in inclusive conjunctivitis of the newborn. Newborn lymphoid tissue cannot form follicles.

NIACIN MACULOPATHY

Niacin (nicotinic acid) is used in the therapy of hyperlipidimias for its serum cholesterol-lowering effects. A major ocular complication of niacin hypervitaminosis is a reversible cystoid maculopathy. A donut-shaped relative scotoma may be shown by Amsler grid testing. Patients may complain of lights with halos and blurred vision in the eye affected.

Pathology

The retina is wrinkled, presenting as a sunburst pattern with a foveola as the center. Small, superficial cysts form triangular patterns with the points directed to the fovea. The fovea may have a bright yellow spot.

Niacin maculopathy is associated with high doses, usually over 3 g per day.

Fluorescein Angiography

No leakage is demonstrable on fluorescein angiography.

No chronic retinal or choroidal changes are seen in these patients.

Incidence

In patients taking high dose oral niacin for hyperlipidemia, the incidence of niacin maculopathy is less than 1%.

NODAL POINT

The nodal point of the eye is that point at which all rays pass through undeviated regardless of the angle to the optical axis. A nodal point of a schematic eye is 5.6 mm back from the cornea and 17.0 mm in front of the retina. Measurements assume that a schematic eye is 22.6 mm long (axial length).

NUTRITIONAL AMBLYOPIA (TOBACCO-ALCOHOL AMBLYOPIA)

Ocular Signs and Symptoms

Nutritional amblyopia is characterized by a visual field defect in and around the point of fixation (centrocecal scotoma). Bilateral decrease in vision occurs in over 50% of patients. The optic disc may appear pale.

Cause

Poor nutrition is the major cause. It is frequently associated with chronic alcoholism. It has also been associated with heavy smoking. Any dietary deficiency that results in inadequate thiamine may predispose to amblyopia.

Course

Although starting on the appropriate diet with good vitamin levels may prevent further damage, degeneration already present is not reversible.

Differential Diagnosis

Chiasmal lesions, multiple sclerosis, toxic changes from methanol poisoning, retrobulbar neuritis, age-related macular degeneration

NVD (NEW VESSELS DISC)

This term is used in proliferative diabetic retinopathy (see page 65) to identify new vessels that occur on the disc or within 1 disc diameter of the optic disc itself. NVD has a poor visual prognosis.

NVE (NEW VESSELS ELSEWHERE)

This term in diabetic retinopathy (compare NVD) refers to new vessels formed more than 1 disc diameter outside the disc. NVE that is nonelevated may remain stable for long periods and is not as severe a risk factor for severe visual loss as NVD (Diabetic Retinopathy).

NYCTALOPIA

Nyctalopia is decreased visual capacity in faint light or at night. It is synonymous with night blindness.

NYSTAGMUS BLOCKAGE SYNDROME

This is an inward deviation of the eyes (esotropia) in the presence of nystagmus. This rare condition of esotropia with nystagmus is thought to develop to decrease the amount of to and fro motion that occurs with nystagmus.

- The esotropia is variable.
- When the turned-out eye fixates the nystagmus is present, but when the turned-in eye fixates the nystagmus is absent or decreased.
- The esotropia may be decreased in lateral gaze.
- With the use of prisms, the nystagmus increases.

O'BRIEN LID BLOCK (O'BRIEN AKINESIA TECHNIQUE)

Anesthetic solution is injected locally to block the action of the facial nerve and prevent lid closure. This technique is used in cataract surgery but is also useful for examining the traumatized eye.

OBJECT DISPLACEMENT

Definition

Displacement of the object is movement of the image. The phenomenon occurs in glasses with a bifocal when the eye looks down from the distance lens into the bifocal lens. Because of optical differences between the two lenses, a prismatic effect results in perceived object displacement. Object displacement causes few, if any, symptoms if both eyes are balanced. However, if there is a difference in the amount of displacement between the two eyes, symptoms do occur.

Technical Consideration

To calculate object displacements, the movement caused by the distance lens must be added to the movement caused by the bifocal lens. In a plus lens, the distance lens has a base-up prismatic effect. The bifocal segment (other than a flat top segment) will have an optical center below the bifocal line and will have a base-down prismatic effect. The Prentice rule (page 343) is used in the calculations of both the distance and the near vision prismatic effects.

For the distant vision prismatic effect, it is assumed that there will be 8 mm of distance between the optical center of the distance lens and the point at which (below that optical center) the visual access will be used for reading. For the bifocal segment, the distance between the edge of the bifocal and the optical center of the bifocal will vary and must be stated or known for that type of lens.

OCULAR BARRIERS

Many substances, such as fluorescein, do not leak into the eye unless there is disruption of an ocular barrier. There are two ocular barriers, the blood-retina barrier and the blood-aqueous barrier.

The *blood-aqueous barrier* is thought to be at the tight junctions between capillary endothelial cells of the iris vessels and in the inner layer of the non-pigment epithelial cells covering the cellular body and cellular processes.

The second barrier is the *blood-retina barrier.* This is found in two places, the tight junctions of the retinal pigment epithelium and the endothelial cells of the retinal capillaries.

Disrupted ocular barriers cause abnormal leakage into the eye in inflammation and after surgery. Signs of uveitis (page 172) and cystoid macular edema (page 281) are a result of altered ocular barriers. Fluorescein angiography is also dependent on differences between intact and disrupted barriers.

OCULOCARDIAC REFLEX

The oculocardiac reflex refers to a decrease in heart rate, a decrease in conduction of nerve impulses in the heart, and an increased muscle contractability that is associated with ocular surgery. The reflex is mediated through divisions of the trigeminal nerve (afferent loop) and the vagus nerve (efferent loop). Although the reflex occurs during a number of ocular procedures, both intraocular and extraocular, it is most often related to extraocular muscle surgery, especially procedures associated with the medial rectus. It is thought that the reflex is initiated by traction on the extraocular muscles. The reflex is blocked by retrobulbar anesthesia.

OCULODERMAL MELANOCYTOSIS OR NEVUS OF OTA

Definition

Oculodermal melanocytosis is pigmentation where it is not usually found on the skin of the face and in structures of the eye (Fig. 16.47). It is classified as a hamartoma.

Pigment cells (melanoblasts) are in the deep layers of the dermis of the face, the

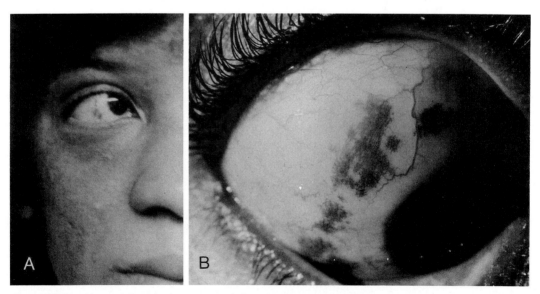

Figure 16.47.   Nevus of Ota (also known as oculodermal melanocytosis). This increase in pigmentation of the skin, the sclera, and the choroid can be variable. It occurs most often in orientals and blacks and is rarely seen in whites. On rare occasions, the nevus may undergo malignant change.

sclera, and other ocular structures. Although the dermis alone (dermal melanocytosis) or the eye alone (ocular melanocytosis) can be involved, oculodermal melanocytosis involves both and is commonly known as the *nevus of Ota.*

Diagnosis

Appearance

The skin pigment is usually limited to one side of the face in the distribution of the first and second branches of the fifth nerve. The skin is discolored with patchy areas of blue or slate gray.

The eye involvement is always unilateral. Many ocular structures can be involved. The sclera is always affected, usually in the superior or outer quadrants of the globe. The discoloration is blue-black. The iris, conjunctiva, and choroid can also be involved. The orbit and optic nerve may have melanocytes. Corneal involvement is rare.

Time of Onset

The pigment is present at birth or soon after. The pigmentation can increase at puberty and during pregnancy, and these may be the times when it is first noted.

Sex

Females are affected more often than males.

Race

Orientals and blacks have ocular melanocytosis more often than whites. The incidence is highest in Japanese.

No definite hereditary pattern is known. The condition has been reported in family members.

Clinical Significance

Glaucoma Rare

Even though the trabecular meshwork and Schlemm's canal are frequently involved with pigment, secondary glaucoma is rare.

Malignant Transformation

Although not common, malignant transformation does occur. The most important points to remember about malignant changes are:

- Whites are more at risk than blacks and orientals;
- Choroid is the most common site of malignancy;
- Orbit is the second most common site;
- Average age at time of malignant transformation is about 50 years.

Differential Diagnosis

The pigment in oculodermal melanocytosis is located in the lower two-thirds of the dermis. The pigment cells are scattered among the collagen fibers without disturbing the normal architecture. *Blue nevi* also have deep pigment but disrupt the normal architecture.

Pigment cells in the superficial dermis are called *dermal nevi*. Pigment cells at the junction of the epidermis and dermis are called *junctional nevi*. A nevus with pigment cells both in the superficial dermis and in the junctional region is a *compound nevus.*

OCULOGLANDULAR DISEASE (PARINAUD'S OCULOGLANDULAR SYNDROME)

This syndrome has three features:

- Large, visible lymph nodes in front of the ear (preauricular adenopathy);
- Conjunctival granulomas; and
- Low grade fever.

In almost all cases, oculoglandular disease is unilateral.

Cause

Cat-scratch disease is most common (page 265).

Other Causes

M-tuberculosis, tularemia *(Francisella tularensis), Treponema pallidum, Pasteurella pseudotuberculosis*

OGUCHI'S DISEASE

Oguchi's disease is a rare type of congenital night blindness (nyctalopia, page 327). It is more common in the Japanese and is transmitted as an autosomal recessive trait. It is not progressive.

A diffuse yellow or gray discoloration of the fundus is characteristic. The normal fundus color will return after 2 to 3 hours of complete darkness. This change in fundus color is known as Mizuo's phenomenon (page 321).

OPSOCLONUS

Clinical Signs

In opsoclonus, there is chaotic, unpredictable movement of the eyes in many directions. The ocular movements are dramatic and characteristic.

Cause

The sign is indicative of cerebellar or brain stem disease. Most often seen in postviral encephalopathic syndrome. In children, it may be associated with a occult neuroblastoma. In adults, it may be associated with visceral carcinoma.

OPTIC ATROPHY IN CHILDREN

Optic atrophy in children is a serious diagnostic sign.

Most common cause—TUMOR

- Glioma—most common tumor
- Craniopharyngioma—second

Second most common cause—INFLAMMATION

- Most commonly optic neuritis
- Also meningitis

Third most common cause—HEAD TRAUMA

OPTOKINETIC DRUM

An optokinetic drum (Fig. 16.48) is a cylindrical drum that is painted with black stripes on a white background. The white and black stripes are of equal width. The drum rotates on a central rod. The drum is held in front of the eyes, which induces an involuntary nystagmus called an optokinetic nystagmus.

ORBITAL ABSCESS

Definition

Orbital abscess is an inflammatory response and suppuration within the orbital fat. Subperiosteal abscess is the same process between orbital bones and the periorbita. Diagnosis is important because antibiotic penetration is poor in these avascular spaces and a surgical approach is often required.

Classification of Complications of Sinusitis

Group I: Preseptal Cellulitis

This is caused by lack of flow through drainage ethmoid vessels. There are swollen eyelids, and the orbital contents may be swollen.

Group II: Orbital Cellulitis

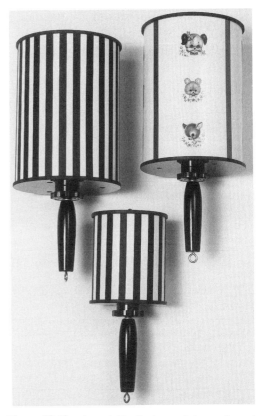

Figure 16.48. An optokinetic drum rotates on the rod that is attached to the handle. This is rotated in front of the patient, eliciting involuntary optokinetic nystagmus. Illustrated are two types of optokinetic drums with stripes and a child's optokinetic drum presenting children's objects to maintain attention. (Credit: DA-Laur, Inc.)

The orbital tissue is infiltrated with cells and bacteria. The eyelids are swollen, and the conjunctiva is chemotic. There is variable proptosis and visual involvement. (Cellulitis may be sterile in some cases.)

Group III: Subperiosteal Abscesses

Purulent material collects between the periorbita and the bony walls. One notes edema, chemosis, and tenderness. Ocular motility, vision, and proptosis are variably affected.

Group IV: Orbital Abscess

There is pus in the orbital fat inside or outside the muscle cone. Exophthalmos, chemosis, ophthalmoplegia, and visual impairment are usually severe. Systemic toxicity may be marked.

Group V: Cavernous Sinus Thrombosis

This is extension of the orbital abscess into the cavernous sinus. There is marked lid edema and an early onset of third, fourth, and sixth nerve palsies bilaterally. General sepsis, nausea, vomiting, and signs of meningeal irritation are seen. In the *orbital apex syndrome,* proptosis, lid edema, optic neuritis, external and internal ophthal-moplegia, and neuralgia of the fifth nerve are caused by sinus disease around the optic foramen and the superior orbital fissure.

Meningitis

Meningitis is the most common intracranial complication of paranasal sinus disease.

Important Diagnostic Signs and Tests

- Lid, orbit, and conjunctival swelling
- Fever
- Elevated white count
- Sinus x-ray films positive
- CT scan

Important Facts

1. Bacteria gain access to the periorbital space by foreign body and direct extention (sinuses, teeth, lids, lacrimal sac).

2. The *sinus is the most important source of infection (84%).* The ethmoids and maxillary sinuses are the most important sites during the first decade of life. Later in childhood, the frontal sinuses are more important. In the adult, the frontal ethmoid and maxillary sinuses are about equally responsible for orbital complications. The sinuses develop progressively during growth: Ethmoids—second trimester; maxillary—2nd year; frontal—5 and 7 years; the sphenoid is present at birth but clinically is not significant. Infection spreads from sinuses through walls and by blood vessels.

3. Orbital abscesses are usually found in children younger than 16 years; many patients are younger than 6 years. The ethmoid is the most common source of infection in children.

Organisms

- Most common
  - *Staphylococcus aureus*
  - *Staphylococcus epidermidis*
  - Streptococci
- Others
  - *Haemophilus influenzae*
  - *Escherichia coli*
  - Diphtheroids

Complications

1. Seven to 50% of patients with orbital abscesses are blind in the eye from:

- Optic atrophy;
- Central retinal occlusion;
- Exposure keratitis.

2. Permanent diplopia occurs even with early intervention.
Delayed surgical intervention increases the risk of serious complications.

Diagnosis

Physical signs may be variable. Orbital swelling is most prominent. Noninvasive diagnostic tools are x-ray films, ultrasound (90% efficiency), and CT scans. CT is the procedure of choice, but it will not differentiate between preseptal cellulitis and eyelid edema. CT will differentiate between preseptal cellulitis and orbital abscess.

ORBITAL APEX SYNDROME

This is a complex of signs that is important because it helps localize disease within the orbit. An orbital apex syndrome has:

- Internal ophthalmoplegia (loss of pupil responses);
- External ophthalmoplegia (loss of eye movement);
- Ptosis (lid droop);
- Decreased corneal sensation; and
- Decreased vision.

The orbital apex syndrome may be associated with bacterial orbital cellulitis or infection due to fungi such as mucormyocosis. It is also associated with trauma and inflammatory processes.

OSCILLOPSIA

Oscillopsia is the illusion of movement of the environment. The illusion is created by movement of the eyes and most often occurs with the back and forth eye movement of acquired nystagmus. It is dependent on both the degree of the nystagmus and the frequency of the nystagmus. It is rarely seen in congenital nystagmus (see Congenital Nystagmus, page 113; Acquired Nystagmus page 112).

PACHOMETER

A pachometer is an instrument that measures corneal thickness. Commonly used is the ultrasound pachometer. A probe is placed directly on the eye. Sound frequency is used to determine distance from epithelium to endothelium.

Optical pachometry is the measurement of corneal thickness by an optical device that fits on a slitlamp. Skill and considerable practice are necessary for optical pachometry.

Specular microscopy can also be used. A specular microscope is focused first on the epithelium and then on the endothelium, and corneal thickness measurements are determined.

The normal thickness of the cornea is about 0.50 mm. A higher value indicates endothelial dysfunction. Epithelial edema and decrease in vision usually do not occur until the thickness of the cornea has increased to 0.65 to 0.75 mm if the intraocular pressure is normal. Higher pressures cause edema at lower thicknesses.

Pachometry gives a general estimate of the reserve of corneal endothelial function. A reading of 0.70 mm represents borderline decompensation.

PANNUS

Pannus is a nonspecific term that refers to tissue on the superficial cornea between the epithelium and Bowman's membrane. The tissue can be an inflammatory membrane or fibrous tissue. At times, the fibrous tissue may be vascularized.

Pannus results from a chronic insult to the cornea. See SLK (page 369) and Trachoma (page 269) for examples of inflammation that are associated with pannus. Trauma to the cornea is another source of pannus formation.

PANRETINAL PHOTOCOAGULATION (PRP)

Panretinal photocoagulation is laser or light burning of the retina of diabetics to impede the progress of proliferative diabetic retinopathy. It has been shown to be effective against the progression of retinopathy by the diabetic retinopathy study (DRS).

Photocoagulation burns are scattered over the entire retina, except the macula, extending beyond the vortex vein ampullae. One uses 800 to 1600 burns. The argon laser, which is most commonly used, is usually set at 500-μm spots of 0.1 second in duration. In addition to the scatter technique throughout the entire posterior retina, focal treatment of new vessel formation is also used.

Harmful effects of this panretinal photocoagulation treatment are constriction of the visual fields and decrease in visual acuity. Dark adaptation is also decreased.

PAPILLOMACULAR BUNDLE

The nerve axons of the retinal ganglion cells that run from the macula to the optic nerve form the papillomacular bundle. These fibers transmit the most discriminating visual information. Recognition of the papillomacular bundle is important in laser therapy. Indiscriminant laser burns in the papillomacular bundle could affect vision more dramatically than burns in the retinal periphery.

PARINAUD'S SYNDROME (PRETECTAL SYNDROME)

Signs

- Loss of voluntary upward gaze
- Loss of pupillary light response with intact near reflex so that miosis occurs
- Convergent retraction movements (nystagmus retractorius) on upward gaze
- Ptosis
- Papilledema
- Third nerve palsy
- Lid retraction
- Loss of convergence and accommodation

Cause

A lesion in the tectal or pretectal area affects the periaqueductal area. Parinaud's syndrome may be caused by infiltrating gliomas, trauma, and pinealomas.

PARS PLANITIS

Other Names

Peripheral uveitis, chronic cyclitis, intermediate uveitis

Clinical Characteristics

Approximately two-thirds of the cases are bilateral. The condition is not uncommon. It occurs in younger individuals, children and young adults.

Symptoms are frequently few. Blurred vision may occur, and floaters may be seen within the visual field. In prolonged, severe cases, reduced visual acuity results from cystoid macular edema (page 281). Also, posterior subcapsular cataracts can occur. In some cases, retinal neovascularization, retinal detachments, and hemorrhages into the vitreous are serious complications.

Signs

The signs are a cellular exudation or membrane over the pars plana (inferior portion). The exudates or membranes are referred to as "snow banks." Periphlebitis of retinal vessels may occur. Edema of the disc and cystoid macular edema occur frequently.

Course

The course is chronic. There are periods of incomplete remissions. The disease may last 1 or 2 decades.

Cause

The cause is unknown. A very small percentage of pars planitis patients have developed multiple sclerosis.

PELLUCID MARGINAL DEGENERATION

Pellucid marginal degeneration of the cornea is bilateral. It is a clear degeneration that occurs inferiorly, usually from 4 to 8 o'clock. There is a narrow band of corneal thinning of approximately 20% of normal corneal thickness. This band is 1 to 2 mm in width. Characteristically, there is an uninvolved area of normal cornea, usually 1 to 2 mm in width, between the thin section and the limbus. Within the area of thinning, the cornea protrudes.

Characteristics

- High and irregular astigmatism
- No known hereditary pattern
- No sex predilection
- Corneal sensation normal
- No iron ring (page 13), no cone, and no lipid deposition
- Descemet's folds or stress lines
- Late complications of inferior edema, ruptures, and Descemet's membrane causing acute hydrops (page 13)
- Scarring and vascularization

Pathology

Abnormal collagen [fibrous long-spacing (FLS) collagen] is found.

PEMPHIGOID

Other Names

Cicatricial pemphigoid, benign mucosal pemphigoid, essential shrinkage of the conjunctiva, ocular pemphigoid

Characteristics

This is a subepithelial blistering disease of older people. It affects skin and mucous membranes and leads to scarring, shrinkage of tissue, and adhesions. Women are more often affected than men. It has no racial or geographic predilection. The conjunctiva is involved in approximately two-thirds of patients.

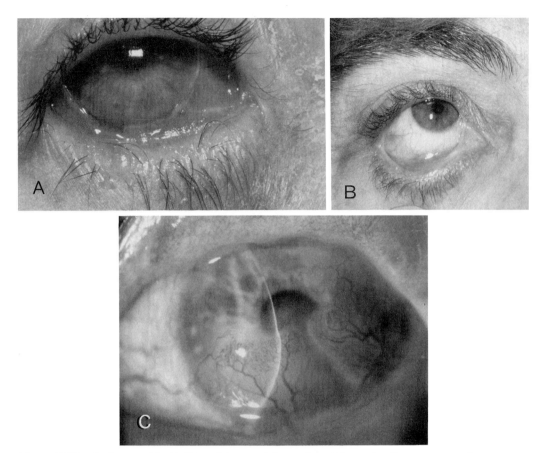

Figure 16.49. Ocular pemphigoid. This autoimmune inflammation of the conjunctiva causes scarring and may progress to cause severe visual loss. **A,** This conjunctival change is symblepharon, especially noted in the inferior conjunctival fornix (see page 19). (Credit: Ted Wojno, M.D.) **B,** Advanced pemphigoid with scarring. (Credit: George Waring, M.D.) **C,** In patients with progressive ocular pemphigoid, corneal changes may result in severe loss of vision. Illustrated are the vascularized changes that can occur in the cornea with pemphigoid. (Credit: George Waring, M.D.)

Clinical Features

This is a chronic progressive shrinkage of the mucous membranes. Blindness is reported in 16%. The condition is usually bilateral, although it may be asymmetrical.

There is progressive conjunctival scarring. Goblet cells are lost from the epithelium, and the epithelial cells become thick and keratinized. Tears become deficient from decreased mucus. The tear deficiency results in corneal epithelial complications; infections, stromal melting, and scarring occur.

The lid margins develop both entropion and trichiasis, which lead to further corneal scarring and damage. The vesicles on the conjunctiva eventually form symblepharon (page 369), with subsequent shrinking and scarring of the conjunctiva (Fig. 16.49). Associated systemic lesions occur in the mouth, nose, esophagus, pharynx, glands, penis, and vagina.

Cause

In cicatricial pemphigoid, hemogloblins and complement components bind to the epithelial basement membrane of skin or oral mucosa. IgG is most frequent, but IgA and IgM are also found.

Bullous Pemphigoid

Cicatricial pemphigoid frequently affects the eye. Bullous pemphigoid, also an autoimmune disease, rarely affects the eye. It is characterized by large bullae over areas of the skin. It is also more common in woman but tends to be a mild, relatively benign, self-limited disease.

PERIOCULAR DRUG SENSITIVITY

Topical ocular medications can produce skin sensitivity reactions. Response to antibiotics is a common cause. There is characteristic periocular redness and edema of the skin that results in puffiness and skin folds (Fig. 16.50). Desquamation may be present. Itching and rubbing of the eyes occurs, and tearing is a common accompanying symptom.

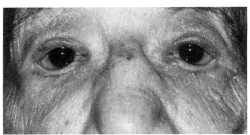

Figure 16.50. Drug sensitivities present a characteristic swelling and reddish to purplish discoloration of the eyelids and the periorbital region. A drug that commonly causes this reaction is the antibiotic neosporin. (Credit: Ted Wojno, M.D.)

PERIPAPILLARY CHOROIDAL ATROPHY

Peripapillary choroidal atrophy (Fig. 16.51), that is, atrophic choroid around the optic disc, can be seen in normal eyes (called the scleral crescent), in myopic eyes (called the myopic crescent), and in presumed ocular histoplasmosis syndrome. A helpful differential diagnostic point regarding choroidal atrophy is the position of a line of pigment (when present). The line of pigment in presumed ocular histoplasmosis syndrome is on the inner portion of the atrophy, that is, toward the disc margin of the peripapillary scarring. In peripapillary choroidal atrophy in normal eyes and in myopic eyes, the pigmentation is at the outer portion, that is, away from the disc.

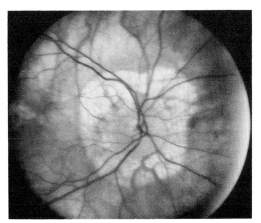

Figure 16.51. Peripapillary choroidal atrophy may be seen in normal and myopic eyes. Here the atrophy is represented as a whitish area where the choroidal vessels seem more prominent. Although this atrophy, which is in myopia, surrounds the disc, often only portions of the area around the disc are involved. (Credit: Paul Sternberg, M.D.)

PETERS' ANOMALY

Other Names

Mesodermal dysgenesis of the cornea, von Hippel's internal corneal ulcer

Ocular Findings

Peters' anomaly refers to a posterior corneal defect that has a scar (leukoma), adherent iris strands, and contact between the lens and the cornea. Because of the anterior positon of the lens, a shallow anterior chamber is present; as a result, peripheral anterior synechiae may cause secondary glaucoma. Primary glaucoma may be present in this condition. These eyes may be small (microphthalmic) and have congenital abnormalities of the vitreous (persistent hyperplastic primary vitreous) and retina (retinal dysplasia).

Associated Systemic Anomalies

Mental deficiency, congenital heart defects, genital and urinary abnormalities, cranial and facial abnormalities, syndactyly or polydactyly, and abnormalities of the external ear may be present.

PHENOTHIAZINE TOXICITY

Toxicity Subclasses

- Piperazine group (e.g., trifluoperazine) does not produce retinal complications.
- Dimethylamine group (e.g., chlorpromazine) rarely produces retinal pigment changes.
- *Piperadine group* (e.g., thioridazine): There is a risk of *retinal toxicity* with this group.

Ocular Changes

Phenothiazines, especially of the piperadine group, cause pigmentary ocular changes. Although pigment deposits can be seen on the corneal endothelium and on the lens capsule, they do not have serious effects on vision and are reversible after the drug is stopped.

It is the *pigmentary retinopathy* that is most important. Pigment deposits cause a diminution of central vision and night blindness. Diffuse narrowing of the retinal arterioles can also be seen with pigmentary changes.

Variable Reversibility

Although some of the pigmentary retinopathy changes are reversible when the drug is discontinued, in some patients the changes and effects are permanent.

Ocular Extrapyramidal Signs Common to All Phenothiazine Drugs

Phenothiazines can produce extrapyramidal signs that involve ocular movements.

PHLYCTENULE

A phlyctenule may occur on the cornea or on the conjunctiva. It is a whitish elevation with hyperemia (Fig. 16.52). In the center of the elevation, a central gray crater may develop. Phlyctenule is secondary to allergic toxins of staphylococcus most commonly but is also associated with tuberculosis. Histologically, lymphocytes and plasma cells predominate.

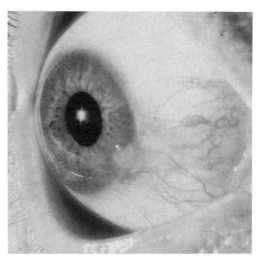

Figure 16.52. Phlyctenule is a localized hypersensitivity reaction most frequently associated with staphylococcal organisms. It is found most often at the limbus or peripheral cornea. Note the signs of acute inflammation.

PHYSIOLOGIC CUP

The physiologic cup is a central depression in the optic nerve (Fig. 16.53). This is seen as depression of the cup in the nerve and as a lighter or whiter coloration differentiating the cup from the surrounding, pinker disc tissue. A physiologic cup is not present in all individuals. The size of the physiologic cup is important in determining the cup/disc ratio (page 45).

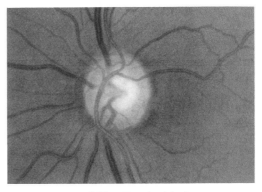

Figure 16.53. The physiologic cup.

PHOTOSTRESS TEST

Basics

The photostress test helps determine macular function by testing the recovery of macular cells after bleaching with a bright light.

The Test

1. Best corrected visual acuity is determined in the eye that is being tested. The opposite eye is occluded.
2. A bright light, either from an ophthalmoscope or from a hand-held muscle light, is directed into the eye at a distance of about 3 to 4 inches. The patient is asked to look at the light. This position is held for 20 seconds.
3. The timer is started when the light is removed.
4. The subject is then asked to read the eye chart. At first, the subject will be able to see only very large letters. As macular function adapts, the ability to read smaller lines will improve. When the subject reaches pretest acuity, the time is checked. The time from light stimulus removal to return to pretest acuity is recorded in seconds.

Results

Most patients will recover their pretest visual acuity after light bleaching in less than 30 seconds. Anything over 30 seconds is suspicious. Anything over 60 seconds is abnormal and should be investigated. The test is useful especially in central serous retinopathy and macular edema with diabetic retinopathy.

PHOTOTOXICITY

Definition

Photochemical damage is not associated with temperature elevation but results from exposure of the ocular tissues to light. Drugs can potentiate photochemical changes.

Snow Blindness

Snow blindness is a superficial corneal photokeratitis caused by high levels of UV radiation. Eighty per cent of UV radiation is reflected by snow, whereas earth and grass reflect less than 5%.

Indirect Ophthalmoscopy

Indirect ophthalmoscopy is known to cause retinal damage in primate eyes. Focal energy applied to the retina can be greater than that from exposure to the sun. The total radiation by indirect ophthalmoscopy is estimated to be one-third visible light and two-thirds infrared radiation.

Operating Microscope

Retinal burns have been associated with cataract surgery and exposure to the operating microscope light. Damage is primarily photochemical. Limiting the amount of light entering the eye and limiting the length of the operating procedure are the best prevention. Ultraviolet filters on the operating microscope have not prevented retinal burns.

Loss of the UV Filtration of the Crystalline Lens

With age, ultraviolet radiation (300 to 400 nm) transmission decreases. Seventy-five percent of ultraviolet radiation is transmitted in eyes under 10 years of age. Over 25 years of age, however, the UV transmission drops considerably. The lens is thought to act as a protective mechanism for the aging retina. Removal of the crystalline lens may result in loss of this protective mechanism.

Pathology

Photochemical damage causes outer segment loss first by changes in the normal lamellar structure and then by breaking off from the inner segment. The retinal pigment epithelium phagocytoses the outer segments, and the inner segments develop pyknotic nuclei. The final result is that photoreceptor cells vanish from the retina while other remaining layers of the retina remain intact.

It has been suggested that UV exposure may potentiate the effects of age-related macular degeneration. In patients who are aphakic (without the crystalline lens), sunglasses that filter UV light under 400 nm are recommended.

PINGUECULA

A pinguecula (plural, pingueculae or pingueculas) occurs as a yellow-white discoloration of the conjunctiva between the lid margins on either the nasal or the temporal side (Fig. 16.54). Pingueculae lack definite shape, are yellow white, and are subepithelial deposits in the conjunctiva. Pingueculae are degenerative lesions and may enlarge gradually over years.

The epithelium that overlies the pingueculae is usually normal. There is a subepithelial change in the collagen fibers, which become fragmented and curled and become more basophilic when stained with hematoxylin-eosin. These collagen fibers take on the staining characteristics of elastic tissue, although they are not actually elastic tissue. The process is referred to as elastoid or elastotic degeneration. Calcification may occur in the pingueculae.

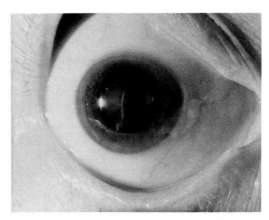

Figure 16.54. A pinguecula is a yellow-white discoloration on the conjunctiva. This one is close to the limbus. Pingueculae usually lack definite shape. They are degenerative changes. They are rarely symptomatic and, although frequent, are rarely removed.

PLACIDO'S DISK

Placido's disk is a flat metal disk that has alternating black and white circles painted on one side (Fig. 16.55). The painted side faces the patient. The examiner looks at the cornea through a hole in the center of the disk. The black and white circles are reflected from the cornea. With a normal cornea, these circles are regular. With abnormal curvatures or an irregular surface of the cornea, the circles are distorted or have irregular spacing. This examination is useful in keratoconus, irregular astigmatism, and corneal scars. Principles of the placido disk and corneal reflections are used with instruments such as the keratoscope and corneoscope, which photograph similar concentric rings on the cornea.

PLATEAU IRIS

Normally, the iris approaches a chamber angle well away from the

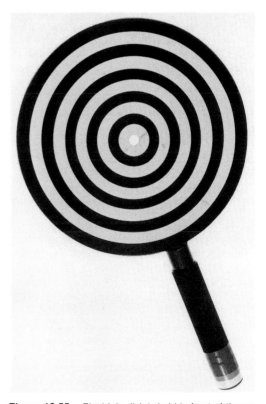

Figure 16.55. Placido's disk is held in front of the examiner, and the examiner looks through the central hole at the patient's cornea. The white and black circles are reflected from the cornea. Irregularities in the cornea can be seen as irregularities in the black and white circles reflected from the cornea. A normal cornea shows regular, smooth circles.

angle structures that allow egress of aqueous fluid. In the plateau iris, there is an anatomical irregularity in the periphery of the iris. This irregularity is a raised configuration at the angle that is in the shape of a plateau (see Fig. 3.17). This abnormal configuration stops the outflow of fluid and results in angle closure glaucoma.

It is difficult to determine clinically the presence of a plateau iris versus angle closure. Plateau iris is usually diagnosed when a peripheral iridectomy, the treatment for angle closure, is not successful. If a plateau iris configuration is present, then the diagnosis of plateau iris is made.

POLYARTERITIS NODOSA

In 20 to 30% of patients with polyarteritis nodosa, the eye is involved, typically the choroidal arteries. In addition, bilateral iritis, vitritis, and retinal vasculitis involving both the retinal arteries and the retinal veins have been described.

POSNER-SCHLOSSMAN SYNDROME

The Posner-Schlossman syndrome is a mild anterior uveitis in one eye of unknown cause that is frequently associated with a transient glaucoma. The preferred term is glaucomatocyclitic crisis (page 295).

POSTERIOR EMBRYOTOXON

See Anterior Cleavage Syndrome and Prominent Schwalbe's Ring (page 252).

POSTERIOR KERATOCONUS

Other Names

Posterior corneal depression, posterior conical cornea

Description

Posterior keratoconus, a posterior corneal indentation, is focal and discretely outlined. It involves the posterior cornea, and the cornea is thinned. The defect may be localized or total. A variable amount of stromal haze is associated with the defect; however, the cornea may be clear in some cases. In most cases, posterior keratoconus involves the central cornea, involves one eye, and has no familial or hereditary tendency. It is congenital.

The anterior corneal curvature is normal, and there is no relationship of this condition with the more common and entirely different anterior keratoconus.

Visual acuity is reduced only moderately, if at all. Glaucoma is not usually seen with this change, and systemic abnormalities are rare.

Posterior keratoconus is a variant of the anterior cleavage syndrome (page 252).

POSTERIOR POLYMORPHOUS DYSTROPHY

Posterior polymorphous dystrophy is a corneal dystrophy that has an onset in early childhood. It is a dystrophy of the endothelium and Descemet's membrane. Plaques of crystals occur in the deep stromal layers, with edema in the deep stroma and vesicular regions in the endothelium. The lesions tend to be round, elliptical, or regular. Inheritance is *autosomal dominant.*

The course tends to be stable, and vision is not severely affected. However, corneal transplantation may be necessary when severe corneal edema is associated.

PREAURICULAR ADENOPATHY

Swelling of the lymph nodes in front of the ears (preauricular adenopathy) is associated with certain infections of the conjunctiva. It can be of diagnostic significance, and the preauricular lymph nodes should be checked for swelling with all ocular infections. Common causes of preauricular adenopathy are:

- Epidemic keratoconjunctivitis (adenovirus);
- Pharyngeal conjunctival fever (adenovirus);
- Chlamydia infection (small nodes and only moderately tender);
- Gonococcal infection;
- Cat-scratch fever;
- Parinaud's oculoglandular syndrome;
- Others.

PREDILECTION FOR RETINAL QUADRANT NEOVASCULARIZATION

Neovascular lesions found in proliferative sickle cell retinopathy and in diabetic proliferative retinopathy have an identical selective preference for the following quadrants in this order: superotemporal, inferotemporal, superonasal, inferonasal. This predilection is similar to that seen in retinopathy of prematurity and retinal branch vein occlusion.

PRENTICE'S RULE

Prentice's rule of decentration is used to calculate induced prism power in a bifocal lens.

P = prism power in prism diopters
d = decentration (distance between the optical center and the line of sight expressed in centimeters)
l = lens power in diopters
$$P = d \times l$$

(See also Object Displacement, page 327.)

PRESBYOPIA

Presbyopia results from changes in accommodation with age. Accommodation is an adjustment of the lens, ciliary body, and zonules to allow focus from far to near. With age, hardening of the lens and decreased elasticity of the lens fibers results in less capacity for accommodation. In the very young, the accommodation is 15 diopters or more. By the age of 40, accommodation is decreased to less than 5 diopters (Table 16.4).

Table 16.4.
Presbyopia: Table of Accommodation

Age (years)	Diopters of Accommodation (diopters)
8	13.8
25	9.9
35	7.3
40	5.8
45	3.6
50	1.9
55	1.3

This lack of accommodation power results in the pushing away of reading material characteristic in middle age and the complaint "my arms are not long enough." Presbyopia is corrected by plus lenses usually given as a reading glass or as a bifocal with distance correction.

PRIMARY INFANTILE GLAUCOMA (CONGENITAL GLAUCOMA)

This developmental glaucoma manifests signs and symptoms at birth or during the early months of life. When the condition exists while the fetus is in the uterus, the effects of high pressure and an immature sclera that is soft and cannot resist expansion causes enlargement of the globe *(buphthalmos)* and enlargement of the corneal diameter. The increased intraocular pressure results in *cupping* of the optic nerves.

In infants, the presence of increased tearing *(epiphora)*, light sensitivity *(photophobia)*, and spasms of the lid *(blepharospasm)* are highly suggestive of primary infantile glaucoma.

Characteristics

Most cases develop within the first 6 months of life. The condition is bilateral in more than 75% of patients. The children often present with cloudy corneas, and infantile glaucoma is one of the prime considerations in the differential diagnosis of cloudy cornea. Frequently, the presence of characteristic breaks in Descemet's membrane (Haab's striae) cannot be seen because of the corneal edema.

Diagnosis

General anesthesia is usually required for intraocular pressure measurement and optic nerve evaluation in an infant suspected of having infantile glaucoma.

Enlargement of the globe, increased diameter of the cornea, corneal edema, and enlargement of the optic nerve cup all point to the diagnosis. Measurement of intraocular pressure is essential at the time of anesthesia.

Confirmation of the diagnosis is by gonioscopy. The following gonioscopy features are characteristic:

- Anterior iris insertion;
- Thickening of the uveal meshwork;
- Translucent and glistening appearance to the meshwork;
- Hypoplastic peripheral iris;
- Iris pulled toward Schwalbe's line.

Differential Diagnosis

- Inherited corneal dystrophies
- Infectious diseases
- Metabolic diseases such as the mucopolysaccharoidoses
- Birth trauma
- Secondary glaucomas due to inflammation or congenital abnormalities of the eye

PRISM DIOPTER

Prism power expresses the amount of deviation of a light ray passing through a prism. One diopter of prism power will cause displacement of the ray (or image) by 1 centimeter at a distance of 1 meter (Fig. 16.56).

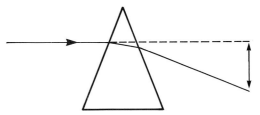

Figure 16.56. A prism diopter (different than a diopter of power of a lens) is the amount of power of a prism that will change the direction of a ray of light 1 cm at a distance of 1 meter from the prism.

PROSOPAGNOSIA

Prosopagnosia is the inability to recognize or distinguish faces. It occurs with bilateral brain lesions. It is a subset of visual agnosia, which occurs with bilateral lesions also. Visual agnosia is the inability to recognize objects by sight while retaining the ability to recognize them by touch.

PROLIFERATIVE DIABETIC RETINOPATHY

New vessel formation in the retina of a patient with diabetes represents the proliferative phase of diabetic retinopathy. Only a small percentage of patients with background retinopathy (page 65) progress to proliferative diabetic retinopathy. However, proliferative diabetic retinopathy can be highly destructive to the eye.

With the proliferation of new vessel formation, vessels leak fluorescein readily. New vessels do not have the same vascular stability as old vessels. As new vessels proliferate, they can break into the vitreous, where vitreous hemorrhage can occur. Hemorrhage can also occur between the retina and the vitreous, causing a contained area of bleeding (preretinal hemorrhage). With proliferation and hemorrhage, a fibrovascular reaction occurs and fibrous, dense scarring causes traction retinal detachments and eventual loss of vision.

New vessel formation can be divided into two areas, which changes the prognosis of individual patients. New vessel formation in the disc area (known as NVD for "new vessels disc") is a term used for any new vessel formation on the disc or within 1 disc diameter of the optic disc. This has a poor prognosis. Outside this area, new vessel formation is known as NVE ("new vessels elsewhere"). NVE seen alone, and not being raised, may remain stable for long periods. It is not a significant risk factor for severe visual loss from proliferative diabetic retinopathy.

PROMINENT SCHWALBE'S RING (POSTERIOR EMBRYOTOXON)

Schwalbe's line is the junction at the periphery of the cornea of the uveal trabecular meshwork and the termination of Descemet's membrane. Schwalbe's line is not visible in most eyes by slitlamp biomicroscopy but can be seen by gonioscopy.

A prominent Schwalbe's ring, also known as posterior embryotoxon, is seen as a whitish, irregular ridge located 0.5 to 2 mm central to the limbus by slitlamp without gonioscopy. It can be seen in 8 to 15% of normal eyes.

Schwalbe's ring (that is, a prominent Schwalbe's line) consists of collagen core-containing reticulin fibers and a basement membrane-like substance. It is surrounded by Descemet's membrane and is covered by a layer of endothelium.

PROGRESSIVE SUPRANUCLEAR PALSY

Ocular Signs and Symptoms

The patient loses the smooth pursuit of ocular motion. There is also loss of Bell's phenomenon (page 260). The patient is unable to fixate on an object, and convergence of the eyes inward is deficient. There may be an inability to open the eyelids (apraxia) and associated spasm of lid closure (blepharospasm).

General Signs

Patients have disturbed balance, which results in abrupt falls. Speech becomes slurred, and there is difficulty swallowing (dysphagia). Personality changes occur, and there is mild loss of mental function (dementia).

Pathology

There is neural loss, gliosis, and demyelination in the brain stem, with relative sparing of the cerebral cortex and the cerebellar cortex.

PSEUDOFACILITY

Pseudofacility is a term used in measuring the total facility of outflow (C-value, see page 264) of aqueous and is measured by tonography. With a tonometer, the eye is indented, and the degree of indentation correlates with the intraocular pressure. Tonography uses tonometry over a number of minutes. The tonometer forces fluid out of the eye, and the difference in intraocular pressure is measured over 4 minutes. Facility of outflow is calculated.

During tonography, the indentation of the plunger not only forces fluid out, resulting in lower pressure, but also decreases aqueous production during the 4-minute period required for tonography. Pseudofacility is that part of total facility outflow that is represented by the decrease of aqueous production during the tonography procedure.

PSEUDOPTOSIS

Ptosis, a drooping of the upper lid, narrows the distance between the upper and lower lids (a smaller palpebral fissure) because the lid cannot be elevated properly. There are conditions, however, that may simulate a ptosis when the lid is normal. Both a congenitally small eye (microphthalmos) and a shrunken globe due to disease or injury (phthisis bulbi) cause pseudoptosis. Because the globe is small in these conditions, the lid has no support and appears to be lower, suggesting a ptosis when the lid is actually normal.

PSEUDOXANTHOMA ELASTICUM

Loose elastic skin changes occur in pseudoxanthoma elasticum. Pseudoxanthoma elasticum is associated with angioid streaks (page 248) in the posterior pole of the eye.

PTERYGIUM

Pterygium is a growth of conjunctival and fibrous vascular tissue that proceeds onto the cornea (Fig. 16.57). It is almost always accompanied or preceded by a pinguecula.

Pathologic changes consist of elastoid degeneration of the collagen and the appearance of subepithelial fibrovascular tissue ingrowth. The epithelium is usually normal but may show some dysplasia over the pterygium. Inflammatory changes may be present. An iron line can be seen at the head of the advancing portion of the pterygium. This is known as *Stocker's line.*

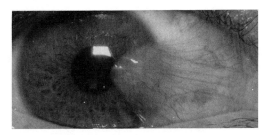

Figure 16.57. Pterygium is a growth that extends from the conjunctiva onto the cornea. These growths are always found between the lids extending from either the nasal or the temporal side. They may be slowly progressive. They are most often associated with ultraviolet exposure and drying. They are found most often in hot, equatorial climates. (Credit: Ted Wojno, M.D.)

It is unknown why some patients develop pterygium and some don't. The prevalence of pterygium is high in a belt around the earth close to the equator. Pterygia are not seen as frequently in colder climates away from the equator. The distribution suggests that one of the major predisposing factors is sunlight (ultraviolet) exposure of the conjunctiva.

Another factor thought to contribute to ptergium growth is localized drying of an abnormal tear film. Because the pterygium is raised above the surface of the cornea, the head of the pterygium may not allow adequate wetting of the cornea by tears distributed by the blink. Localized drying of the cornea at the head of the pterygium may occur. Growth of the pterygium may result as a tissue repair reaction to this drying.

PTHIRUS PUBIS (PUBIC LOUSE) INFECTION

The pubic louse can be seen not only on pubic hairs but also on lid margin lashes. Adult organisms or nits (which are ova-shaped) can be found on the eyelashes, a finding that is diagnostic. Itching is a frequent complaint.

The pubic louse secretes feces that are toxic to the conjunctiva. The conjunctival reaction to this toxin is (*a*) follicular in children and (*b*) papillary in adults.

PUPILLARY BLOCK GLAUCOMA

Pupillary block glaucoma is a secondary glaucoma. In pupillary block glaucoma, there is a backward pressure of aqueous behind the iris because of the resistance to flow of aqueous between the lens and the iris. The increase in pressure in the posterior chamber causes the thin peripheral iris to bulge forward in the anterior chamber angle and close off the trabecular meshwork. With the apposition of the iris to the meshwork, the pressure rises (Fig. 16.58). The maximal area that tends to bring on an acute attack of pupillary block glaucoma occurs when the pupil is at the size of 3.5 to 6 mm.

Peripheral iridectomy, to allow aqueous to flow from the posterior chamber to the anterior chamber freely, corrects pupillary block glaucoma. Pupillary dilation also reverses an acute attack.

Certain anatomical factors predispose the eye to pupillary block: a thick, anteriorly displaced lens, a smaller diameter and shorter posterior curve of the cornea, and a short axial length of the globe. These factors may be influenced by hyperopia, advancing age, and hereditary predisposition.

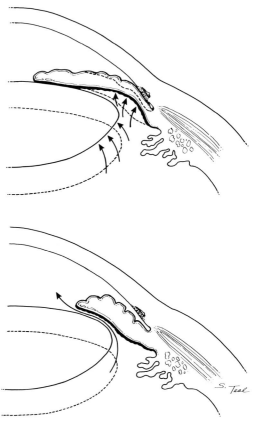

Figure 16.58. Pupillary block occurs when the iris is pushed forward against the trabecular meshwork, causing a decrease in the outflow of aqueous and a secondary rise in intraocular pressure (glaucoma). Pupillary block can be broken by dilating the pupil, allowing the iris to fall back because the aqueous that has been trapped behind the pupil (pushing it forward) is now released.

RADIATION CATARACT

Ionizing radiation, even low concentrations, can cause lens damage. After exposure of the human lens to irradiation, changes that are clinically apparent may not occur for up to 20 years. This latency, from exposure to lens change, relates to the patient's age as well as the dosage of radiation. Patients who have more actively growing lens cells are more susceptible to damage. The threshold dose is 500 to 600 r.

These cataracts are first seen as small, very fine, anterior subcapsular opacities. Posterior subcapsular opacities then occur, which are granular or appear as vacuoles.

RAMSAY-HUNT SYNDROME

The Ramsay-Hunt syndrome is herpes zoster involvement of the facial nerve. Diagnosis is established by seeing vesicles over the tympanic membrane and along the posterior aspect of the external auditory meatus, a distribution that corresponds to the sensory distribution of the facial nerve. This facial nerve involvement is often associated with severe pain.

RED REFLEX

Description

By shining a light into the pupil so that the choroidal blood and retinal pigment epithelium provide a reddish glow from within the eye, a red reflex can be produced. This is helpful in diagnosis.

Technique

The most common technique to produce a red reflex is by dialing plus lenses in the direct ophthalmoscope. Standing at approximately arm's length from the patient, the examiner shines the light in the pupil and the pupil fills with a reddish orange sunset color. To help focus, keep details of the eye sharp. The lenses usually needed are +5 to +9.

Opacities of either the vitreous or the lens show up as black. Irregularities of the cornea and some irregularities of the lens (keratoconus in the cornea, for example, and lenticonus in the lens) show up as variations and irregularities in the intensity of the light reflex (see Fig. 1.15 page 12).

(See also Bruchner's test, page 263.)

REIGER'S ANOMALY (PRIMARY DIGENESIS MESODERMALIS)

Characteristics

Reiger's anomaly is a prominent Schwalbe's ring with attached iris strands and a hypoplastic anterior iris stroma. The superficial iris stroma is absent, and there are no crypts or furrows. As a result, the posterior iris stoma, which consists of delicate radial fibers, gives the iris a gray-brown, stringy appearance. The iris sphincter can be seen easily at the pupillary ring. The pupil is abnormal in shape and size in almost 75% of these cases. A prominent Schwalbe's ring, with variable appearance, is present.

Other Findings

When facial and dental abnormalities accompany the ocular findings of Reiger's anomaly, it is called Reiger's syndrome. Nonocular changes include maxillary hypoplasia, telecanthus, and small or absent teeth. Malformation of the limbs and spine occur. Congenital heart defects, mental retardation, cerebellar hypoplasia, and deafness have also been reported.

Heredity

Reiger's anomaly is autosomal dominant in the majority of cases and has a very high penetrance with extreme variation in the clinical presentation.

REIS-BUCKLER DYSTROPHY

Inheritance

Autosomal dominant

Clinical Appearance

Reis-Buckler dystrophy presents with a number of ring-like opacities that form a network at the level of Bowman's layer and protrude into the epithelium, causing distortion of the anterior corneal surface.

Onset

Reis-Buckler dystrophy begins at about 5 years of age.

Course

The course is progressive with recurrent epithelial erosions that become more frequent as the dystrophy progresses. Anterior scarring causes a loss of visual acuity. Corneal sensation is decreased.

Histopathology

Destruction of Bowman's layer, irregular scar tissue, microfilamentous aggregates, and the absence of hemidesmosomes are characteristic.

RELATIVE SCOTOMA

A relative scotoma is a functional defect in the visual field. If you stimulate with a large enough or bright enough test object, the object can be seen in a relative scotoma. This is in contrast to an absolute scotoma, where no vision is possible. (A scotoma is an area of reduced or absent vision within the visual field.)

RETINAL HEMORRHAGE

Hemorrhages in the retina may make a variety of clinical presentations (Fig. 16.59). Those superficial in the retinal layers (that is, most internally), which are in the nerve fiber layer, present as flame-shaped hemorrhages. Round or dot-blot hemorrhages are deeper hemorrhages in the outer layers of the retina. Preretinal hemorrhages occur between the hyaloid of the vitreous and the retina.

RETINAL PIGMENT EPITHELIAL HYPERPLASIA

Congenital retinal pigment epithelial hypertrophy appears as a jet-black lesion with pigmentation that may not be uniform. There are focal lacunae of hypopigmentation. Borders are frequently distinct and scalloped (Fig. 16.60). In contrast, choroidal melanocytic lesions appear slate-gray to black or brown.

RETINAL TELANGIECTASIS

Retinal telangiectases are aneurysms on the retina that leak fluores-

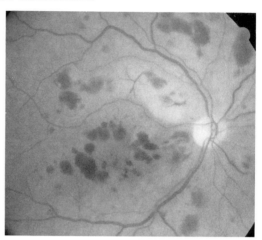

Figure 16.59. Retinal hemorrhages can occur in the nerve fiber layer or in the deeper (outer) layers of the retina. They are easily seen by direct or indirect ophthalmoscopy.

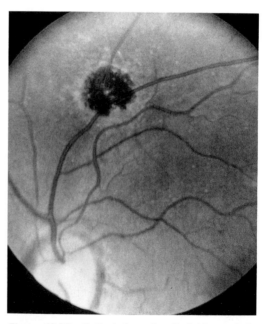

Figure 16.60. Retinal pigment epithelial hyperplasia. Note the distinct borders and the vessel passage over the top of the lesion without distortion.

cein readily and are associated with exudates. They tend to form along the retinal vasculature and are associated with ischemic areas. They should be differentiated from cavernous hemangioma (see page 265). Systemic changes associated with retinal telangiectasis are cystic cerebellar hemangiomas, renal cysts, renal cell carcinoma, and pheochromocytomas.

RETINAL VENOUS BEADING

Retinal venous beading is a vascular disorder characterized by marked beading of the retinal veins. To a lesser agree, the conjunctival veins may also be involved. The inheritance pattern is autosomal dominant. Patients also have an associated retinopathy including microaneurysms, exudates, new vessel formation, and hemorrhage into the vitreous. The cause is unknown. No systemic findings are consistently associated with the retinal findings.

RETINOSCOPY

A retinoscope is a hand-held instrument. It uses a light that is reflected from a mirror into the pupil of the subject. The examiner views the light reflex in the pupil that is created by the light. Movement of the reflex is seen with movement of the retinoscope.

By placing lenses in front of the patient's eye, the patient's focal point is altered. This alters the character of the retinoscope reflex. In this way, an objective refraction can be completed that is very accurate in the hands of a skilled retinoscopist.

ROSACEA

Rosacea is a hyperemic disease of the skin. It affects primarily the middle third of the face, involving the skin of the forehead above the nose, the skin on the nose, and the cheeks. It is characterized by erythremia, telangiectasia, papules, pustules, and hypertrophic sebaceous glands. In advanced cases, rhinophyma occurs. This is hypertrophy of the nose, increased vascularity, and increased size of the sebaceous glands.

Ocular rosacea is diagnosed when skin rosacea is also present (Fig. 16.61). In ocular rosacea, blepharoconjunctivitis, keratitis, and episcleritis occur.

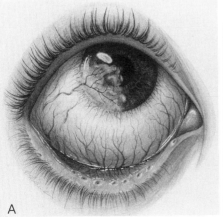 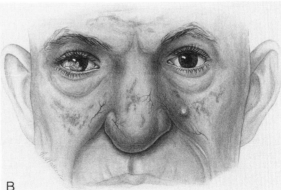

A   B

Figure 16.61.   Ocular rosacea. Changes on the eyelids and in the eye are commonly associated with the skin changes of rosacea. The skin changes include a flushing redness of the nose, upper face, and forehead area. There are also spider-like telangiectatic vessels on the nose and face. The eye changes can become severe and may vascularize. Illustrated is a corneal lesion secondary to ocular rosacea associated with skin rosacea.

Blepharoconjunctivitis is most common. It is characterized by thickening of the lid margin. The margins are red and have telangiectasia. Chalazia are frequently associated with rosacea. Rosacea is twice as common in patients with recurrent chalazia as in those who have had only one episode of chalazion.

The conjunctivitis associated with rosacea is usually diffuse hyperemia and engorged vessels. It is characteristic for both the palpebral and the bulbar conjunctiva to be involved. The discharge tends to be watery.

Nodular conjunctivitis is unusual, but it does occur. Vascularized nodules appear on the bulbar conjunctiva, especially near the limbus. These have a rapid onset and also clear rapidly.

Rosacea may also be associated with meibomitis, and the meibomian gland orifices may characteristically protrude. Meibomian gland secretions also may be cloudy and thickened.

The second most common associated ocular change with rosacea is keratitis. This may be associated with foreign body sensation, pain, and light sensitivity. Subepithelial infiltrates, which are small, round, and sharply delineated, occur near the limbus. Larger subepithelial infiltrates of grayish coloration are also seen. Heavy vascularization is not uncommon.

Punctate epithelial erosions occur on many corneas in patients with rosacea. Usually, the inferior one-third of the cornea is involved.

Episcleritis and scleritis are the least frequent developments with rosacea. Nodules that are highly vascularized may be seen.

ROSENMÜLLER'S VALVE

Rosenmüller's valve is a small valve that prevents the reflux of tears from the lacrimal sac back into the canaliculus (see Fig. 11.1 page 195). With inflammation, edema, or distortion, the valve may become tight and prevent reflux of material from the lacrimal sac through the canaliculus. Examination of the function of this valve is a common diagnostic technique to determine the status of the lacrimal system.

ROTH'S SPOTS

Roth's spots are seen best on examination with direct ophthalmoscopy. They are hemorrhages with white centers that correspond to an area of infarction. They are most often associated with subacute bacterial endocarditis; however, they are a nonspecific observation and are seen in patients with a variety of other conditions, including anemia and other hematologic disorders.

RUBEOSIS (RUBEOSIS IRIDES)

Definition

Rubeosis is new vessel formation on the surface of the iris.

Clinical Features

In the early stages, the new vessels are seen at the pupillary border. Later, all of the iris and the angle may be involved, and secondary glaucoma that is difficult to control can occur. Bleeding into the anterior chamber (hyphema) is not unusual.

The two most important causes of rubeosis are:

- Diabetes (page 65);
- Retinal vein occlusion (page 84).

There are many other causes of rubeosis, all of which relate to reduced oxygen to the retina:

- Aortic arch syndrome;
- Carotid occlusive disease;
- Radiation effects;
- Anterior ocular segment ischemia; and
- Others.

SALMON PATCH

Salmon patch is a descriptive term applied to the corneal changes seen in congenital syphilis. The corneal edema, which is vascularized, has a pinkish hue on the background gray-white corneal edema (see Congenital Syphilis, page 14).

SALUS SIGN

Salus sign is associated with high blood pressure. It is due to a rigid retinal arteriole that occurs with arteriosclerosis. There is retinal vein deflection as the artery crosses over the vein. This change is noted as Salus sign (see Hypertensive Retinopathy, page 160).

SALZMANN'S NODULAR DYSTROPHY

Salzmann's nodular dystrophy is a condition that is always preceded by corneal inflammation. Most commonly associated are trachoma or phlyctenular keratoconjunctivitis.

Clinical Appearance

Gray-white lesions in the cornea are round and raised above the epithelium but involve the stroma and Bowman's layer. Although the lesions are most often isolated, either singular or multiple, they may occasionally appear in chains.

Pathology

This is a *degeneration* of the superficial layers of the cornea.

SAMPAOLESI'S LINE

Sampaolesi's line is associated with glaucoma and the *exfoliation syndrome.* Pigment deposited anterior to Schwalbe's line (page 253) forms Sampaolesi's line. Also, there is often an unusual amount of pigment in the trabeculum.

SANFILIPO'S SYNDROME

Carbohydrate storage disorders include the mucopolysaccharidoses types I–VII. Sanfilipo's syndrome characterizes type III, with a progressive systemic storage of herparan sulfate.

Four clinically indistinguishable forms are found. They are separated biochemically by their specific enzyme deficiencies:

- Type A—heparan sulfate sulfaminidase
- Type B—*N*-acetyl-*α*-*β*-glucosaminidase
- Type C—*α*-glucosaminidase *N*-acetyltransferase
- Type D—*N*-acetylglucosamine 6-sulfatase

Heredity

Autosomal recessive

Ocular Findings

The ocular findings of mucopolysaccharidosis type III include corneas that are clinically clear (in contrast to types I, IV, VI, and VII, where clouding can occur). Ultrastructurally, however, the corneal cells show mucopolysaccharide deposits. These deposits are also seen in the iris, lens, ciliary body, and sclera. The involvement of the retina looks like retinitis pigmentosa (page 75) and leads to visual loss. The massive storage of the heparan sulfate within the retinal pigment epithelium is thought to disturb retinal metabolism and lead to photoreceptor damage.

Symptoms usually appear before 5 years of age. Death occurs in the 20s or 30s.

Diagnosis

A mucopolysaccharide urine spot test is required for diagnosis. The urine contains high levels of heparan sulfate. The definitive diagnosis is made by specific enzyme assay.

Sanfilipo's syndrome is differentiated from the other mucopolysaccharidoses by more severe mental retardation and less skeletal involvement. The genetic pattern also helps establish the diagnosis.

SCHIÖTZ TONOMETER

The Schiötz tonometer is a metal device that measures intraocular pressure by a footplate that fits directly over the cornea (Fig. 16.62). In the center of the footplate is a hole though which a plunger moves. As the plunger indents the cornea, a pointer records readings on a scale. The plunger, when flush to the footplate on the cornea, produces a reading of zero.

The plunger and its weight (the weight can be adjusted by adding heavier or lighter metal disks) indent the cornea. The amount of indentation of the cornea depends upon the intraocular pressure. The higher the pressure, the less indentation; the lower the pressure, the more indentation.

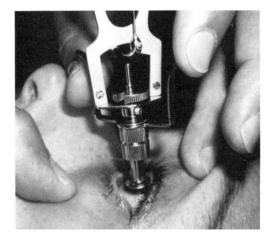

Figure 16.62. Schiötz tonometer in position on the cornea. The Schiötz tonometer is a tonometer with a central plunger and a footplate that fits directly on the cornea. At the top is a scale that has absolute numbers that are converted into millimeters of mercury (see Fig. 3.1 page 40).

Scale Reading

On the scale, a zero reading shows high pressure. Higher scale numbers correspond to lower pressures. With each tonometer, a chart for converting scale readings to intraocular pressures in millimeters of mercury is provided.

If the Schiötz tonometer is placed on the eye and the scale reading is zero, additional weight is added until a numerical scale reading is obtained. Conversion charts for these additional individual weights are provided.

Technique of Tonometry

Local anesthesia, proparacaine or tetracaine, is dropped in the eye. The patient is usually placed in a supine position so that the eye is looking straight up. The patient fixates on a point (with the eye not being examined) either on the ceiling or on his thumb with his arm extended.

The examiner separates the lids with his thumb and forefinger (see Fig. 16.62). He keeps the lids away from the eyeball to avoid pressure and is sure not to exert pressure directly on the globe. The Schiötz tonometer is placed in a vertical position directly on the cornea. The plunger inside the footplate is allowed to exert its full weight. The appropriate weight is tested by moving the support sleeve, held by the hand, up and down.

The starting weight (5.5 g) is baseline. Scale readings above 3 are converted to millimeters of mercury and recorded. If the scale reading is below 3, a 7.5-g weight is added. The procedure is then repeated for scale readings, which are converted. If the scale reading is below 3 with a 7.5-g weight, a 10-g weight is used.

Sources of Error

If the eye is very elastic (low ocular rigidity), it may expand more with the action of the plunger and give a falsely low intraocular pressure reading. If, however, the globe is very rigid (high ocular rigidity), the excursion of the plunger in the footplate may be inhibited and a falsely high intraocular pressure may be recorded.

Schiötz tonometry may be less accurate in myopic patients and patients with thyroid ocular disease. In these patients, applanation tonometry is more accurate.

Important Note

Most tonometers are sterilized with alcohol after a reading. An alcohol wipe is used to wipe the footplate and the plunger. Most effective sterilization occurs with removal of the plunger and a separate wiping of the plunger itself. Because certain viruses, especially epidemic keratoconjunctivitis (adenovirus 9), can be transmitted by Schiötz tonometry, it is important to take additional cleansing care between patients and especially when treating patients with red eyes or suspected infections. Mechanical cleansing is important because there is no known effective method of sterilization for all viruses and bacteria.

AIDS virus and antibodies have been detected in tears. Soaking tonometers in hydrogen peroxide or Hydrochlorite for 5 minutes has been recommended. However, transmission of AIDS by tonometry has never been reported.

SCHISTOSOMIASIS (*SCHISTOSOMA HAEMATOBIUM*)

Regional Distribution

This is endemic in Egypt, especially around the Nile basin.

Clinical Appearance

This is a granulomatous conjunctivitis with small tumors that appear smooth on the surface and are pinkish-yellow.

Diagnosis is made by examination of biopsy material. Granulomas contain lymphocytes, plasma cells, and giant cells plus eosinophils. These cells surround the *bilharzial ova.*

SCHNABEL'S OPTIC ATROPHY

Schnabel's or cavernous optic atrophy occurs after long-standing glaucoma. It is associated with accumulation of hyaluronic acid in the anterior portion of the optic nerve.

SCLERAL CRESCENT

In most eyes, the pigment epithelium, which provides the color background of the fundus, runs to the edge of disc. In some eyes, this approximation of the pigment epithelium is not complete. Without the reddish or red-brown pigment epithelium, sclera shows through the transparent retinal tissue as a white crescent (Fig. 16.63). The shape and position of the crescent can be variable.

The myopic crescent also appears at the disc margin because the pigment epithelium fails to approximate the disc edge. Unlike scleral crescents, however, myopic crescents progress as the myopic eye elongates.

Because scleral crescents are very common, the beginner with the ophthalmoscope should identify crescents to avoid confusion with other, more serious conditions such as optic atrophy, papilledema, and disc hypoplasia (see Myopic Crescent, page 324).

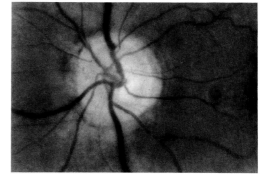

Figure 16.63. The scleral crescent is a common finding and is variable in appearance. It is a whitish ring or partial ring around the optic disc. It may be pigmented. In this illustration, the optic disc edge shows as a faint, pale white. The scleral crescent to the *right* is fairly uniform and that to the *left* is more irregular, with some pigment.

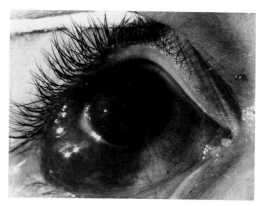

Figure 16.64. Scleral rupture is an important diagnosis that can almost always be made clinically, although CT scanning is frequently used to confirm the diagnosis. Conjunctival edema, a deep anterior chamber, hyphema (blood in the anterior chamber), and a faint corneal haze are common findings.

SCLERAL RUPTURE

Scleral rupture is due to blunt trauma (Fig. 16.64). With injury, the pressure against the outside of the globe increases pressure internally until the globe ruptures. The most common sites of rupture are the limbus and the equator. There is a special predilection to positions under the rectus muscle, where the sclera tends to be the thinnest.

There are classic clinical signs of scleral rupture:

- Decreased vision;
- Chemosis of the conjunctiva, localized or generalized; .
- Deep anterior chamber;
- Low intraocular pressure (although pressures may be normal or even increased on occasion);

- Hyphema (blood in the anterior chamber);
- Faint corneal clouding.

CT scanning can help establish the diagnosis, as can other diagnostic techniques such as ultrasound. Classic CT signs are:

- Scleral discontinuity;
- Scleral thickening (probably due to blood in the region);
- Flattening of the normal posterior curve of the eye;
- Blood in the vitreous;
- Air in the eye.

SCOTOMA (BLIND SPOT)

Scotoma is a non-seeing area in the visual field. It can be caused by damage anywhere in the visual system, from the retina to the occipital cortex. There are many adjectives used with the word scotoma.

Absolute Scotoma

This is an area where a test object, regardless of its size or brightness, *cannot* be seen.

Relative Scotoma

This is a scotoma where objects can be seen with bright or large stimuli but cannot be seen with smaller, dim objects.

Arcuate Scotoma

This is an arc-shaped scotoma caused by nerve fiber bundle damage, which is common in patients with glaucoma.

Bjerrum Scotoma

This is an arc-shaped defect in the paracentral area of the visual field that is caused by damage to the retinal nerve bundle fibers and is common also in patients with glaucoma.

Seidel's Scotoma

This is an extension of the normal physiologic blind spot into a comma shape. As it continues to enlarge, it becomes an arcuate scotoma of the Bjerrum type. It is seen with glaucoma.

Central Scotoma

This is loss of the central 5° of the visual field.

Centrocecal

This is a blind spot involving the central portion of vision, which includes the fixation area as well as the physiologic blind spot. It is most often seen with toxicity to the optic nerve.

Junction Scotoma (Page 310)

This is a scotoma characteristic of a lesion in the *chiasm,* where the optic nerves meet and then separate into the optic tracts. It is a lesion that interrupts the lower nasal fibers as they cross through the chiasm. Its characteristics are changes in both eyes; one eye has a loss of central vision, and the other eye has a visual field defect in the other half of the visual field.

Negative Scotoma

This is a scotoma of which the patient is not aware.

Positive Scotoma

This is a scotoma of which the patient is aware. It is seen as an area of decreased illumination within the visual field.

Ring Scotoma

This is a scotoma that is ring-shaped and surrounds the area of fixation. It is usually located about 20 to 40 degrees from the central area. It is associated with degeneration of the retina. It also may be an artifact of certain types of glasses with high plus powers that are used after cataract extraction (aphakic correction).

SEA FAN SIGN

Sea fan sign is associated most often with the ischemia of sickle cell retinopathy (page 83). In the early stages of neovascularization, new blood vessel formation adopts a fan-shaped configuration. This lies flat on the internal surface of the retina and is two-dimensional. In the initial stages, the sea fan is supplied by one major feeding arteriole and drained by one major venule.

Sea fans leak fluorescein dye profusely when dye is injected into the venous system. This may be observed by direct ophthalmoscopy, indirect ophthalmoscopy with a cobalt filter, or with fluorescein angiography.

Sea fans are most commonly observed in sickle cell C disease and in sickle cell thalassemia patients. They are uncommon in other sickle cell hemoglobinopathies.

SEBORRHEIC BLEPHARITIS

This is a noninfectious blepharitis of the lid margins. It is associated with seborrheic dermatitis, most commonly of the scalp (dandruff). Oily lid margins are seen, with crusting on the lashes and lids. The course is chronic and protracted. Approximately 15% of patients will have an associated keratitis. A papillary or follicular conjunctivitis with bulbar injection may also be seen. The cause is thought to be sebaceous gland dysfunction.

SECONDARY MALIGNANT NEOPLASMS IN PATIENTS WITH HEREDITABLE RETINOBLASTOMA

Secondary malignant neoplasms (SMN) are known to occur in survivors of bilateral retinoblastoma. Such patients have an increased risk of developing osteogenic sarcomas as well as other secondary cancers. Malignant melanoma has also been reported as an important SMN in survivors of hereditary retinoblastoma.

The risk of SMN in survivors of retinoblastoma increases with age. It is estimated to be 2% at age 12 and as high as 90% at age 30.

SECTOR PALSIES OF THE PUPIL

When the pupil is dilated and reacts poorly or not at all to light, the possibility of Adie's pupil (syndrome) should be considered. A characteristic contraction of the pupillary margin is seen with Adie's pupil. On stimulation with light and viewing with magnification of the slitlamp, segmental contractions of the pupillary margin are seen. These are also called *vermiform* movements (see Adie Syndrome and Adie's Pupil, pages 94 and 359).

SENSORY EXOTROPIA

Sensory exotropia is an outward deviation of the eyes that results from decreased vision in one eye. Decreased vision in one eye might be due to a difference in refractive error between the eyes, cataract, corneal scars, or any opacity of the ocular medium.
(See Exotropia, page 151.)

SERPIGINOUS CHOROIDOPATHY

Characteristics

Serpiginous choroidopathy is a bilateral involvement of the choroid around the disc area (peripapillary) and of the retinal pigment epithelium. It occurs later in life in the 4th, 5th, and 6th decades. It has a long course with recurrent episodes. Fluctuations of vision may occur during exacerbations and remissions. There is a slight male preponderance.

Ophthalmoscopy

Gray or creamy lesions develop beneath the retina in the retinal pigment epithelium. These may be adjacent to previous scars. Active inflammatory signs are rare.

The lesions last for several weeks and then resolve, showing extensive atrophy of the pigment epithelium and the choriocapillaris. Pigment proliferation and dispersion occur. Fibrous tissue also forms.

Prognosis

Macular vision is often lost with progression of the disease. The visual loss is secondary to direct involvement of the macula.

SHERRINGTON'S LAW (SHERRINGTON'S LAW OF RECIPROCAL INNERVATION)

If you are looking to the right, a muscle pulls the right eye out. The muscle that would normally be pulling the eye inward has to pull less. Sherrington's law states that, if a muscle is pulling an eye in one direction, the other muscle, which would normally pull in the opposite direction (the antagonist), has decreased innervation.

SIDEROSIS (OCULAR SIDEROSIS)

Ocular siderosis is a term given to changes in the eye that occur from oxidation of an iron-containing intraocular foreign body. Use of the electroretinogram (ERG) may be helpful. In the early stages, an increase in the A wave may be generated, but characteristically the A wave gradually progresses to extinction as the siderosis advances.

The iris may become dark and produce heterochromia (page 301). Cataract may also form; typically this is an anterior subcapsular cataract. Retinal pigment epithelial atrophy may surround an iron-containing intraocular foreign body accompanied by pigment migration and retinal arteriolar narrowing. Iron foreign bodies that cause siderosis occur in many ocular structures including the retina, vitreous, lens, iris, ciliary body, and anterior segment.

SILICONE

Liquid silicone has been used in vitreoretinal surgery to assist in the management of diabetic retinopathy patients and other patients with retinal detachments from other causes. Silicone liquid is injected into the interior of the eye. It is used to help dissect membranes, to hold (tamponade) the retina in position where adhesions will form, and to eliminate the cavity that occurs with vitreous removal, causing a physiologic difference in the fluid balance of the eye.

There are a number of complications of silicone liquid in the eye.

- Emulsification of the liquid may occur.
- Glaucoma of the pupillary block type may develop, unless surgical iridectomy (hole in the iris surgically created) is used.
- Band keratopathy occurs when the silicone oil goes into the anterior chamber (see Band Keratopathy, page 15).
- Low grade subclinical inflammation may occur.
- Cataracts develop when the lens is still in the eye: 50% after 6 months, 100% after 1 year.

SKEW DEVIATION

Definition

Skew deviation is vertical misalignment of the eyes that cannot be explained on the basis of extraocular motor muscle dysfunction or oculomotor nerve palsies. To differentiate it from trochlear (fourth) nerve palsy, skew deviation does not generally have the torsional or cyclodeviation movements that are seen with fourth nerve palsy.

Skew deviations may be constant in all positions of gaze (concomitant) or occur only in certain positions of gaze (nonconcomitant). A unilateral internuclear ophthalmoplegia (see page 117) may be seen with skew deviation.

Cause

Skew deviation is associated with brain stem lesions and is often associated with other signs of brain stem dysfunction.

SLITLAMP

Definition

A slitlamp is a microscope that allows examination of the eye under various magnifications. The view is binocular and is therefore three-dimensional. The variable shape and intensity of the illumination source is a key to making the slitlamp a useful diagnostic tool. The light source can be changed from a small pinpoint spot to a slit beam or to broad illumination. The color, intensity, and position of the beam can be changed for complete diagnostic illumination of the anterior or posterior of the eye (Fig. 16.65).

Use of the Slitlamp

Position the patient's head so that the eye is at the level of the line on the instrument. To adjust the chin rest, use the knob (Fig. 16.66). Turn on the slitlamp at the switch, usually located on the left side of the stand (Figs. 16.67 and 16.68). Adjust the oculars for the distance between your eyes. Both oculars swing out or in, and this should be done while viewing. Be sure that the patient's head is positioned against the

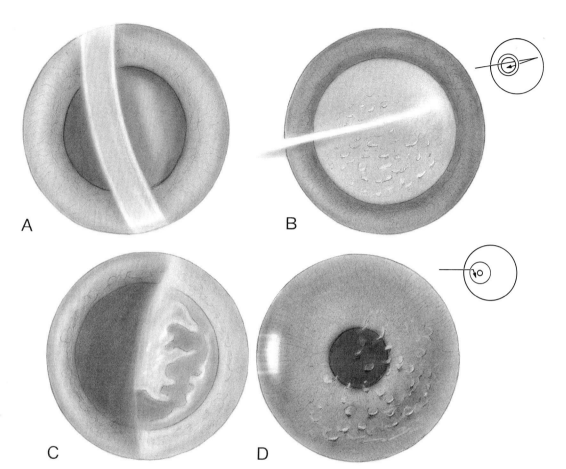

Figure 16.65. The slitbeam is a narrow, elongated beam of light. The slitlamp allows adjustment of this beam to be very thin. The illumination can also be adjusted. **A,** The slitbeam is useful in evaluating an optically clear structure such as the cornea. To see a rising column of smoke in a room is difficult with overhead fluorescent lights. However, if the lights are turned off and a small pen light is used, the smoke can be seen in the clear air more easily. This is similar to the way in which opacities can be seen in certain areas of the clear cornea. **B,** Using retroillumination to evaluate corneal structures. When a bright but narrow beam of light is shown through the pupil at an angle, the posterior pole shines with a red reflex. (There is a similar principle that is observed at night when an animal is caught in the dark by the headlights of an automobile. The pupils frequently shine a greenish color.) This red reflex can also be seen on photography with flash where the human pupil shows a bright red. Using these principles at the slitlamp, opacities can be shadowed and more easily delineated and described by the red reflex. The illustration shows the principle of retroillumination. **C,** Broad illumination. Some conditions, such as basement membrane dystrophy, are best seen with broad illumination. Here, the slitbeam is not used; the beam is widened to provide a broad light source. This is helpful in showing fingerprint lines, microcysts, and other subepithelial changes. **D,** Retroillumination using the iris as a background. The red reflex from the posterior portion of the eye can be used for retroillumination. However, this may not always be easily elicited and may provide too bright an illumination. The iris can be used as a backdrop illumination for corneal evaluation. By shining a light on the iris and using the reflected light from the iris as a posterior light source, subtle changes can be seen. This technique is frequently useful in the evaluation of guttata and other lesions in the area of Descemet's membrane. Illustrated is a light beam on the iris with the retroillumination showing lesions on the cornea.

chin rest and the front forehead strap (Fig. 16.66).

The slitlamp is moved back and forth and from side to side by a joy stick (Figs. 16.67 and 16.68). This allows focus by movement of the entire optical column. To move the slitlamp, one must release a lock. This is a small screw on the right side (Figs. 16.67 and 16.68).

The width of the slitbeam is controlled by a knob on the optical portion of the lamp. If you do not find a light source, this is the first place to check to be sure that the beam has not been turned down so small that it is not providing light.

Once the light source has been turned on, the light is placed in the general direction of the eye and the joy stick is used while looking through the oculars to bring the beam into focus (Figs. 16.66 and 16.69). The light source swings in an 180° arc, and you can move this from left to right while viewing (Fig. 16.70).

To change the color of the beam [cobalt or red-free (green)] filters or to change size or illumination, you adjust the knob at the top of the slitlamp (Figs. 16.67 and 16.68).

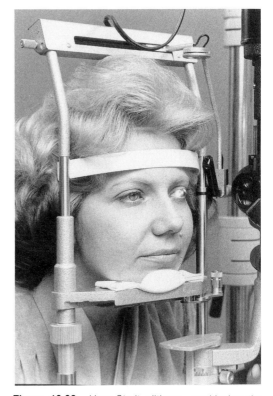

Figure 16.66. Haag-Streit slitlamp—positioning the patient. Once the subject's chin has been placed on the chin rest and the forehead has been brought against the forehead restrainer, the eye level is aligned on the Haag Streit slitlamp to the black line marked on the support to the patient's left. To adjust the height of the eye, the chin rest can be moved by turning the grooved wheel on the support to the patient's right just below the chin rest.

Types of Slitlamps

The two most common slitlamps in use now are the Haag-Streit (Fig. 16.67) and the Zeiss (Fig. 16.68). Other slitlamps are available but are frequently modeled after these two basic types. Familiarity with the slitlamp will provide a new world of diagnostic techniques. In the color section, see the examples of flare (Fig. C.5), gutattae (Fig. C.7), Kayser-Fleischer ring (Fig. C.8), Krukenberg's spindle (Fig. C.2), and herpes simplex (Fig. C.43).

Figure 16.67. Haag-Streit slitlamp. A slitlamp is a biomicroscope that allows visualization of the eye with increased magnification and with a variable light source. The light source can be adjusted in intensity, size, and direction.

Illustrated is a Haag-Streit slitlamp. In the lateral view (**C**), patient would sit to the *right* and the examiner would be to the *left*. The *right column* supports the patient's head and provides a fixation light. It is immobile. The column on the *left* is entirely mobile front and back. The runners can be seen *below*, where the housing has been taken off to show the wheel mechanism on a spiked track. The L-shaped bar that supports the oculars also rotates around the central column.

1, Lamp housing, where a light bulb provides a source of light that is projected downward and then with a mirror at a right angle toward the patient. *2,* Adjustment for various filters. White light, cobalt blue,

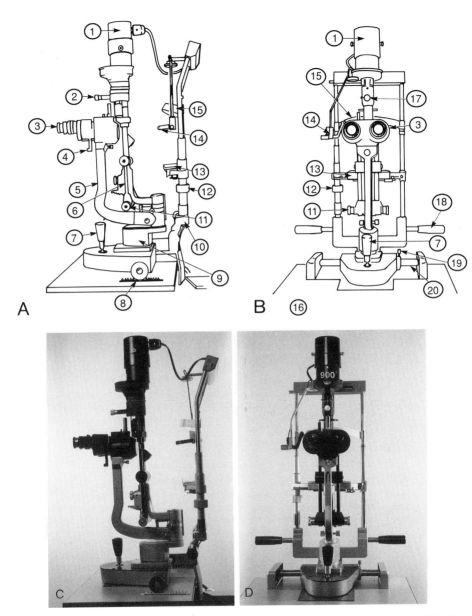

and green filters are all obtainable with this adjustment. This knob also adjusts the character of the beam. *3*, Oculars. *4*, Adjustment knob for changing magnification. *5*, Movable support for the oculars. Rotation is around the central axis. *6*, Column of light support that is also movable around a central axis. *7*, Joy stick, which provides movement forward, backward, and side to side. *8*, Track on which the central column movement depends. *9*, Central support for oculars and light source. *10*, Column, which is fixed, for patient support. *11*, Knob to adjust characteristics of the beam for different functions. *12*, Adjustment knob for raising and lowering the chin rest. *13*, Chin rest. *14*, Movable fixation light to allow the patient to fixate with the eye not being examined. *15*, Forehead strap. The patient's head must be placed against this strap. *16*, Approximate location of the on and off switch for the slitlamp. This may vary from lamp to lamp depending upon installation. *17*, Filter and light size adjustment knob. *18*, Handles that the patient can grasp for support. *19*, Tightening screw which, when tightened, will prevent movement of the lamp when not in use. This screw must be loosened for the slitlamp to function. *20*, Bar that slips through the base of the movable portion of the sliplamp. This bar moves the slitlamp backward and forward and allows movement from side to side.

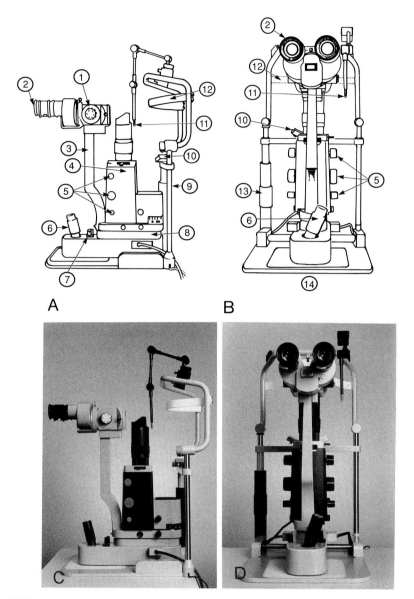

Figure 16.68. Zeiss slitlamp. Side and front views are provided. Compare the general features with the Haag-Streit slitlamp in Figure 16.67. *1,* Knob for changing magnification. *2,* Oculars. *3,* Support column for oculars, which rotates around a central axis. *4,* Lamp housing and source of light that is projected upward and then by mirrors toward the patient. This portion also rotates independently from the ocular source around a central point. *5,* Adjustment knobs for changing light characteristics. *6,* Joy stick for moving the entire ocular and lamp mechanism forward and backward. *7,* Release button. This button is tightened to prevent motion when the slitlamp is not in use. *8,* Base support for oculars and light source. *9,* Support column for patient, which is fixed. *10,* Chin rest for patient. *11,* Fixation light, which is used in front of the eye not being examined. *12,* Forehead strap. Patient must place forehead against this strap. *13,* Adjustment knob, which allows movement of the chin rest up and down. *14,* Approximate location, either to the left or the right, where an on-and-off switch is mounted.

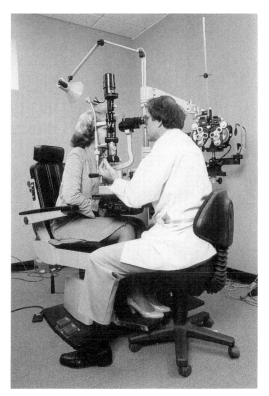

Figure 16.69. To align the slitlamp so that it can be used effectively in diagnosis, one must place both the patient and the observer at the appropriate height. The slitlamp should be mounted on a movable stand, the observer should be sitting in a chair that is mobile and adjustable in height, and the patient's chair should also be adjustable. (Credit: George Waring, M.D.)

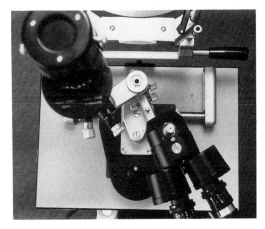

Figure 16.70. Haag-Streit slitlamp, top view. Looking down on the slitlamp (Haag-Streit), one can see a number of features. There is a central core going up and down, which has supports that will rotate both the oculars *(lower right)* and the source of light *(upper left)*. Just to the *left* of the oculars is the joy stick, which allows movement in all directions. The silver bar in the metallic casing below allows motion of the slitlamp forward and backward. The black footplate posteriorly in this view moves along the metallic rod to allow free right-to-left motion. The design allows complete freedom of motion for focusing and, once focused, scanning of ocular structures.

SNELL'S LAW

In a vacuum, light travels at 186,000 miles per second. In any other medium, light travels more slowly. The denser the medium (that would mean a higher refractive index), the more slowly the wavelength travels. Refraction is based on this concept.

Snell's Law states that a change in the direction of light occurs when a light ray moves from one medium to another (Fig. 16.71). For example, a light ray traveling in air and entering glass will be bent away from its path. The direction and degree of bending of the ray depend upon the density of the glass and the angle at which the light beam enters at the glass interface (Table 16.5).

Only oblique rays that enter from one medium to another medium are bent and therefore refracted. Those rays that enter the medium perpendicular to the interface of the two media progress unrefracted, although they change speed.

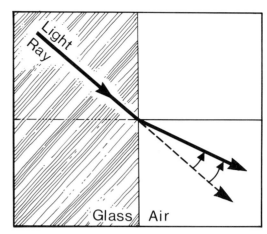

Figure 16.71. Snell's Law states that light traveling from a denser medium to a less dense medium will be altered in direction. There is no deviation if the light ray is perpendicular to the surface between the two media. However, a light ray approaching the interface at an angle will be deviated because of the change in speed of the light ray. This is important in understanding total internal reflection as it relates to gonioscopy (page 44).

Table 16.5.
Velocities and Refractive Indices of Various Substances

Substance	Velocity (m/sec)	Refractive Index
Air	2.9×10^8	1.00
Water	2.25×10^8	1.33
Cornea	2.19×10^8	1.37
Crown Glass	1.97×10^8	1.52
Diamond	2.9×10^8	2.42

SPHEROID DEGENERATION

Other Names

Climatic droplet keratopathy, Bietti nodular dystrophy, Labrador keratopathy, proteinaceous degeneration, corneal elastosis, keratinoid degeneration

Appearance

Spheroid degeneration involves the anterior stroma and at times the conjunctiva. Translucent, golden brown spherical deposits appear in the superficial corneal stroma and in the conjunctiva. These are extracellular proteinaceous deposits. Deposits may extend across the cornea in the interpalpebral zone, appearing as a noncalcific band keratopathy.

Characteristics

The condition is usually bilateral and is seen more frequently in male patients.

Cause

The proteinaceous deposits have no known cause. Exposure to sunlight, age, exposure to certain environments other than sunlight, and a genetic predisposition have all been suggested as contributing to the cause of spheroidal degeneration.

SPHINCTER TEAR

The iris sphincter may be disrupted by blunt injury. This is almost always associated with hyphema. The injury is usually moderate to severe when this occurs.

Sphincter tears may also be associated with angle recession (page 53). Angle recession may result in glaucoma. Late unilateral glaucoma with or without a history of previous trauma years before, may present as a diagnostic problem. Careful evaluation for a sphincter tear may help establish a diagnosis of trauma and glaucoma.

SPHINGOLIPIDOSES

Sphingolipidoses are characterized by enzyme deficiencies that interfere with hydrolysis of certain sphingolipids. Abnormal amounts of lipid are found in the central nervous system.

Tay-Sachs Disease

This is the most commonly known of the sphingolipidoses. It is seen in patients primarily of Ashkenazic Jewish ancestry. First signs develop during the 1st seven months of life. Infants are usually normal in the 1st year of life.

Characteristic Ocular Changes—the Cherry-Red Spot

A cherry-red spot may be seen early in the disease process. It is caused by the accumulation of ganglioside in the ganglion cells of the retina. These cells are greater in number around the macula. In the center foveola, however ganglion cells are not present. The result is whitish opacification of the retina with the center foveola maintaining the normal reddish background, creating a cherry-red spot (page 268). (See Krabbe's disease, page 311, and Fabry's disease, page 291.)

SPIRAL OF TILLAUX

The spiral of Tillaux is a theoretical line that connects the four insertions of the four rectus muscles on the globe.

SPLIT FIXATION

Split fixation is when a visual field loss cuts across the area of fixation in either the horizontal or the vertical meridian. It can be detected only by very careful visual field testing.

SPORTS INJURIES TO THE EYE

In certain sports, there is a incidence of ocular injury. Racket sports, especially squash, racquetball, and tennis (particularly net play), are frequent causes of minor and severe ocular injuries. Protective glasses with resin polycarbonate lenses are recommended in these sports. The nonracket sports, hockey and golf, are also high risk.

In children, BB rifles are a significant cause of severe injuries and loss of sight. BBs can be propelled at high velocity and are capable of through and through penetration of the globe and deep penetration into the orbit.

STEVENS-JOHNSON SYNDROME

See Erythema Multiforme (page 288).

STILES-CRAWFORD EFFECT

In the photoreceptors of the eye, how a ray strikes the photoreceptor will dictate how the receptor reacts. Oblique rays striking the photoreceptors are not as efficient as axial rays. This is true for both acuity and color perception. This results in the Stiles-Crawford effect.

Significance

The Stiles-Crawford effect is thought to be the explanation for decreased vision in conditions such as retinal detachment or chorioretinal scars where the orientation of the cones, and therefore the photoreceptor elements, has been altered.

STOCKER'S LINE

Stocker's line is a vertical line of iron deposited at the edge of a pterygium (see Iron Lines, Pterygium).

SUBCONJUNCTIVAL HEMORRHAGE

Description

Spontaneous subconjunctival hemorrhage appears as bright red hemorrhage under the subconjunctiva. It may be localized but also on occasion may completely surround the cornea. Although painless, the dramatic appearance of subconjunctival hemorrhage usually makes the patient immediately aware of its presence. The visual acuity with subconjunctival hemorrhage is unchanged.

Most subconjunctival hemorrhages are spontaneous and without known cause. They are frequently associated with certain predisposing historical features such as cough, sneezing, or straining. Blood dyscrasias are frequently mentioned as a cause but are clinically a very infrequent reason for subconjunctival hemorrhage. Workup for blood dyscrasia is not indicated unless hemorrhages are recurrent.

Simultaneous bilateral subconjunctival hemorrhages are unusual. They are most often seen in strangulation.

Subconjunctival hemorrhage may be associated with disease processes such as infections but is easily differentiated from spontaneous hemorrhage by lack of additional signs and symptoms.

Differential Diagnosis of Infectious Causes

There are four important disease processes associated with infectious conjunctivitis with subconjunctival hemorrhages:

- Acute hemorrhagic conjunctivitis;
- Epidemic keratoconjunctivitis;
- *Staphylococcus pneumoniae;*
- Koch-Weeks bacillus (hemophilus).

SUPERIOR LIMBIC KERATOCONJUNCTIVITIS (SLK)

Diagnosis

The conjunctiva superiorly at the cornea is hyperemic and will have punctate staining (Fig. 16.72). Under the upper lid there is a velvety papillary hypertrophy. Changes at the corneosleral limbus are micropannus and punctate staining. Filaments may be seen on the upper limbus and adjacent conjunctiva.

Cause

The cause is unknown. An association between SLK and thyroid dysfunction is not uncommon. However, the course or extent of the thyroid disease does not seem to affect the course of SLK.

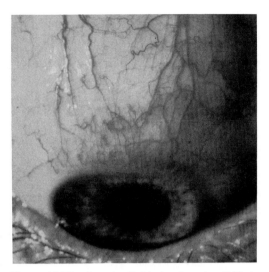

Figure 16.72. Superior limbic keratoconjunctivitis is an inflammatory condition of unknown etiology, although it has been associated with thyroid disease in some patients. It is at the superior limbus and may have extension onto the cornea (micropannus).

Symptoms

Irritation, foreign body sensation

Course

Self-limited. Exacerbations and remissions occur with or without treatment.

SWIMMING POOL WATER, EFFECTS ON CORNEA

More than two-thirds of swimmers in chlorinated pools will see halos or rainbows. It takes 5 to 30 minutes in the water for these symptoms to develop. The halos are probably due to corneal edema. These symptoms disappear in all swimmers 30 minutes after they leave the water.

Nine of 10 swimmers will also show corneal epithelial damage that stains with fluorescein. Punctate erosions on the lower one-third of the cornea are the most common finding, but linear, wavy erosions also occur. These changes do not decrease vision.

The cause for the corneal staining is unknown. Suggested important factors are: (*a*) chlorine (effects unknown); (*b*) monochloramine (formed from chlorine in the pool and ammonia from swimmers), which is known in the laboratory to cause ocular irritation; (*c*) pH; (*d*) hypotonicity of the water; and (*e*) disruption of the tear film.

SYMBLEPHARON

A symblepharon refers to scar adhesions between two conjunctival surfaces (Fig. 16.73). The cause of these adhesions may be general reactions such as Stevens-Johnson syndrome, inflammation due to conditions such as ocular pemphigoid, trauma including chemical burns such as lye burns, and previous surgery such as retinal detachment surgery.

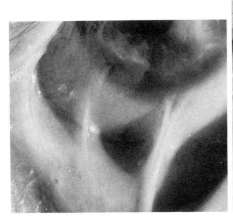 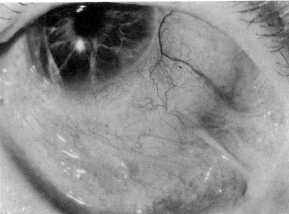

Figure 16.73. Symblepharon is conjunctival scarring that bridges the fornices, as illustrated in both of these photographs. Symblepharon can occur with a number of conditions but is most often associated with ocular phemphygoid (page 335) and chemical burns (page 139).

SYMPATHETIC OPHTHALMIA

Sympathetic ophthalmia is a bilateral uveitis that occurs after injury to the eye or after intraocular surgery. Surgery or injury to one eye occurs. After that occurrence, the other eye develops an inflammation. It is usually within a few months after injury but almost never before 14 days. (Rarely, sympathetic ophthalmia has been noted to occur decades after the initial injury or surgery.)

Terminology

The eye that responds after trauma to the opposite, injured eye is called the sympathizing eye.

Characteristics

There is no external inflammation. Uveitis occurs in either eye or both. The first symptom may relate to loss of accommodation, a frequently quoted fact but rarely seen clinically. The first signs in the sympathizing eye may be patches of choroiditis that appear as yellow-white areas of inflammation. The iris may show edema and deep nodules, and inflammation of the optic nerve are not uncommon. Yellow-white spots on the fundus are known as Dalen-Fuchs nodules. There may be associated general signs of vitiligo, poliosis, and alopecia.

Treatment

Enucleation of the traumatized eye will prevent sympathetic ophthalmia if done within 9 to 10 days after the injury.

Cause

The cause is unknown. The condition is rare. However, there is an increased incidence of sympathetic ophthalmia after vitrectomy for trauma.

SYNCHYSIS SCINTILLANS

Other Names

Cholesterolosis, hemophthalmos

Characteristics

Synchysis scintillans is found in eyes that have had surgery or ocular trauma and in which there has been extensive hemorrhage.

Diagnosis

Highly refractile cholesterol bodies are seen in the anterior chamber and in the vitreous. The vitreous is degenerated, and liquid and the crystals settle interiorly. Although the crystals are yellow-gold to yellowish white, their refractile properties often give them multiple colors of oil-on-water as they float in the aqueous or vitreous.

SYNECHIAE, POSTERIOR

A synechia is a scar formation in the eye. Posterior synechiae occur between the iris and the lens. This results in a pupil irregularity and an inability to dilate or constrict the pupil in the area where the scar occurs. Extensive posterior synechiae may block aqueous flow from the posterior chamber to the anterior chamber. A build-up of aqueous may occur behind the iris, causing a pupillary block glaucoma. Posterior synechiae are due to inflammation with conditions such as sarcoid or uveitis of unknown cause and may also be associated with inflammation after trauma.

T-SIGN

T-sign is a thickening of the posterior sclera near the optic nerve, which can be seen by ultrasound or CT scanning. It may be seen in pseudotumor or posterior scleritis.

TELECANTHUS

Telecanthus is an anatomical defect: wider-than-normal distance between eyes (intercanthal distance), accompanied by normal distance between pupils (interpupillary distance).

TERRIEN'S MARGINAL DEGENERATION

Clinical Symptoms

This is a rare, bilateral, symmetrical condition that is characterized by thinning of the cornea, especially in the upper nasal quadrants. There is opacification of the outer margin of the area of thinning, which may look like arcus senilis. The thinned area vascularizes.

Onset

This degeneration begins during the 3rd or 4th decades of life.

Sex Predominance

The condition is seen more frequently in males than in females.

Prognosis

On occasion, Terrien's marginal degeneration may perforate and the iris may prolapse. The progression tends to be slow, and observation is usually sufficient. The central cornea is spared. There is difficulty with irregular astigmatism as the condition progresses. This can be a significant cause of symptoms.

Cause

Unknown

Histopathology

Areas that are affected reveal vascularized connective tissue. There is fibrillary degeneration of the collagen fibers. Fatty infiltration is seen.

TERSON'S SYNDROME

Terson's syndrome is the occurrence of (*a*) subarachnoid hemorrhage and (*b*) vitreous hemorrhage. The syndrome is described in all types of intracranial bleeding that are associated with vitreous hemorrhage. The ocular hemorrhage can include retinal and preretinal hemorrhages. With the syndrome, papilledema may or may not be present. The death rate in patients with intracranial bleeding is higher when secondary vitreous or retinal hemorrhages are present.

TESSIER CLASSIFICATION

This classification is useful for understanding the facial cleft syndromes. The partitioning of the facial clefts both in ocular soft tissues and in the skeletal structures is outlined in this classification.

THREE-MIRROR PRISM (GOLDMANN)

This is a contact lens used for examination of the chamber angle (gonioscopy) and the posterior pole. Three mirrors are present. Each mirror is a different shape and serves a different purpose. The dome-shaped mirror is for gonioscopy, and the mirrors that are rectangular are for evaluation of the retinal periphery and equatorial regions. This prism is good for glaucoma, retinal examination, and examination of the disc and macula. It does give a three-dimensional view. It requires a slitlamp for use. It also requires the examiner to practice and develop skill (see Fig. 3.8).

THYGESON'S SUPERFICIAL PUNCTATE KERATITIS

Diagnosis

Slitlamp examination reveals coarse, punctate, snowflake-shaped opacities in the corneal epithelium. There may be a slight subepithelial haze, but the stroma is not involved. Signs are almost always bilateral.

Symptoms

Irritation, light sensitivity, tearing, and foreign body sensation are symptoms.

Course

The condition is self-limited. However, it may persist with exacerbations and remissions. It leaves no permanent damage to the cornea.

Cause

The cause is unknown. A viral etiology is suspected.

TOXOCARIASIS

Characteristics

Toxocariasis occurs in older children and may present as a chronic general inflammation (endophthalmitis) or as a focal inflammatory or postinflammatory mass in the retina, in subretinal areas, or in the vitreous. Although systemic toxocariasis causes fever, hepatomegaly, leukocytosis, and hyperglobulinemia, the ocular form of the disease is rarely associated with these changes.

Ophthalmoscopy

The focal retinal lesion may present as a whitish mass about 1 disc diameter in size. It may be within the posterior pole or the periphery. It has been confused with retinoblastoma. Changes around the inflammation may produce fibrous traction bands, and retinal detachment may develop.

Diagnosis

- Serum. A positive enzyme-linked immunosorbent assay (ELISA) is 90% sensitive with a titer of 1:8 in patients with ocular disease.
- Histopathology. The lesion is an eosinophilic granuloma.
- History. Possible exposure to young puppies should be sought.

Cause

Toxocariasis is caused by the nematode *Toxocara canis.* Children contract the organism by eating soil where dogs have deposited the ova. In the larval stage, *Toxocara canis* lodges in the eye and subsequently causes an inflammatory reaction. Finally, it becomes encased in a fibrous inflammatory mass. The reaction is predominated by eosinophils and polymorphonuclear leukocytes, but epithelioid cells and giant cells are also seen.

TOXOPLASMIC RETINOCHOROIDITIS

Symptoms

Patients present with floaters and blurred vision.

Diagnosis

One or more white lesions with indistinct borders are seen in the retina. After the acute phase, these lesions heal within 3 weeks to 6 months. After healing, a choroidoretinal scar with a variable amount of pigmentation is seen.

Congenital Form

Toxoplasmic retinochoroiditis can be transmitted across the placenta from an infected mother to her fetus. The eye and brain are the most frequent sites. The infection usually passes the placenta during the first 90 days. Newborns with the disease show atrophic retinal scars, usually in the macular region. It is the congenital choroidoretinal scar that becomes most activated in adult life. Acquired choroidoretinitis from toxoplasmic organisms is rare in later life.

Diagnosis

- Sabin-Feldman toxoplasma dye test
- Fluorescent antibody test
- Enzyme-linked immunosorbent assay (ELISA)
- Hemagglutination test

Cause

The retinal choroiditis is caused by *Toxoplasma gondii*. The host for *Toxoplasma gondii* is cats, and the organism is shed in feces.

Prognosis

Loss of vision is associated with macular changes. Traction retinal detachment, distortion of the retina by traction bands, and vitreous debris may also cause visual decrease.

TRACHOMA

Characteristics

Trachoma causes a follicular conjunctivitis and is usually on the upper tarsal conjunctival plate (Fig. 16.74).

Cause

Trachoma is a chlamydial organism. In the early stages, follicles are seen on the tarsal plate. These follicles then mature, and papillary hypertrophy may be prominent. Scarring then begins to occur on the conjunctiva. In the final stages, the follicles regress and severe scarring is left on the conjunctiva. Scarring that traverses the tarsal plate is described as *Arlt's line*.

The cornea is also involved. An epithelial keratitis, marginal and

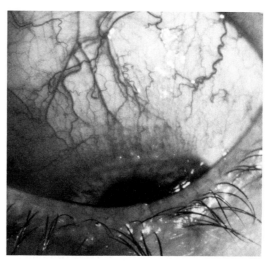

Figure 16.74. Trachoma with a superior pannus and Tranta's dots. Tranta's dots are collections of lymphocytes along the junction between the sclera and the cornea. Note the increase of vessels in the area of inflammation. Trachoma is a leading cause of blindness in the world, although it is rarely seen in the United States.

central corneal infiltrates, superficial vascularization of the cornea, and a fibrovascular pannus may be present. Follicle formation on the cornea occurs superiorly near the limbus and, when these follicles regress, depressions are left; these are known as *Herbert's pits*.

The conjunctival changes have been classified in MacCallan's Classification (page 316).

Epidemiology

Trachoma is a major cause of blindness throughout the world. It is a disease of undernourished, underprivilidged populations. Trachoma is associated with poor hygienic conditions. Cycles of reinfection occur so that the conjunctival and corneal changes become blinding.

In the United States, trachoma is seen in American Indian tribes, especially in the southwest. Because trachoma is common in the Middle East, natives from that area may present in the United States with evidence of previous infection.

TRACTION TEST (FORCED DUCTION TEST)

Principle

A traction test demonstrates restriction rather than a neurologic cause of abnormal ocular motility.

Technique

Anesthetic eye drops are instilled in the eye. Using a cotton swab, one applies a potent anesthetic (such as 4% cocaine) over the area where the test will be conducted. The conjunctiva and Tenon's capsule are then grasped with forceps at the corneal limbus in the area of restriction. For example, if the inferior rectus is suspected, the limbus is grasped at 6 o'clock. An attempt is then made to rotate the globe up and down. Lack of movement indicates a constrictive component of the ocular motility abnormality.

Use of the Traction Test

- Graves' ophthalmopathy (thyroid ophthalmopathy)
- Blow-out fracture
- Duane's syndrome
- Differential diagnosis of nerve palsy
- Brown's syndrome

TRANSILLUMINATION OF THE IRIS

Technique

Direct Application

Direct application of a light source is accomplished by placing the light directly on the sclera 8 mm behind the limbus. This avoids the ciliary body, where deep pigmentation and thickness would prevent the entrance of light into the eye. Light through the sclera illuminates the eye, and the pupil and the iris can be observed by internal illumination.

Slitlamp

By arranging a small circular or rectangular beam on the slitlamp to shine directly in so that the pupil fills with red reflex from the anterior illumination, the iris can be transilluminated.

Principle

Transillumination of the iris determines the degree of pigment on the posterior part of the iris. In most normal individuals, pigment on the posterior portion of the iris prevents light from shining through. This will be in contrast to the reddish glow seen in the pupillary area.

Conditions in Which Transillumination of the Iris Can Be Important

Albinism

In albinos, loss of pigment may be generalized, allowing the entire iris to transilluminate.

Pigmentary Dispersion Syndrome

In the pigmentary dispersion syndrome, the pigment is lost in the mid-periphery of the iris. The transillumination pattern may appear linear, like flower petals.

Exfoliation Syndrome

In the exfoliation syndrome, pigment is lost on the surface adjacent to the pupil, causing a characteristic transillumination pattern.

Transillumination of the Iris after Cataract Surgery

During cataract surgery, manipulation of the iris, removal of the cataract, or insertion of the intraocular lens may disturb part of the posterior pigment on the iris. This will produce localized, round or oval patches of irregular pigment loss and subsequent area transillumination.

TRICHIASIS

Definition

A misdirection of the eyelashes from their normal position results in trichiasis. This condition is acquired and may be a result of chronic inflammation from infection, drug effects, injury to the eyelids, or previous surgery.

Complications

Trichiasis not only causes irritation to the globe but also results in corneal damage and loss of vision. The lashes rub against the corneal epithelium, disrupting normal integrity. Corneal staining with fluorescein helps reveal the extent of corneal changes. Secondary infections may occur.

TRIGEMINAL NEURALGIA (TIC DOULOUREUX)

Characteristics

Severe pain lasts a few seconds. The pain is in one or more of the divisions of the trigeminal nerve. The pain may be triggered by touching the skin in the involved areas.

Frequency may vary. Early in the disease, the attacks may be spaced weeks or months apart. However, the frequency may increase with time.

Cause

Trigeminal neuralgia is thought to be due to microvascular compression of the trigeminal root of the nerve as it exits from the pons.

Cautions

If the pain is constant or if there is an associated sensory deficit, a structural lesion is probable. Under these circumstances, a complete workup is indicated.

TRILATERAL RETINOBLASTOMA

Trilateral retinoblastoma refers to the association of bilateral retinoblastoma simultaneously with a midline intracranial tumor, usually in the pineal region. The tumor originates from photoreceptor-like cells in ocular tumors and from vestibular photoreceptor cells in the pineal body. The pineal neoplasm displays histologic features that are similar to those of ocular retinoblastoma. The pineal tumor is a primary tumor rather than a metastasis.

UHTHOFF'S PHENOMENON

This is a temporary worsening of vision and other neurologic function typical in patients with multiple sclerosis just after exertion or in situations where they are exposed to heat. The phenomenon is of interest to ophthalmologists because multiple sclerosis may present as an optic neuritis (see Optic Neuritis, page 101), and diagnostic clues can be helpful.

ULTRASONOGRAPHY

Diagnostic ocular ultrasonography uses the differential reflection of high frequency sound waves through soft tissue. The reflected waves create echoes and are displayed on a oscilloscope screen. The resultant picture can be used for clinical interpretation (Fig. 16.75).

The A-mode of ultrasonography is a one-dimensional time amplitude representation of echoes. The B-mode takes the echos produced in A-mode ultrasonography but presents them as dots instead of spikes. In the B-mode, there is a two-dimensional representation. In the B-mode, the configuration of structures and the size and location of changes are readily apparent.

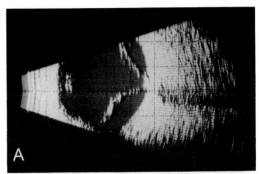

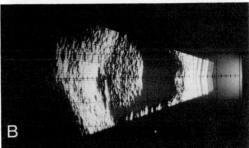

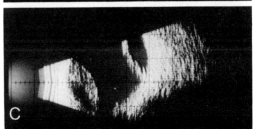

UNILATERAL CONJUNCTIVITIS ASSOCIATED WITH LID CONDITIONS

Molluscum lesions on the lid margins can be associated with conjunctivitis. Removal of the molluscum lesion cures the conjunctivitis. Warts (verruca vulgaris) on the eyelid, which go away on their own, can produce a unilateral conjunctivitis.

USHER'S SYNDROME

Characteristics

Association of retinitis pigmentosa and partial complete congenital deafness

Figure 16.75.   A, Retinal detachment illustrated by B-scan ultrasound examination. The detachment shows as two curved lines in the dark circle that represents the interior of the eye. **B,** A malignant melanoma demonstrated by B-scan ultrasound. The melanoma shows as a whitish mass in the dark cavity that represents the interior of the eye. **C,** Ultrasound evaluation of a scleral rupture that has been repaired. The elevation on the retina surface is a portion of the repaired globe. Ultrasound examination can be helpful in determining the degree of injury when direct visualization with the ophthalmoscope is not possible. (Credit: Peter Forgach, M.D.)

Heredity

Autosomal recessive

Four Subtypes

All of the subtypes have retinitis pigmentosa changes. Type 1 is associated with total deafness and no vestibular function. Type 2 includes partial deafness and intact vestibular function. Type 3 has complete deafness that was vestibular ataxia and sometimes psychosis. Type 4 has total deafness and mental retardation. The genetic association with these types is unclear.

UVEAL EFFUSION

Uveal effusion (ciliochoroidal effusion) is a collection of fluid in the choroid. It is most commonly seen in male patients. The following features are characteristic:

- Intraocular pressure usually normal;
- Dilated episcleral blood vessels;
- Thickened and detached choroid;
- Retinal detachment (nonrhegmatogenous);
- Course of remissions and exacerbations.

(See Ciliochoroidal Effusion.)

VACCINIA

Cause

In smallpox vaccination, the vaccinia virus may be transmitted from the vaccination site to the eyelid. (This is rarely seen since smallpox vaccination is rarely done.)

Clinical Appearance

Focal inflammation develops on the eyelid. This lesion may have a central area of depression. Conjunctivitis may be papillary. The discharge has mucus plus pustular characteristics.

The cornea may be involved, and small dendrites (Fig. C.43) may appear (see Dendrites of Herpes Simplex and Herpes Zoster). Extensive corneal changes may occur, including ulceration and inflammation in the stromal area.

VALVE OF HASNER

The valve of Hasner is a mucosal fold beneath and lateral to the inferior turbinate in the nose. This mucosal fold (valve) partially covers the ostium through which the nasal lacrimal duct, and therefore the contents of the nasal lacrimal sac, empties. Obstruction of this nasal lacrimal duct at the valve of Hasner is often present at birth. It usually clears within the first few months of life. However, symptoms of tearing and lacrimal blockage may occur before the obstruction clears.

VERTEX POWER

The vertex power is the reciprocal of the focal length. Vertex measurements from the back of the lens to the eye are made during refraction so that compensation can be made for changes in the vertex distance (and power) when lenses are ground.

VISUAL ACUITY AND THE SNELLEN CHART

Visual acuity is measured by the size of a letter that subtends an angle of 5 minutes of an arc (each stroke of the letter subtends an angle of 1 minute of the arc) (Fig. 16.76**A**). In the Snellen chart, each letter on the chart subtends an angle of 5 minutes of an arc at a specific distance.

In a 20/20 notation, the first 20 represents the testing distance. The second 20 represents the distance at which this letter subtends an angle of 5 minutes. In 20/40, this is a letter size that subtends an angle of 5 minutes of an arc at 40 feet. On the Snellen chart, Snellen notations of letter size are based on the minimal visual angle and the distance that the letter subtends that minimal visual angle (Fig. 16.76**B**).

VISUAL FIELD TESTING

Concept

Visual field testing shows peripheral visual perception. (The fovea represents the area of central visual acuity. In the fovea, the cones are most concentrated and 20/20 vision is achieved.) In visual field testing, the peripheral retina is stimulated. To study the measurements of central visual acuity, see Snellen Chart (page 379), Amsler Grid (page 247), and Color Vision Testing (page 276.

A
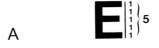

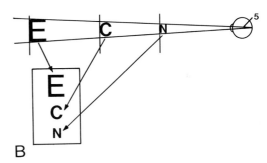

Figure 16.76. Visual acuity is dependent upon a minimal visual angle. This figure illustrates the construction of an eye chart based on visual acuity.

A, A letter is constructed based on a size of 5 minutes of an arc. The spaces and bars of the letter are each 1 minute of the arc, as illustrated.

B, Taking a visual angle of 5 minutes of an arc illustrated at the eyeball and projecting the lines of the angle outward, the lines diverge. The farther away from the point of origin, the farther apart the lines. If letters are placed within these lines at certain distances, the letter size can be measured as a function of the distance from the originating point. For example, the large E might be 200 ft from the origin. In Snellen acuity, 20/200 means that, at a testing distance of 20 ft (first number), the smallest letter that can be seen is a letter subtending the minimal visual angle at 200 ft. The normal visual acuity is 20/20, which simply states that at a testing distance of 20 ft a letter can be seen that subtends the angle 20 ft from the point of origin. The chart in **B** is almost always tested at a distance of 20 ft, and the size of the smallest letter that can be read becomes the visual acuity for the eye being tested.

VOGT'S LIMBAL GIRDLE

See Limbal Girdle of Vogt (page 314).

VON HIPPEL'S INTERNAL CORNEAL ULCER

Von Hippel's internal corneal ulcer is one of the classifications of the anterior cleavage syndrome (page 252). When active inflammation is associated with Peters' anomaly [that is, a posterior corneal defect associated with scarring and sometimes iris or lens attachments to the cornea], it is known as von Hippel's internal corneal ulcer.

VOSSIUS' RING

Vossius' ring is a ring of pigment on the anterior lens capsule. It is usually under the iris or near the pupillary border, and one may have to dilate the pupil to see the ring. Vossius' ring is diagnostic of previous blunt injury to the eye. It is formed by the pigment epithelium at the sphincter region impacting against the lens during concussion.

WAARDENBURG'S SYNDROME

Clinical Features

Ocular Features

Waardenburg's syndrome is important to ophthalmologists because it is a rare cause of heterochromia iritis. The heterochromia is frequently only in a sector of the iris that is light-colored. Examination of the fundus often shows a corresponding sector of hypopigmentation.

Facial Features

The eyebrows tend to be thick and heavy, and there is wide separation of the eyes. There is a broad nasal root, and a white forelock may be seen.

Heterochromia is seen in 25% of patients with Waardenburg's syndrome. Also seen is a white forelock (20 to 40% of patients) and unilateral or bilateral deafness (20% of patients). The syndrome is inherited in an autosomal dominant pattern.

Inheritance

Irregular autosomal dominant

WAGNER'S HEREDITARY VITREORETINAL DEGENERATION (DEGENERATIO HYALOIDEORETINAS HEREDITARIA)

This is a degeneration of the vitreous associated with retinal and choroidal changes. It has the following characteristics:

- Usually bilateral;
- Autosomal dominant with 100% penetration;
- Affecting both sexes;
- Progressive;
- Associated cataract in 60% of cases; onset of cataract in the 30s to 40s;
- Onset at birth or during the first few years of life;
- Mild myopia;
- Electroretinography showing weak or subnormal response;
- Color vision normal;
- Dark adaptation usually normal;
- Visual fields variable, possibility of slight contraction or ring scotoma.

The vitreous becomes abnormal early in these patients. The vitreous loses its gel characteristics and becomes more fluid. The posterior vitreous may detach, leaving large areas of nonvitreous fluid. Fibrils are found in the vitreous. The vitreous becomes loose and broken, and there is much free-floating debris. A gel is often observed on the retina, and fibrous bands may cause traction.

In the periphery, the vessels become whitish with sclerosis and pigment collects along arterioles. Choroidal atrophy may appear as whitish patches with prominent choroidal vessels.

The condition is progressive. Retinal breaks do occur and tend to be difficult to treat. Visual acuity may be decreased by cataract, by the vitreous changes, or by retinal detachment.

WARBURG SYNDROME

This rare syndrome emphasizes the embryologic similarities of the brain and the eye in a unique way. Essentially, both the brain and the eye arrest in development during the first trimester of gestation. Postmortem examination reveals abnormalities limited to the neural tube. The brain fails to develop gyri and sulci, leaving a smooth surface not unlike that of lower animals and reptiles and appearing like the brain of a 3-month-old fetus. With this abnormality, the development of the subarachnoid space may also be affected, resulting in hydrocephalus in some patients.

Similarly, the eye arrests in development. There is an inferior coloboma consistent with arrest before the 7th week because the embryonic fissure closes at this time. Concomitant with this timing is the failure of the retina to attach to the pigment epithelium, a normal finding only until the 8th week of gestation. The lens changes—persistence of lens epithelium, absence of lens bow, and posterior lenticonus—also support arrested development in the 2nd month.

The ophthalmologist sees bilateral leukocoria and microphthalmia. There is no inflammation. Most important, unlike trisomy 13 (which also presents with leukocoria), the congenital abnormalities are limited to the head. Hydrocephalus occurs with or without an encephalocele. The condition is lethal in infancy. The characteristic brain findings establish the diagnosis.

The condition is thought to be autosomal recessive.

WEILL-MARCHESANI SYNDROME

General Features

These patients have short, stubby fingers and broad hands, with reduced joint mobility.

Ocular Findings

They may have microspherophokia (page 58), which is important because of its association with angle closure glaucoma and high refractive myopia.

WELCH-ALLEN OPHTHALMOSCOPE

This is a direct ophthalmoscope (Fig. 16.77). The power source, usually batteries or a battery pack, is housed in the handle. The light bulb is directed upward and then the path of the light changes so that the light is directed through the pupil and into the patient's eye. The observer looks along the path of the light to examine the interior of the eye.

WESSELY RING

A Wessely ring is an immune corneal ring.

Composition

The ring is made up of antigen-antibody complex, complement, and polymorphonuclear leukocytes. The reaction occurs in the corneal stroma as a ring because the

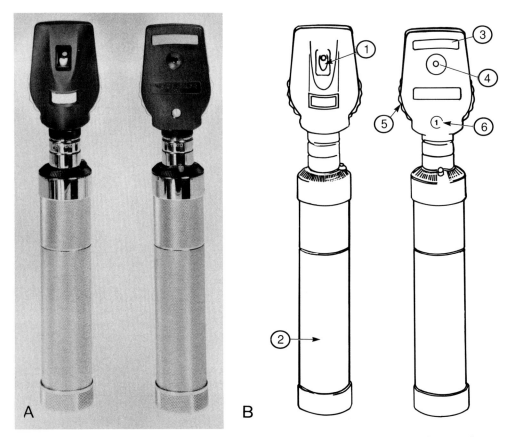

Figure 16.77.   The ophthalmoscope is turned on by pushing the small button on the top of the handle and rotating the black ring with the serrated edge. This is a rheostat and allows intensity adjustment of the light source. *1,* Mirror that reflects light into the patient's eye with a viewing hole above, through which the examiner looks. It is in this viewing hole that positive or negative lenses can be superimposed to adjust focus. *2,* Handle where battery power is supplied. On top of the handle base is a rheostat for light adjustment. *3,* Headrest bar, which goes against the examiner's forehead. *4,* Viewing hole through which the examiner looks. It is this hole that lenses may superimpose for focus. *5,* Focusing wheel. While holding the ophthalmoscope, one's index finger can move this wheel to adjust the lenses in the hole at *4. 6,* As the dial wheel (*5*) is moved, the power of the lens is indicated in this small window. Red numbers indicate minus lenses, and black numbers indicate plus lenses.

antigen is central and antibody diffuses from the limbus toward the antigen. The ring usually clears with no sequela.

Causes

- Herpes simplex virus antigen
- Severe corneal burns (attributed to altered corneal protein becoming antigenic)
- Antigenic fibers, such as insect
- Experimentally—injection of antigen directly into the cornea
- Bacterial products, as from *Staphylococcus aureus*

WHIPPLE'S DISEASE

Ocular Characteristics

Patients lose the ability to make vertical movements. Eyes become totally immobile (total ophthalmoplegia). Inflammation of the vitreous may be present (vitritis).

General Characteristics

This occurs primarily in middle-aged men. There is weight loss, edema, fever, steatorrhea, and abdominal pain. Joint pain may occur. There is lymphadenopathy. Jejunal biopsy shows macrophages filled with a PAS-positive material. Diagnosis may be important because this disease, which has severe complications, can be treated with tetracyclines.

WHITNALL'S LIGAMENT

This ligament is a condensation of the sheath of the levator muscle, which lifts the upper lid. It functions as a support for the upper eyelid and the orbital tissues. It attaches where the levator muscle transforms into the levator aponeurosis (page 200). The ligament then goes medially, where it attaches to connective tissue around the trochlea. Laterally, it goes through the stroma of the lacrimal gland to attach to the inner aspect of the lateral orbital wall. Additional attachments are found on the roof of the orbit. A similar suspensory ligament is found in the lower lid and is called Lockwood's ligament (page 315).

WILSON'S DISEASE (HEPATOLENTICULAR DEGENERATION)

Ophthalmic Orientation

This disease can present to the ophthalmologist as a greenish yellow or golden ring best seen with the magnification of the slitlamp—Keyser-Fleischer ring. It occurs in the deepest layers of the cornea around the periphery. It extends 1 to 2 mm in from the periphery and fades as it comes closer to the center (Fig. C.8). In the early stages, the ring can be seen only by gonioscopy, primarily in the superior and inferior corneal regions.

Cause of the Ring

The ring is a collection of copper granules that are deposited in the deep layers of the cornea. The copper deposition is in two parallel zones close to the endothelial surface. Other structures (other parts of the cornea, Bowman's membrane, stroma, and endothelium) are normal and show no deposition of copper.

Systemic Signs

Wilson's disease is an inborn error of copper metabolism. It is autosomal recessive. The onset is before 30 years of age. A decrease in ceruloplasmin is found in 90% of affected patients.

WYBURN-MASON SYNDROME

Other Names

Racemose hemangiomas, cirsoid aneurysms

Ophthalmologic Findings

Markedly dilated and tortuous retinal blood vessels project from the retina. Arteries and veins may be impossible to differentiate.

Characteristics

Wyburn-Mason syndrome shows arteriole-venous malformations of both the retina and the central nervous system. The condition is congenital. It is thought to occur during embryologic development in the 6th week. The condition does not progess.

XANTHELASMA

Xanthelasma occurs in middle-aged or elderly individuals with normal serum cholesterol. Multiple lesions are yellowish plaques on the inner aspects of the upper and lower eyelids. They demonstrate clusters of foam cells, which are found in the superficial dermis. Cells contain a lipid material (Fig. 16.78).

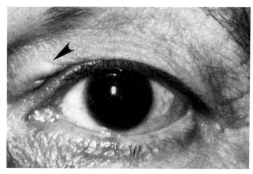

Figure 16.78. Xanthelasma. This deposit of lipid in the eyelids is fairly common. Here the yellowish white deposit is on the nasal portion of the upper lid *(arrow)*. The condition does not represent, in older patients, any serious disease process. (Credit: Ted Wojno, M.D.)

XANTHOPSIA

Xanthopsia is a shift in color perception so that objects appear yellow. It is most commonly described in digitalis toxicity but has also been reported with chlorothiazide diuretic intake.

XERODERMA PIGMENTOSUM

Patients with xeroderma pigmentosum have increased sensitivity to ultraviolet radiation and also defective DNA repair. *Ocular abnormalities* occur in 40% of patients. Patients are susceptible to ultraviolet radiation exposure—inflammation of the eyelids, conjunctiva, and cornea. Less commonly, ectropion, corneal opacification, and neoplasms of the skin on the eyelids are seen.

Cutaneous Changes

One-half of patients wtih the condition will have basal cell carcinoma or squamous cell carcinomas of the skin.

Characteristics

There is no sex predilection. Sun sensitivity and freckling are usually recognized between 1 and 2 years of age. The general prognosis is poor, and there is only a 70% probability of survival at age 40.

YOKE MUSCLES

When we consider the action of both eyes together, it is obvious that when one eye is looking in one direction the other eye is adjusted to the same direction to keep the eyes aligned. In any field of gaze, there is a muscle acting on the right eye and another muscle acting simultaneously on the left eye. Looking right, the right lateral rectus and the left medial rectus are in prime action. These are called yoke muscles. This is true of any field of gaze. In looking up and to the right, the right superior rectus pulls the right eye up and the left inferior oblique pulls the left eye up (see Motility, page 143).

INDEX

Page numbers in *italics* indicate figures, those followed by *t* denote tables.
Boldface entries indicate major topics. *Italic* roman numerals indicate color section.

Boldface entries indicate major topics. *Italic* roman numerals indicate color section.

Boldface entries indicate major topics. *Italic* roman numerals indicate color section.

Boldface entries indicate major topics. *Italic* roman numerals indicate color section.

Page numbers in italics *indicates figures, those followed by* t *denote tables.*

Boldface entries indicate major topics. *Italic* roman numerals indicate color section.

Boldface entries indicate major topics. *Italic* roman numerals indicate color section.